Rebuild Your Bones

Rebuild Your Bones

*The 12-Week
Osteoporosis Protocol*

Mira Calton, CN, and Jayson Calton, PhD

RODALE.

NEW YORK

The information given here is designed to help you make informed decisions about your health. It is not intended as a substitute for any treatment that may have been provided by your doctor. You should speak with your doctor before administering any suggestions made in this book.

Mention of specific companies, organizations, or authorities in this book does not imply endorsement by the author or publisher, nor does mention of specific companies, organizations, or authorities imply that they endorse this book, its author, or the publisher.

All rights reserved.
Published in the United States by Rodale Books, an imprint of Random House, a division of Penguin Random House LLC, New York.
rodalebooks.com

RODALE and the Plant colophon are registered trademarks of Penguin Random House LLC.

Library of Congress Cataloging-in-Publication Data has been applied for.

ISBN 978-1-63565-372-4
Ebook ISBN 978-1-63565-373-1

PRINTED IN CANADA

Illustrations on p. 39 by iStock/Leontura
Jacket photograph by Shironosov/Getty Images

10   9   8   7   6   5   4   3   2   1

First Edition

We dedicate this book to the women and men around the world who have overcome the prejudices and false beliefs of the past and are now empowered to stand up, demand truth, and retake control of their health.

Contents

Our Osteoporosis Journey

> All the adversity I've had in my life, all my troubles and obstacles, have strengthened me. . . . You may not realize it when it happens, but a kick in the teeth may be the best thing in the world for you.
>
> —WALT DISNEY

We are so excited to take this journey to better bone health with you. People always ask us how we became so impassioned about micronutrients and healing osteoporosis. The truth is that we've been right where you are now—frightened by a diagnosis but determined to heal. After years of research, trial and error, and innovation, we know the way out. And we want to share it with you.

Mira's Story

When I turned thirty I was diagnosed with advanced osteoporosis—and from that moment on, everything in my life changed. My bustling New York City life came screeching to a halt when I simply could no longer ignore the pain in my hips and lower back. It was time to face the fact that the pain I had been experiencing for almost a year couldn't simply be due to my high heels and long hours of stressful work—I had come to the reality that something was wrong with my body.

My doctor diagnosed me with advanced osteoporosis. He told me my bones had deteriorated to those of an eighty-year-old woman.

I was only thirty years old and had been living what I believed to be a healthy lifestyle! How could this be happening? The most devastating part of all was that my doctor didn't think my bones would get any better. It seemed I was fated to live a life filled with prescription medications with a host of detrimental side effects that at best would keep my bones from getting worse.

I can honestly say that being diagnosed with osteoporosis scared me to death—and I don't scare easily. I had so many fears—from losing my job, to losing my independence, to being constantly in and out of the hospital with broken bones. It felt like the best days of my life were behind me. I felt useless, ashamed, embarrassed, and helpless and my future was looking like a nightmare I was terrified to live.

But I am a fighter, and if you're reading this right now, you're a fighter too. After the fear and depression passed, I wanted to face my osteoporosis head-on. I wanted the truth about what osteoporosis was, how I got it, and most importantly, how to reverse it. After spending months thoroughly researching the negative side effects of the medications I had been prescribed (which will be shared with you in Chapter 2), I decided to forgo taking medication. I took my health into my own hands and began to search for an alternative, natural treatment. However, after several years, and a small fortune later, my efforts were not proving successful. I was discouraged and was beginning to fear that my decision to say no to medication had been a mistake. I was afraid that my fight, determination, and quest for knowledge had been in vain.

That's when fate stepped in. I was introduced to a pioneer in the field of nutrition and lifestyle medicine, known for his cutting-edge, out-of-the-box theories, who was willing to look at my osteoporosis from a completely new angle.

Jayson's Story

When I first met Mira, I was shocked to find out that such a young, vibrant woman had such an advanced form of osteoporosis. She told me that she had refused to take the medication her doctor had prescribed and instead was looking for an alternative, natural treatment for her condition, and I was immediately intrigued.

Over the last decade, I helped thousands of clients with a wide variety of health conditions and diseases through a unique low-carbohydrate (ketogenic) diet and lifestyle program that I had developed. It focused on whole foods, specific exercises, and supplementation with vitamins, minerals, essential fatty acids, and amino acids. Although much of my work had been focused on weight loss, my clients often reported back to me other amazing health benefits—from lower cholesterol to alleviated chronic headaches. By the time I met Mira, the program had either improved or reversed more than twenty different health conditions beyond weight loss. Because of this, I was hopeful that I could help Mira find a way to reverse her osteoporosis.

Although I knew that a ketogenic diet and a weight-bearing exercise program would be an essential part of Mira's recovery, I also knew that these two factors would not be enough on their own. Mira was a special case; I suspected that severe micronutrient deficiencies had played a central role in the development of her advanced osteoporosis. We needed to determine the cause of her deficiencies and then figure out a way to successfully get her body to absorb the vitamins and minerals necessary to rebuild her bones. This forced me to shift my attention away from the macronutrient side of food (carbohydrates, fats, and proteins), which I had been focusing on for most of my career (as macronutrients are the key component to a ketogenic diet). Instead, I took a much deeper look at essential micronutrients (vitamins, minerals, essential fatty acids, and amino acids), and how they interacted with one another.

Coincidentally, when I met Mira in 2003, I had been researching a little-known discovery in supplemental science: the fact that certain minerals compete with one another for absorption sites in the gastrointestinal tract. This competition prohibited the absorption of certain minerals, leading to deficiencies. I felt that by applying this knowledge to Mira's supplementation program, and by separating the minerals that were crucial for her body to absorb into multiple doses throughout the day, we could eliminate their competition for absorption pathways. Although I was unsure whether this method to increase the absorption potential of the minerals would work, it just made sense to me. I had high hopes that this new "anticompetition" method of supplementation would yield the benefits we were looking for.

Mira and I worked to pinpoint specific diet and lifestyle habits that may have contributed to her disease. Mira thought that her daily routine was healthy: a low-fat muffin and black coffee for breakfast, spinach salad for lunch, and steamed chicken and vegetables for dinner. So she was shocked to discover that all of these dietary habits had, in their own ways, *contributed* to her micronutrient deficiencies and ultimately her osteoporosis. Most of the foods she was eating were micronutrient-poor foods, filled with what we call *naked calories*—foods that have been stripped of their essential, health-promoting micronutrients and are therefore "naked." Her diet was also filled with *antinutrients*—naturally occurring substances in certain foods that can reduce the body's ability to absorb micronutrients. She was getting plenty of these naked calories and antinutrients but very few of the vitamins, minerals, essential fatty acids, and amino acids her body needed to maintain strong bones.

Her life in the big city didn't help matters either—her days had been filled with stress, excessive caffeine and alcohol consumption, carbon monoxide inhalation, poor sleep patterns, extreme exercise, and frequent dieting. This lifestyle and environment further sabotaged her body's ability to absorb and properly allocate the micronutrients necessary for healthy bones.

We changed Mira's eating habits to reduce as many antinutrients as possible and replace the micronutrient-poor foods with micronutrient-rich alternatives. We also eliminated many of her micronutrient-depleting lifestyle habits and began a daily weight-bearing exercise program. Perhaps most importantly, we developed and implemented a micronutrient therapy protocol based on our new anticompetition theory. Slowly, after a lot of hard work, Mira began to feel better. However, we knew that only a DEXA scan, the common test given to measure bone mineral density (BMD), would give us proof that she was healing. I joined Mira on her return visit to her doctor's office to hear the test results. The news couldn't have been any better: after two years of following the protocol we had developed, Mira's advanced osteoporosis was completely reversed.

Our Success Spawns New Questions

As you can imagine, we were elated. Our years of searching through scientific research for any information we could find on the causation, prevention, and reversal of osteoporosis had paid off. We had done what Mira's doctors had said was impossible—we safely and naturally reversed her advanced osteoporosis. Without drugs, she had achieved a bone density of a normal thirty-four-year-old. By harnessing the benefits of a micronutrient-rich and low-carbohydrate diet, implementing healthy lifestyle habits, following a weight-bearing exercise program, and introducing a strange yet effective supplementation program, we had been able to promote an environment where Mira's body could absorb and use the essential micronutrients required to rebuild her lost bone.

It seemed to us that we had discovered something important, and we were eager to explore our idea further to see where it would lead us. Our intense research and mutual respect for one another had also given us something beyond the results of Mira's DEXA scan to celebrate. After months of working so closely and passionately together, we had also fallen in love. Now, working as a couple and inspired by our success in reversing Mira's osteoporosis, we turned our complete attention to investigating micronutrient deficiency. We wanted to know everything—what caused it, how prevalent it was, and most importantly, was it a primary causative factor in other common health conditions and diseases beyond osteoporosis?

Could the dietary, lifestyle, and supplementation protocols we had used to improve Mira's health help others with osteoporosis or osteopenia? Could others delay, prevent, or even reverse advanced stages of osteoporosis through the same protocol? Our investigation into the causation and prevention of micronutrient deficiency led us on an incredible journey—a quest for knowledge that spanned both many years and many miles.

The Calton Project

In 2005, we got married and set off on a six-year around-the-world expedition with one goal in mind: to observe cultures around the globe and discover how different dietary and lifestyle habits affected the prevention and development of disease. Simply reading research studies performed at acclaimed institutions and universities no longer satisfied our desire for knowledge. Instead, we wanted to sit with, eat with, and question people from diverse cultures in an attempt to relearn what has been forgotten about both the healing and the disease-producing power of nutrition. We would follow in the tradition of Weston A. Price, who had explored the diets and health of native peoples back in the 1930s. For us, the knowledge would be in the discovery, and we would use that knowledge to rethink how we look at the causation and prevention of disease in America and around the world.

We called this adventure to more than 135 countries on all seven continents the Calton Project. Our quest for a fresh perspective on nutrition sent us traveling from the low-lying Sepik River in Papua New Guinea to the heights of the Andes in Peru and the Himalayas in Tibet. Our observations of these diverse cultures led us to a unique global understanding of nutrition and its ability to both prevent and cause disease.

Our discoveries on the Calton Project and diligent exploration of mainstream research studies have driven us to one final conclusion: *The primary causative factor of almost every one of today's most debilitating health conditions lies in a preventable "hidden" pandemic.* We're talking about diseases like osteoporosis, cancer, heart disease, diabetes, Alzheimer's, and obesity, to name but a few. This same causative factor gave Mira her advanced osteoporosis and is likely doing the same to you and millions of other people worldwide. *It is called micronutrient deficiency, and we believe that it is the most widespread and dangerous health condition of the twenty-first century.*

But as you've seen with Mira's story, there's hope. And it starts here.

CHAPTER 1

Micronutrient Deficiency

The Hidden Pandemic Keeping Us Tired, Fat, and Brittle

I can't reiterate this enough: The fate of your health is a choice—
not a destiny dictated by your genes.

—DAVID PERLMUTTER, MD

O ur belief that micronutrient deficiency is the most widespread and
dangerous health condition of the twenty-first century has become the foundation of our nutritional philosophy, and it is at the heart
of the Rebuild Your Bones osteoporosis protocol you are about to start.
Let's take a moment to dissect this statement and explore the facts that
led us to this conclusion.

Let's start with this fact: According to U.S. Department of Agriculture (USDA) published statistics, only 7 percent of the entire U.S.
population over the age of two has an adequate intake of vitamin D,
an essential fat-soluble vitamin whose deficiency has been shown to
greatly increase the risk of osteoporosis. Otherwise stated, 93 percent
of all Americans are deficient! Additionally, the data also reveals that
92 percent of the U.S. population is deficient in potassium, 86 percent is
deficient in vitamin E, 70 percent is deficient in calcium, and approximately 50 percent is deficient in vitamin A, vitamin C, and magnesium.
Although these statistics alone are disturbing to say the least, it gets
worse when you realize that deficiencies in any of these micronutrients
have been scientifically proven to either increase the risk of osteoporosis or lead directly to bone loss. In fact, Americans were found to be at
least somewhat deficient in all eighteen of the essential micronutrients

the USDA examined. There wasn't a single micronutrient for which all Americans met the government's minimum standards.

Although this shows us that at least 93 percent of Americans are deficient in at least one essential micronutrient (vitamin D), the USDA neglects to publish the percentage of the population deficient in more than one micronutrient, or all eighteen for that matter. However, according to Mehmet Oz, MD, of *The Dr. Oz Show*, when an independent research team investigated this question, their study of three million people revealed that less than 1 percent of the participants got enough essential micronutrients from diet alone. With approximately 325 million people in the United States, this means that depending on which statistic you use, between 300 million and 321 million Americans have a micronutrient deficiency.

To get a little perspective on the sheer magnitude of this number, consider the fact that when you take the total number of Americans affected by the world's most prevalent and deadly diseases (including osteoporosis, heart disease, cancer, and diabetes), it totals up to just over 194 million people—*combined*! And although we are in no way trying to downplay this devastating statistic, it's just over half of the 300-plus million Americans who have a micronutrient deficiency. This makes micronutrient deficiency the most widespread health condition of the twenty-first century.

Micronutrient Deficiency Spreads Globally

Micronutrient deficiency is not just a problem in the United States. According to the World Health Organization (WHO), more than two billion people in both developing and developed countries have micronutrient deficiencies. According to a 2010 study in the journal *Public Health Reviews*, "These are silent epidemics of vitamin and mineral deficiencies affecting people of all genders and ages, as well as certain risk groups. They not only cause specific diseases . . . such as osteoporosis, osteomalacia, thyroid deficiency, colorectal cancer, and cardiovascular diseases . . . but they act as exacerbating factors in infectious and chronic diseases, greatly impacting morbidity, mortality, and quality of life."

In Great Britain, researchers determined that *every person residing in the United Kingdom (UK)* was at risk for micronutrient deficiency to some degree. In fact, the number of British children diagnosed with the bone disease rickets, due to a vitamin D deficiency, is on the rise, with figures quadrupling in the last ten years.

In the United Arab Emirates (UAE), 90 percent of residents are deficient in vitamin D, and in China, research shows that 84 percent of men and 89 percent of women are deficient in vitamin D, and 40 percent are deficient in vitamin B9. Researchers caution that this may leave a large percentage of these populations at risk not only for bone-related conditions such as osteoporosis, but also for diabetes, cancer, cardiovascular diseases, infectious diseases, multiple sclerosis, and other autoimmune disorders.

In India, research found that 75 percent of the population shows alarming levels of deficiency. And according to the World Health Organization (WHO), the number of countries affected by a vitamin A deficiency nearly tripled from 39 to 122 between 1987 and 2005.

All these statistics point to the fact that America is not alone in this micronutrient deficiency pandemic. We, as a global community, must recognize micronutrient deficiency as the silent and harmful pandemic that it is, and take steps to reverse it—before it is too late.

Micronutrient Deficiencies Bring Danger

Now that we have proven to you that micronutrient deficiency is the most *widespread* health condition of the twenty-first century, it's time to show you why we believe that it's also the most *dangerous* health condition of our time. Here is a scientific fact to consider: **Micronutrients are so powerful that being deficient in even one can kill you.** It's the truth. Take scurvy (a deficiency in vitamin C), beriberi (a deficiency in vitamin B1, or thiamine), and pellagra (a deficiency in vitamin B3, or niacin): these diseases killed millions of people all around the world until medical science discovered that they were the direct result of a single micronutrient deficiency.

In 1912, scientists Casimir Funk and Sir Frederick Hopkins examined the relationship between micronutrient deficiencies and disease. After studying the effects of deficiency on disease, they released their *vitamin hypothesis of disease*, which stated that certain diseases are caused by a dietary lack of specific vitamins. Today, approximately one hundred years later, nothing has changed regarding the causation of disease.

However, many people want to believe that our modern health conditions and diseases are somehow different from those of the past, and that our current epidemics of osteoporosis, cancer, blindness, heart disease, diabetes, dementia, and obesity (to name a few) are caused by "age" itself or something other than a micronutrient deficiency. But thousands of peer-reviewed studies over the last century show that in most cases, these diseases are not infectious or genetic and are instead caused by a deficiency in essential micronutrients. Most medical and nutritional professionals agree that genetics play a very small role in determining your overall health. Even when it comes to cancer, one of the deadliest diseases in the world, only 5 to 10 percent of all cases can be attributed to genetic defects. This is fantastic news because it means that the remaining 90 to 95 percent of cases are directly affected by factors you can control.

Let's start with a statement from the *Journal of the American Medical Association* (AMA): "Insufficient vitamin intake is apparently a cause of chronic diseases. Recent evidence has shown that suboptimal [below standard] levels of vitamins, even well above those causing deficiency syndromes, are risk factors for chronic diseases such as cardiovascular disease, cancer, and osteoporosis. A large proportion of the general population is apparently at increased risk for this reason." As you can see, the AMA is fully aware of the fact that micronutrient deficiency is a risk factor for modern diseases, including osteoporosis, and that a large proportion of the general population is vulnerable.

Do other prominent doctors agree that diseases can be directly linked to micronutrient deficiencies? Dr. Mark Hyman, *New York Times* bestselling author and director of the Cleveland Clinic Center for Functional Medicine, puts it this way: "[Today] vitamin deficiency does not cause acute diseases such as scurvy or rickets, but [it does] cause what have been called 'long-latency deficiency diseases.' These include conditions like blindness, osteoporosis, heart disease, cancer, diabetes, dementia, and more. Most conventional doctors have it completely backward when it comes to vitamins and minerals—doctors tend to only use vitamins if medications don't work, when they should be prescribing the vitamins in the first place. Imagine a drug that could cure a fatal disease within days or weeks, using a very small dose, without toxicity and with a 100 percent success rate. Such a drug does not exist and will never exist. But that is the power and potential of nutrients."

The AMA and Dr. Hyman agree that micronutrients really are powerful and that their deficiencies can serious health implications. Could these deficiencies be the missing factor we have all been searching for on our quest for disease prevention? Here are several studies highlighting the connection between a variety of health conditions and diseases and micronutrient deficiencies:

- In a study published in the *Proceedings of the National Academy of Sciences*, researchers determined that the severity of heart disease correlates with the severity of CoQ10 deficiency and concluded, "CoQ10 deficiency might be a major if not the *sole cause* of cardiomyopathy [heart disease]."
- Michael Holick, MD, of Boston University School of Medicine, found that women who are vitamin D deficient have a 253 percent increased risk for developing colorectal cancer and a 222 percent increased risk for developing breast cancer.
- In a study published in the *European Journal of Neurology*, researchers concluded that individuals with elevated homocysteine levels caused by a vitamin B12 deficiency had more than twice the risk of developing Alzheimer's disease.
- Researchers at Erasmus University Medical Center in Rotterdam, Netherlands, studied 4,807 men and women for over seven years and determined that supplementation with vitamin K2 improved cardiovascular health by reducing arterial calcium accumulation by 50 percent and slashed the risk of a cardiovascular event by 50 percent.
- According to a 2012 study out of Harokopio University of Athens in Greece, participants using vitamin K2, calcium, and vitamin D supplementation showed significantly lower markers for bone loss and significant increases in total-body BMD.

We could go on and on, but all the evidence points to the fact that a lack of essential micronutrients increases the risk of a wide variety of health conditions and diseases, including osteoporosis. Micronutrient deficiency has been shown to be a causative factor for nearly every health condition and disease we are all trying to avoid.

Being passionate about the true power of micronutrients, in 2012, we published a new hypothesis in our book *Naked Calories*—exactly 100 years after Funk and Hopkins's vitamin hypothesis of disease. We call it the *micronutrient sufficiency hypothesis of health*. It states:

If a condition or disease can be directly linked to a micronutrient deficiency, then it can be prevented and/or reversed through sustained sufficiency of the deficient micronutrient(s).

Our hypothesis is different from Funk and Hopkins's in that it includes all micronutrients, not just vitamins. Perhaps most importantly, it points to the ability to prevent and reverse deficiency diseases through sustained micronutrient sufficiency. That's the goal of *Rebuild Your Bones:* to show you how to create and sustain a state of micronutrient sufficiency. By identifying which micronutrients you are likely deficient in and exploring how you became deficient in those micronutrients, you can take the necessary steps to fill in the gaps and begin to heal your bones naturally. Our Rebuild Your Bones twelve-week protocol not only guides you to naturally reverse your osteoporosis, it also puts you on the path to prevent future disease and improve any other health problems you may have. We believe our way is way better than the pharmaceutical path, where the chance of improvement usually comes with a high likelihood of devastating side effects. Based on the research presented so far, we feel that we have proven the statement on which we founded our nutritional philosophy: *Micronutrient deficiency is the most widespread and dangerous health condition of the twenty-first century.*

Osteoporosis and You

Let's talk about you. If you are reading this book, then there is a very high likelihood that you or someone you love has been diagnosed with osteoporosis or osteopenia. The first thing we want to tell you is that *you are not alone.* Millions of people just like you are suffering from this debilitating disease. In fact, over fifty-four million men and women in the United States (two hundred million worldwide) either already have osteoporosis or are at an increased risk for developing osteoporosis due to low bone mass. This represents more than 50 percent of the people over age fifty in the United States. However, less publicized and potentially even more concerning are these facts:

Fact: About one in two women over age fifty will fracture a bone because of osteoporosis.

Fact: Women over age forty-five spend more days in the hospital for osteoporosis than for diabetes, heart attacks, and breast cancer *combined.*

Fact: Up to one in four men over age fifty will fracture a bone because of osteoporosis. In fact, these same men are more likely to fracture a bone because of osteoporosis than they are to get prostate cancer.

Fact: Twenty-four percent of women and men age fifty and over who fracture a hip die within twelve months of the injury.

Fact: Because of the lack of focus on preventive bone health, the rising number of baby boomers, and the increased cases of men with osteoporosis, the number of hip fractures in the United States could triple by 2020.

Fact: Around the world, osteoporosis causes more than 8.9 million fractures annually, resulting in an osteoporotic fracture every 3 seconds.

Those are some pretty frightening statistics. Although it is true that osteoporosis is much more prevalent with women, contrary to popular belief, men are not immune to osteoporosis. In fact, more men than ever in their forties, thirties, and even twenties are being diagnosed. According to the International Osteoporosis Foundation, "In 2025, the estimated number of hip fractures occurring worldwide in men will be similar to that observed in women in 1990." And yes, although it pains us to say it, children are getting osteoporosis too!

As the global population ages and diets and lifestyles everywhere are slowly becoming more Westernized, osteoporosis-related fractures worldwide are rising. For example, the worldwide incidence of hip fractures is projected to increase 310 percent in men and 240 percent in women by 2050 when compared to rates in 1990. In Finland, the total number of hip fractures increased by 70 percent within a ten-year period (1992–2002). In Switzerland, osteoporosis is ranked the number one disease in women and number two in men. In the European Union (EU), the annual number of fractures will rise from 3.5 million in 2010 to 4.5 million in 2025 (a 28 percent increase). And in China, the percentage of the population age fifty and over with osteoporosis has more than doubled from 15.7 percent in 2006 to 34.65 percent in 2016 and is expected to double again by 2035.

So as we can see, osteoporosis is a widespread global disease that is affecting both men and women of all ages. Now let's explore what osteoporosis is and how you get it.

What Is Osteoporosis and How Do You Get It?

Although the definition of osteoporosis is pretty clear, there are several theories about the cause. Let's start with what it is. Osteoporosis, which literally means "porous bone," is a disease in which the *quality* and *density* of bone are reduced, causing an increased risk of fracture. More specifically, WHO defines osteoporosis as bone density that is 2.5 standard deviations (SDs) or more below the young adult mean value (T-score < −2.5). Patients with bone density between 1 and 2.5 SDs below average (T-score −1 to −2.5) are said to have osteopenia.

As bone density decreases, the more porous and fragile a bone becomes and the greater the risk of fracture—pretty simple, right? For many, the loss of bone occurs silently and progressively, creating no symptoms until the first fracture occurs. However, for others a great amount of pain is associated with the bone loss, which is what ultimately drives them to have a DEXA scan revealing the condition.

Bones themselves are living, growing tissues that are constantly changing. Bone is made up of a type of protein called collagen, which provides a soft framework, and a mineral called calcium phosphate, which adds strength and hardens the bone. The combination of calcium and collagen makes your bones strong and flexible enough to withstand stress. There are two types of bone: cortical (or compact) bone and trabecular (or spongy) bone. Cortical bone forms the hard outer layer of the bone and is dense and compact. Trabecular bone is found on the inner layer of the bone and has a spongy, honeycomb appearance. From birth until young adulthood, bones are developing and strengthening, reaching their maximum density in our early twenties—called peak bone mass. From then on, our bones go through a self-repair process known as remodeling. In simple, nonscientific terms, these repairs are carried out by two types of bone cells, which you will hear a lot about as we go through this book. There are the **osteoclasts**, which dissolve or break down old, worn-out bone and clear it away, and the **osteoblasts**, which build new bone where the old bone was. When everything is working properly, this amazing ballet between the osteoclasts and osteoblasts keeps your bones strong and flexible. The problem occurs when old bone is removed more quickly than new bone is built. For people with osteoporosis, bone loss simply outpaces the growth of new bone.

Causes of Osteoporosis

Now that we understand what osteoporosis is and how our bones work, let's jump into how we get osteoporosis. The medical community divides osteoporosis into two main types—primary and secondary osteoporosis.

Primary osteoporosis is defined as a bone disorder that occurs with aging (accelerating at menopause) and has no direct or singular cause. Basically, the idea is this: if we start with the accepted theory that we all lose approximately 1 percent of our total bone density annually after we reach our peak bone density in our early twenties, and add to it the idea that our ability to build bone decreases as we age, then, given enough time, it's no surprise that a sixty- or seventy-year-old person would find themselves with osteoporosis. When you look at osteoporosis from this point of view, there's really no reason to look into what caused it or why a person got it—it just happens.

Secondary osteoporosis, on the other hand, is defined as osteoporosis that has a direct root cause, meaning that it's not natural and it's caused by something that can be fixed. It's called secondary because it is "secondary to" or caused by, something other than old age. **There are four commonly accepted potential causes of secondary osteoporosis:**

1. Nutritional deficiencies (from poor diet or processed junk foods)
2. Lifestyle factors (such as stress or use of sunscreen)
3. Pre-existing medical conditions (such as secondary hyperparathyroidism or celiac disease)
4. Medications (such as Prevacid or prednisone).

THE TRUTH ABOUT PRIMARY OSTEOPOROSIS

Although both types of osteoporosis are being diagnosed around the world every day, the big question is: does "primary" osteoporosis even exist, or is it *all* secondary osteoporosis? This is an important question. The mindset with primary osteoporosis is that since there is no real cause, it can't really be prevented and the only treatment option is drugs. In contrast, with secondary osteoporosis, since there is a cause, the cause can be eliminated and the osteoporosis can theoretically be prevented or reversed.

Today, aging is not what it used to be. We now know that by exercising, eating healthy, drinking more water, and reducing stress, we can completely change the rate at which we age. In fact, there are devices that will look at certain physiological factors and give you something called your "real age." For example, your biological age may be sixty, but based on your heart rate, body fat, bone density, lean muscle tissue, and so on, your real age may be only fifty, or even forty! If we all know that a poor lifestyle can negatively affect our health and a healthy lifestyle can positively affect our health, then why is it so hard to believe that the same is true of bone health?

And how can we blame osteoporosis on aging when we are now seeing bone deterioration at younger and younger ages? Do you remember how type 2 diabetes used to be called *adult-onset diabetes*? Now, anyone can get type 2 diabetes, including children—whereas twenty years ago, children having type 2 diabetes was almost unheard-of. Today, more than 132,000 children have "adult-onset" type 2 diabetes, with more than 5,300 newly diagnosed cases in the United States each year! If we aren't careful, it won't be long until we see the same thing happening with osteoporosis. In fact, osteoporotic fractures in children have increased dramatically in the past few decades. According to Laura Bachrach, MD, a pediatric endocrinology professor at Stanford University, "separate studies carried out in the United States and Scandinavia showed that fracture rates in children increased in the past 40 years by 35 percent in boys and 60 percent in girls and the likely culprit is weak bones." The scary thing is that the medical community is now experimenting with giving bisphosphonates to children with juvenile osteoporosis. (You will find out how dangerous that could be in Chapter 2.)

The fact that osteoporosis is more common than ever, among more demographics than ever, should be enough to tell us that osteoporosis does not come from nothing—osteoporosis is caused by *something*!

Understanding Secondary Causes of Osteoporosis

Almost universally, when someone is diagnosed with osteoporosis, they are told to take calcium and vitamin D. More and more frequently now, they may also be told to take vitamin K2 and magnesium. All are essential micronutrients. That's because at the very root of it all, osteoporosis is a micronutrient deficiency disease! Let's look back at the list of potential causes of secondary osteoporosis and quickly touch on how each ultimately leads back to micronutrient deficiency—we'll go into greater detail in the coming chapters.

NUTRITIONAL DEFICIENCIES BRING ABOUT MICRONUTRIENT DEFICIENCIES

The first potential cause of secondary osteoporosis is nutritional deficiencies. A nutritional deficiency could mean an insufficient amount of food, which would in turn restrict the amount of essential micronutrients (vitamins, minerals, essential fatty acids, and amino acids) you are receiving from your food. Or it may mean poor-quality food such as processed junk food, which has been stripped of its essential, health-promoting micronutrients. Over time, these deficient foods can lead to any number of micronutrient deficiencies, all of which will set you up for osteoporosis.

However, even if these examples don't seem to apply to you, don't be too quick to brush by this first category. Nutritional deficiencies can also come from eating a seemingly "healthy" diet (like Mira was eating) that includes plenty of fresh fruits, vegetables, and whole grains. Take our word for it—by the time you finish Chapter 3, you will have a completely different view of what a "healthy" diet is in terms of avoiding micronutrient deficiencies and preventing or reversing osteoporosis. For now, all you need to know is that both *how much* you eat and *what* you eat (both "healthy" and "unhealthy") can lead to a micronutrient deficiency, which can then lead directly to the development of osteoporosis.

LIFESTYLE FACTORS CAN CAUSE MICRONUTRIENT DEFICIENCIES

Now let's examine the second category—lifestyle factors. Seemingly unrelated things like stress or the use of sunscreen can lead to micronutrient deficiency. With these two examples, we see two different ways micronutrients can become depleted through everyday lifestyle factors. We all get stressed, right? Some of us more than others. Although some people "stress eat" (usually deficiency-inducing junk food), science shows us that stress itself actually causes deficiencies in your essential micronutrients by using your available micronutrients at a faster rate. This is why de-stressing is one of the things we will teach you to do to improve your bone health. (You will get a lot more information regarding safeguarding yourself against this bone thief in Chapter 5.)

Our other example of a lifestyle factor, sunscreen, works in a different way to create a micronutrient deficiency. Although sunscreen is designed to block ultraviolet (UV) rays and prevent sunburns, it also blocks vitamin D—the only vitamin that we can get without eating food or taking a supplement. Because vitamin D is naturally produced by the skin when it is exposed to sunlight, the more often someone uses sunscreen and the better and more thoroughly they apply it, the more likely it is that they are blocking their body's ability to make vitamin D. Although it's important to protect yourself from skin cancer, moderate levels of unprotected sun exposure can be healthy and very helpful in boosting vitamin D. Completely limiting your sun exposure can, over time, lead to a deficiency in vitamin D, one of the most important vitamins in the fight against osteoporosis. These are just two examples, so don't be too quick to discard the idea that lifestyle factors have played a role in the development of your osteoporosis if they don't seem to apply to you. We'll introduce you to many more potential lifestyle factors that contribute to micronutrient deficiency in Chapters 4 and 5.

PRE-EXISTING MEDICAL CONDITIONS CAN CAUSE MICRONUTRIENT DEFICIENCIES

The next possible cause of secondary osteoporosis is pre-existing medical conditions. We will use secondary hyperparathyroidism and celiac disease in our examples here, but almost any condition can lead to the same conclusion, as you'll learn later. In the case of secondary hyperparathyroidism (not primary) we see that micronutrient deficiency itself is the root cause of this condition, as it is actually caused by low levels of calcium in the blood. A person with secondary hyperparathyroidism is more likely to get osteoporosis because they are already deficient in calcium, but there is also an increased risk because higher levels of the parathyroid hormone cause increased osteoclast activity, which breaks down bone in order to release more calcium into the blood. Eliminate the calcium deficiency and you eliminate the hyperparathyroidism and the subsequent micronutrient deficiency, which could lead to osteoporosis.

In the case of celiac disease, this cause-and-effect process is reversed. Celiac disease is a genetic autoimmune condition, which causes an allergylike response to gluten and related proteins, causing inflammation and intestinal damage, which leads to a reduction in the ability to absorb essential nutrients from food. It's really no surprise that a person with celiac disease may be deficient in essential micronutrients that are required to build and maintain strong, healthy bone, and that those deficiencies could eventually lead to the onset of osteopenia or osteoporosis.

Is this all starting to become clear? You don't get osteoporosis because you have secondary hyperparathyroidism or celiac disease or any other medical condition—you get osteoporosis because either the micronutrient deficiencies that caused your pre-existing medical condition also caused your osteoporosis (as in the case of secondary hyperparathyroidism) *or* created the micronutrient deficiencies that caused your osteoporosis. Either way your osteoporosis was induced by one, primary root cause: a micronutrient deficiency!

MEDICATIONS CAN LEAD TO MICRONUTRIENT DEFICIENCIES

To illustrate the link between medications and micronutrient deficiencies, we'll use the examples of Prevacid and prednisone. (Chapter 5 covers many more medications far more thoroughly.) Almost every single medication you can think of depletes your essential micronutrients to some extent, and some a lot more than others. This does not mean that all medications will cause osteoporosis on their own, but there is a good chance your medications are contributing to your osteoporosis in one way or another. Prevacid, for example, is a popular drug for heartburn because it blocks stomach acid. But what most people don't know is that low stomach acid significantly increases the risk of osteoporosis. Stomach acid is necessary to absorb many of our essential micronutrients, which play a role in bone health.

With prednisone, which is a corticosteroid commonly prescribed for inflammatory or autoimmune diseases such as rheumatoid arthritis, we again see that using this drug increases the risk of osteoporosis because it depletes a wide variety of micronutrients. These include beta-carotene; vitamins B6, B9, C, and D; and the minerals calcium, magnesium, phosphorus, potassium, selenium, zinc, and melatonin. (Don't worry if you can't identify exactly what role each of these essential micronutrients plays in bone health right now—we don't expect you to—but rest assured that in Chapter 2 we will explain how each micronutrient can help you strengthen your bones and reverse osteoporosis.) The takeaway here is clear: if you bring home a prescription medication, be aware that there's a chance you could also bring home a micronutrient deficiency.

THE REAL ROOT CAUSE OF OSTEOPOROSIS

What have we learned about the cause of osteoporosis? Although the aging process is inevitable and bone mass does decline with age, osteoporosis does not have to be inevitable. Age is just a number if we keep ourselves healthy. Our goal is to thrive well past our thirties and forties and well into our older and far wiser years. Age does not cause osteoporosis—or every elderly man and woman would have it. No, age as the primary cause of osteoporosis cannot be the answer. Something else has to be turning on the osteoporosis switch.

And what about those well-accepted secondary causes of osteoporosis? We have proven that all four commonly accepted potential causes of secondary osteoporosis have been shown to be caused by or to cause deficiencies in your micronutrients. After examining all this evidence, it seems clear to us that **micronutrient deficiencies are the primary root cause of osteoporosis**.

Time to Get to Work

Isn't this fantastic? Knowing that micronutrient deficiencies are at the root cause of osteoporosis is truly empowering news, because now you can address it straight on—and that means learning how to turn the disease-producing state of micronutrient deficiency into a health-producing, bone-strengthening state of micronutrient sufficiency.

We wrote this book because we wanted to give everyone the vital information that Mira wished she had the day she was diagnosed, so that you can save yourself the years of wasted effort she experienced. We wanted to cut through all the confusion and bring you the newest, most up-to-date science concerning what causes osteoporosis, as well as what has been scientifically proven to prevent and reverse it. Now, we will examine evidence showing you how your diet, lifestyle, and supplementation habits can all influence your level of sufficiency. Along your journey with us, we will reveal the forty healing habits that Mira used to reverse her osteoporosis. (You can find newly introduced healing habits at the end of each chapter so you can easily keep track.) Each habit has been scientifically proven to benefit your bones, so imagine their combined power when you harness them all! They work in unison to make sure your body is flush with powerful micronutrients, creating an environment for your bones to flourish.

We've been through what you are going through from both the patient side and the practitioner side. The complete twelve-week osteoporosis protocol that we outline for you in Chapter 8 mimics what we did to reverse Mira's osteoporosis. We've helped other people get through what you are going through, and we want to help you get through it too if you'll do the work. Yes, there's a lot of work ahead. We don't want you to turn ahead to Chapter 8 and skip all the information that comes before it. It's vital to carefully read (and reread) every chapter with the intention of truly understanding each topic we will cover. And you have to incorporate as many of the healing habits as you possibly can into your daily routine. Rebuilding your bones and beating osteoporosis will not be quick—it's not a sprint; it's a long, hard, grueling marathon. But it is possible, and it is worth it.

Our goal is to get you ready, just as if you were running a real race. Think of reading this book and practicing our forty healing habits as the training phase in preparation for your marathon. The only difference is that a real marathon can't reverse your osteoporosis and would be over in a day. Your marathon to rebuild your bones will be the most important race of your life and will likely last the rest of your life.

In the days following your pantry purge (yes, there will be a pantry purge), or after your first week without sugar or wheat (yes, that's coming too), you may feel like you just ran five miles for the very first time. You may feel frustrated and ask yourself if it's worth it, or question what you have read. Your friends and family may look at you lovingly and tell you to take a day off—to give yourself a break. But true life changes require day-in and day-out commitment, and you will succeed only if you push through. Don't give up! You will survive the coming changes, we promise you that. And after you experience them for a couple of weeks, it will be as if you are hitting the road for a run you have done many times before. You'll find your pace and it will become part of your daily routine. And by the end of your twelve-week protocol, it will all feel like second nature—and you won't want to go back.

So put on your training shoes and lace up; you are about to embark on the most important race of your life—the journey to rebuild your bones and beat osteoporosis. You can totally do this! Let's get started.

Join us On the Couch for an in-depth chat about Chapter 1

One more thing before you run off! We want to be your personal micro-nutrient marathon coaches and guide you every step of the way. At the end of each chapter, you will find an invitation to join us for an "On the Couch" chat where we will personally coach you on that chapter's key points. These bonus videos are designed to make the main points of each chapter easy to understand—kind of like CliffsNotes—and give you additional bonus material we couldn't fit in the book that will make your journey to beating osteoporosis even faster. These videos will be one part encouragement, one part science and strategy, and 100 percent not to be missed. Join us now for our first "On the Couch" chat at RebuildYourBones.com.

CHAPTER 2

Osteoporosis Treatment

Time to Take the Right Steps

One of the first duties of the physician is to educate the masses
not to take medicine.

—SIR WILLIAM OSLER, MD, FOUNDER
OF JOHNS HOPKINS HOSPITAL

Now that you understand that micronutrient deficiency is at the
root cause of osteoporosis and that there is a great likelihood that
you are deficient in your essential micronutrients, it's time to decide
the path you will take to reverse your osteoporosis. As you're about
to see, the paths are very different. In this chapter, we will explore
the pharmaceutical path and ultimately expose it for what it is—Big
Pharma's feeble attempt to manipulate natural bone formation that can
bring about numerous adverse effects. The second path, the one that we
hope you will embark on, works quite differently, by supplying your
body with everything it needs to remodel bone naturally without any
potential health risks.

The Pharmaceutical Approach

The global osteoporosis drug market is a huge business, expected to
be valued at $8.9 billion by the year 2020. Osteoporosis medications
including bisphosphonates, RANK ligand inhibitors, and synthetic
hormone fragments are being marketed and prescribed to millions of
people each year to treat osteoporosis. We know that the promise of an

instant and simple cure is alluring, but these medications often come with unwanted side effects that can have unforeseen health and financial implications. Let's examine a few of the drugs on the market today and their potential adverse effects.

BISPHOSPHONATES

Bisphosphonates (Fosamax, Binosto, Actonel, Reclast, and Boniva) are the most widely prescribed of the osteoporosis drugs and are taken by approximately 190 million people globally. The fact that these drugs are still prescribed by *any* doctors today is astonishing to us, for the following four reasons.

Reason #1: Bisphosphonates Have Been Proven to Be Ineffective

Bisphosphonates, whether delivered in a pill or injectable, work by attaching themselves to the bone matrix. This alters the normal function of the matrix by affecting the replacement of old bone with new bone. Although bone loss will be reduced, inhibiting bone loss also inhibits new bone formation. This makes bones thicker but does not make bones better. In fact, these thicker, more brittle bones are *more* prone to fracture. This is not a new realization. In fact, back in 2015, a meta-analysis of more than thirty studies was published in the prestigious *BMJ* (the former *British Medical Journal*) confirming that bisphosphonates are totally ineffective at preventing fractures.

In 2017, scientists at Imperial College London found evidence that the use of bisphosphonates was linked to microscopic cracks, making bones more fragile and prone to break. In these bone biopsies, researchers also saw that bisphosphonates caused unusual mineralization crystals to form in the bone cavities that ordinary bone minerals would normally fill. These crystals impede the development of new bone tissue and lead to the deterioration of the quality of bone. They also give you false hope. Although bisphosphonates make bones appear to have increased in density on a DEXA scan, don't be fooled: bisphosphonates produce visually denser, stronger bones, but they are of lesser quality and more prone to fracture.

Reason #2: Bisphosphonates Cause Horrible Side Effects

According to the National Osteoporosis Foundation (NOF), "side effects for all the bisphosphonates (alendronate, ibandronate, risedronate and zoledronic acid) may include bone, joint or muscle pain. Side effects of the oral tablets may include nausea, difficulty swallowing, heartburn, irritation of the esophagus and gastric ulcer . . . Side effects that can occur in a minority of people shortly after receiving an IV bisphosphonate include flu-like symptoms, fever, headache and pain in muscles or joints . . . There have been rare reports of osteonecrosis of the jaw with bisphosphonate medicines. Osteonecrosis of the jaw (ONJ) occurs when the jaw bone is exposed and begins to starve from a lack of blood." This terrible, difficult-to-treat disease is marked by pain, infection, abscesses, and rotting bone. As you can see, the side effects of taking bisphosphonates are pretty bad—so bad, in fact, that a 2017 report in the medical journal *BMJ* found that approximately 1 in 5 people who started this drug cited adverse side effects as their reason for not continuing treatment.

As if these side effects were not bad enough, bisphosphonates have also been shown to cause an increased risk of serious atrial fibrillation (AF), a disease that has been linked to an increased risk of heart failure, dementia, and stroke. In 2008, scientists at the Maimonides Medical Center in New York analyzed data from nearly two hundred thousand individuals taking bisphosphonates and determined that bisphosphonate use increases the risk of serious atrial fibrillation by 40 percent.

Finally, if jaw erosion and heart failure are not enough to sway you away from bisphosphonates, then how about cancer? There have been constant complaints that oral bisphosphonates caused acid reflux and esophageal inflammation since these drugs were introduced in the mid-1990s. And although your doctor may advise standing for an hour after taking this "magic pill" to reduce the acid reflux, they may not warn you that those who have taken oral bisphosphonates for five years or more are twice as likely to develop esophageal cancer as those who have not. This means that your likelihood of getting esophageal cancer, a cancer with low survival rates compared to other cancers (with seven out of ten people dying within a year of diagnosis), is doubled compared to those who refuse this commonly prescribed osteoporosis drug.

Reason #3: You Are Pretty Much Stuck on Them Forever

Those choosing to stop the prescriptions will actually increase their risk of fracturing. According to findings presented at the 2017 annual meeting of the American College of Rheumatology, women who discontinued use of bisphosphonates for more than two years after long-term use were up to 39 percent more likely to have hip fractures compared to those who continued treatment. So, according to this study, individuals who started taking bisphosphonates and want to stop because of their adverse effects or possible long-term disease risks actually increase their fracture risk further. This is a serious prescription protocol, and you need to think long and hard about this consequence before beginning it. For those already on bisphosphonates, the risks increase the longer you stay on, so speaking to your doctor about stopping should be a priority.

Reason #4: Bisphosphonates Cause Essential Micronutrient Deficiency

Although prescription drugs may make you "feel better," like a Band-Aid covering and protecting a wound, they likely will not fix the underlying problem. In fact, at a micronutrient level, they may be making matters quite a bit worse. Prescription medications can sabotage your ability to achieve and maintain a state of micronutrient sufficiency by directly depleting micronutrients from your body. In other words, the simple act of taking a prescription medication can rob you of specific micronutrients—creating deficiencies in the same micronutrients whose deficiencies are at the root cause of your osteoporosis.

Have you ever heard that grapefruit juice should not be taken with specific prescription drugs, high-cholesterol and high-blood-pressure medications, or antidepressants? Or perhaps you may have heard that calcium needs to be taken away from thyroid medications such as Synthroid? Did you ever ask yourself why? The scientists that created these drugs realized that specific substances (such as foods, supplements, or other drugs), when taken together or within a certain window of time, can react with one another in a negative way. This is called antagonism or competition. The noncompatible elements may compete for absorption, or perhaps bind together to form insoluble materials, ultimately reducing the effectiveness of one or both.

Bisphosphonates also have similar reactions. They can interfere with the absorption of calcium, antacids, and other oral medications. The labels for certain bisphosphonates, like Fosamax, admit this, and suggest taking the drug *at least* "one-half hour before the first food, beverage, or medication of the day with plain water only."

The antagonistic relationship between bisphosphonates and calcium is so severe that the NOF states, "When low levels of calcium in the blood are present, bisphosphonates should not be given. Low calcium levels must be corrected or the problem will worsen." The NOF recognizes that it is not only the bisphosphonates' bioavailability that is hindered when taken with calcium or before or after taking calcium. Their warning shows that bisphosphonates also reduce calcium levels and that having low calcium levels while taking a bisphosphonate is potentially so dangerous that if you are deficient in calcium, you should not take this drug.

It's bad enough that bisphosphonates could actually cause you to be more deficient in calcium than you were when you were diagnosed with osteoporosis, but the real issue here is that doctors are prescribing oral bisphosphonates to millions of people around the world *when more than 70 percent of people in the United States have been shown to have inadequate calcium intakes.* And it's not just calcium—it turns out that when bisphosphonates come into contact with specific minerals such as calcium, magnesium, iron, copper, and zinc, they may bind to each other in your stomach and become insoluble, preventing your body from absorbing bisphosphonates as well as properly metabolizing all these different minerals. This is why the Linus Pauling Institute takes Fosamax's recommendation a step further and cautions you not to eat, drink, or take any oral supplement containing these additional minerals for at least two hours before or after taking bisphosphonates, and up to six hours after calcium or a calcium-rich meal.

When bisphosphonates and minerals compete, not only do the bisphosphonates become ineffective, but the competition also greatly reduces the ability of the minerals and antioxidants you thought you were getting from your food or supplements to help heal your body.

However, it is not just your minerals that are risk from these prescription drugs. Your antioxidants are also in danger. In a study published in the *Journal of Clinical Endocrinology and Metabolism*, researchers determined that bisphosphonates interfere with the production of CoQ10, a fat-soluble vitamin-like antioxidant that is present in practically all cell membranes. New research suggests that CoQ10 plays an active role in osteoclastogenesis (the formation of osteoclasts) and inhibits osteoclast activity by limiting oxidative damage and supporting bone formation by osteoblasts. Research shows that this reduction in CoQ10 levels then causes a domino effect through the antioxidant family. Both vitamins C and E, as well as other powerful antioxidants, are now at risk because the new pharmaceutically induced deficiency in CoQ10 puts a greater antioxidant burden on these vital nutrients. This results in deficiencies that can limit your body's ability to heal itself—yet again, the drug does more harm than good.

By now, it should be pretty clear that there are numerous reasons you want to strongly reconsider treating your osteoporosis with bisphosphonates. To recap—these drugs have not only been proven ineffective, they have also been shown to cause a slew of side effects including pain, nausea, difficulty swallowing, heartburn, osteonecrosis of the jaw (ONJ), atrial fibrillation, and esophageal cancer. Additionally, stopping this drug has been shown to increase the likelihood of fracture—although staying on it can cause numerous essential micronutrients to become depleted. In the long run, this may cause a worsening of your osteoporosis or may cause new health conditions to arise, possibly requiring yet more medications to treat. Next time your physician suggests bisphosphonates, remember that they are not handing out a harmless, candy-coated cure. This is a serious medication that can cause you serious harm.

RANK LIGAND INHIBITORS

Now let's move on and examine a second class of drugs called RANK ligand inhibitors (aka Prolia), which is not proving to be much safer than bisphosphonates. RANK ligand inhibitors are far newer and their long-term consequences have been far less studied.

Denosumab (trade names Prolia and Xgeva)

Denosumab, sold under the trade names Prolia and Xgeva, works by different methods than bisphosphonates, but toward the same goal of interrupting normal bone remodeling. Whereas bisphosphonates destroy already mature osteoclasts, denosumab prevents osteoclasts from forming by manipulating their precursors. So by what process does denosumab work? A short science lesson is needed here because it will come into play a bit later in our discussion of omega-3, but we will try to keep it brief. Denosumab, being a RANK ligand inhibitor, binds to a RANK ligand (RANKL) and prevents it from doing its job, which is to bind to a cell receptor known as RANK (receptor activator for nuclear factor kappa-B). RANK can be found on many different cell types, one of which is a cell that is a precursor for osteoclasts. Normally, in the absence of the drug denosumab, RANKL would activate RANK receptors on the precursor cells for osteoclasts, telling these "osteoclasts in waiting" to develop into full-blown osteoclasts and perform their function of removing old and damaged bone. However, when denosumab binds to RANKL, it blocks the binding of RANKL to RANK, thus reducing the formation and performance of osteoclasts. This is how denosumab inhibits RANKL from doing its job.

You can imagine why the team of scientists that invented this drug thought this was a perfect way to build bone. Think about it: if you create a system where the osteoclasts can't perform their function of removing old bone, while at the same time still allowing the osteoblast to build new bone, it sounds like a great way to slow down bone loss and get an increase in bone density. But messing with the natural process of bone remodeling was very shortsighted. We already revealed how bisphosphonates, by disturbing osteoclast function, opened the door to a slew of unwanted side effects. So it should not surprise you that this new injectable osteoporosis drug, which causes the same disturbances to your osteoclasts, has also been proven to do the same. A few of the side effects listed on the Prolia website include serious allergic reactions; severe jawbone problems (osteonecrosis); unusual thigh bone fractures; increased risk of broken bones after stopping the drug; severe bone, joint, or muscle pain; and increased risk for developing serious infections.

You can see from this list that these newer RANK ligand inhibitors have just as many horrific side effects as bisphosphonates. However, what you may not have caught earlier in this discussion on denosumab is that we mentioned that RANKL has other non–bone-related jobs. It is because of these non–bone-related jobs being jeopardized that we question how long-term studies (of which none are yet available) might pan out. For example, did you notice at the bottom of Prolia's list of side effects that Prolia may affect your body's ability to fight infections? Not only will your natural bone remodeling process be altered by inhibiting RANKL, but so will your immune system. You see, immune cells are generated when RANKL binds to cell receptors on their immune cell precursors. So when denosumab inhibits RANKL, your immune cells can't be generated. This could have a huge spectrum of health implications over time, many of which have yet to be reported or studied.

TERIPARATIDE (TRADE NAME FORTEO)

Unlike bisphosphonates and RANK ligand inhibitors, Forteo does not attack osteoclasts in an attempt to stop the breakdown of bone. Instead, Forteo increases osteoblast activity, striving to make them work harder and longer. Forteo, which the U.S. Food and Drug Administration (FDA) has approved for limited use (up to twenty-four months), is a synthetic fragment of the human parathyroid hormone (PTH). The natural form of PTH regulates both calcium and phosphate metabolism in our bones and kidneys. Under normal conditions, if PTH stays elevated, as it might with hyperparathyroidism, then bone loss can occur because of increased osteoclast activity. However, if PTH is elevated intermittently, as it might be when you inject Forteo, your osteoblasts get a boost, which should in turn create super-fast bone growth.

Sounds good, right? What could go wrong with trying to artificially stimulate bone growth? You know by now: debilitating side effects, including nausea, leg cramps, low blood pressure, fainting, constipation, low energy, and pain and muscle weakness. An increased PTH level has also been associated with cognitive decline and dementia (Alzheimer's). This is because researchers have concluded that chronic elevation of PTH in the brain increases the risk of calcium overloading, which leads to impaired blood flow in the brain and brain degeneration. As with bisphosphonates, this "super shot" also wreaks havoc on your micronutrient levels by increasing the risk of both life-threatening hypercalcemia (excessively high blood levels of calcium) and hypomagnesia (low blood levels of magnesium).

Forteo and Your Micronutrient Levels

Lilly Medical, the maker of Forteo, is well aware that taking this injectable negatively effects the levels of micronutrients in your body. On their website, under side effects, they state, "Forteo may also cause increased calcium in your blood. Tell your healthcare provider if you have nausea, vomiting, constipation, low energy, or muscle weakness . . . These may be signs there is too much calcium in your blood." And although we know that calcium is important in the bone-building process, too much of a good thing can quickly turn into a really bad thing. According to the Mayo Clinic, "Too much calcium in your blood can weaken your bones, create kidney stones, and interfere with how your heart and brain work." Excess calcium, or hypercalcemia, if left untreated, can be dangerous and can result in what is called a life-threatening hypercalcemic crisis. Although the risk for life-threatening hypercalcemia from Forteo is very small, it's important to know the risk exists.

Although we have just seen that Forteo can cause increased levels of calcium in the blood, it was also found to do the exact opposite to study subjects' magnesium levels. The drug was found to cause hypomagnesia, or low blood levels of magnesium. Making matters worse, the individuals to whom Forteo is most commonly prescribed are men and women age fifty and older, who are already likely deficient in magnesium. Doctors all over the world are supplying this already deficient population with a prescription that has been shown to cause hypomagnesia, a serious condition that can result in disturbances in nearly every organ system and can cause potentially fatal complications (including ventricular arrhythmia, coronary artery vasospasm, and sudden death) in nearly 36 percent of the subjects.

With every Forteo shot, you're digging yourself into a deeper and deeper deficiency of magnesium. This mineral is involved in over six hundred important metabolic reactions in the body, including the transmission of muscular activity and nerve impulses, temperature regulation, and detoxification reactions. It is also involved in the synthesis of DNA and RNA, energy production, and healthy bones. In fact, 60 percent of the magnesium in the human body is found in bone, where it is a key constituent of the bone matrix and is required for osteoblast production, development, and activity. In addition to all these important roles, magnesium also assists in calcium absorption by being a co-factor for the enzyme in the kidneys that converts vitamin D to its active form (25(OH)D to 1,25-D), so that vitamin D can increase calcium absorption.

Low levels of magnesium means your bones will be bombarded with inflammation. Low magnesium levels cause pro-inflammatory prosta-glandins (PGE2 series), highly destructive free radicals (e.g. peroxyni-trite, superoxide), substance P, C-reactive protein (CRP), and TNFα levels, to increase and work as a team to activate osteoclasts and destroy your bone. So you can see how many different things could go wrong if you were deficient in this super-powerful micronutrient.

Forteo and Increased Cortisol

Teriparatide (Forteo) has been found to increase blood and urine levels of the stress hormone cortisol when given to postmenopausal women with osteoporosis. This is not surprising since teriparatide causes a spike in PTH, and one of parathyroid hormone's effects is to increase the adrenal glands' secretion of cortisol. In studies, after only six months of standard teriparatide treatment (20 mcg), women's cortisol levels had increased above baseline. After twelve months, the increase in cortisol levels was deemed scientifically significant. What do higher cortisol levels mean to you? Researchers found that cortisol indirectly acts on bone by blocking calcium absorption, which decreases bone cell growth. This disruption to serum calcium homeostasis increases bone resorption and ultimately reduces BMD. Even a short bout of elevated cortisol secretion may cause a decrease in BMD. High cortisol levels also increases stress levels (as if you weren't stressed enough worrying about your osteoporosis), high blood pressure, type 2 diabetes, increases in unhealthy visceral fat (the dangerous form of fat that is concentrated around abdominal organs), and vertebral fractures. To make matters worse, researchers are unsure if cortisol levels will revert back to normal if teriparatide treatment is stopped. But they do know that the increases seen in bone density after several weeks of teriparatide treatment disappear within four weeks of stopping teriparatide. So you lose the benefits, but you may keep the negative side effects for life.

Teriparatide and Bone Cancer

Research shows that teriparatide's dramatic stimulation of bone formation peaks at six to twelve months of use. Perhaps this is why it is approved for safety for only up to twenty-four months. But the FDA's reason for limiting its approval of this drug could be a little more serious. Today, more than 430,000 patients have been treated with short-term teriparatide injections, but before FDA approval, there was concern that teriparatide might increase a patient's risk of developing osteosarcoma (bone cancer). We feel this concern is well founded since almost 45 percent of the research rats treated with this drug developed this aggressive form of bone cancer. In case you missed it, nearly *half* of the rats treated with this drug were diagnosed with bone cancer, and the FDA still approved it. To be fair, the FDA did mandate a "black box" warning revealing this potential side effect and has been monitoring the situation. Only a couple of cases of humans taking teriparatide injections and being diagnosed with osteosarcoma have been documented, but there's still cause for concern. This drug received FDA approval for use (for a *maximum* of twenty-four months) in 2010, and cancer can take years or even decades to develop. Currently the only studies done on humans have been short-term, to a maximum of thirty-six months.

ABALOPARATIDE (TRADE NAMES TYMLOS, ELADYNOS): TAKING A STEP IN THE *SAME* DIRECTION

Abaloparatide is a newcomer to the osteoporosis drug market, approved by the FDA in 2017. It's a small tweak on teriparatide that the pharmaceutical companies are hoping brings them a big monetary reward. Because of their chemical similarities, these two drugs have similar adverse effects. However, there are some pluses and minuses to choosing abaloparatide vs. teriparatide. First, and this is a plus, your odds of getting hypercalcemia are less. On the minus side, although the initial increases in the bone formation marker were similar for abaloparatide and teriparatide within the first month, by month three, bone formation began to decrease in the abaloparatide group compared with the teriparatide group. Basically, it's not as good at building bone. Both cause plausible increases in cortisol and calcium levels, as well as decreases in cognition and magnesium levels. Here, again, the main issue is cancer. Radius Health, the pharmaceutical company that owns the patent on Tymlos, states, "It is unknown whether Tymlos will cause osteosarcoma in humans." It's concerning that the FDA approved this drug with no long-term data on its effects, and regulators from across the pond seem to share these concerns. When Radius Health applied for the opportunity to market abaloparatide in the European Union under the name of Eladynos, they were rejected. The Committee for Medicinal Products for Human Use (CHMP) and the scientific committee of the European Medicines Agency (EMA) stated that from a safety point of view, they were concerned about the medicine's negative effects on the heart. Because most postmenopausal women are at an increased risk of heart problems, the CHMP could not identify a group of patients for which the benefits would outweigh the risks. Therefore, the committee recommended that the medicine be refused marketing authorization. Three cheers for the European committee—we suggest you take their advice and reject it as well.

Nature + Science Reaps Rewards

We hope by now your mind is made up: that except in the most extreme cases, the risky adverse effects of these drugs greatly outweigh the rewards—especially because many of them are shown to be ineffective. Although bisphosphonates, RANK ligand inhibitors, and synthetic hormone fragments may sound promising, the only thing they are promising is a big income for Big Pharma. Now it's time to reclaim your health and to embark on a journey that will undoubtedly be safer and more successful.

THE MICRONUTRIENT THERAPY APPROACH

Our goal is to show you how supplying your body with all of the essential micronutrients it needs to thrive will naturally and safely help you prevent and reverse bone loss. Everything we recommend in this book is backed by science. So much so, that you may even get sick of seeing all the studies we list by the time we are through. But both modern science and ancient wisdom agree on this topic: healthy foods that supply essential nutrition, coupled with lifestyle habits that promote micronutrients, topped off with properly formulated supplements to fill in nutritional gaps, will carry you to the finish line with a healthy body that you can be proud of. Your fear and embarrassment of osteoporosis can turn into pride in your ability to take control of your own health and naturally and safely increase your bone mass. Your feelings of being a burden can transform into satisfaction as you use your new knowledge to help others fight their illnesses. Deciding to battle your osteoporosis naturally without the crutch of potentially harmful medication is not easy, but we believe you will be walking tall on your road to being free of osteoporosis.

Our micronutrient therapy approach to reversing osteoporosis addresses the numerous underlying causes of bone loss and provides a safe and natural means of improving bone quality and strength. Your body will benefit from becoming sufficient in the diverse family of vitamins, minerals, essential fatty acids, and amino acids, each playing their unique role in creating an environment where your bone density can improve naturally.

The Orchestra Analogy

It is about time that we learn a bit more on how micronutrients work with a quick little story we call the orchestra analogy. You may have heard us reference this analogy in our last book, *The Micronutrient Miracle*, or in one of our lectures, as we have used it for years. It is the best and most illustrative analogy that we have found where micronutrient interactions are concerned, and it has made their unique relationships clear to many who have heard it before. So, as the saying goes: if it ain't broke, don't fix it.

Imagine that each micronutrient (calcium, vitamin D, magnesium, etc.) is like a different instrument in the orchestra. In order to successfully play a piece of music (the equivalent to the body carrying out an essential function such as bone building or hormone production), all the instruments (or micronutrients) that are required for that piece of music must be present. When one or several instruments (micronutrients) are missing, the orchestra (body) will not be able to play the piece of music (carry out the essential function), and this will lead to a subpar performance (a health condition or disease, such as osteoporosis).

Just as a standard orchestra generally has four sections—woodwinds, brass, percussion, and strings—the human body uses four types of micronutrients: vitamins, minerals, essential fatty acids, and amino acids. And like the orchestra, each of the four sections is made up of similar yet vastly different instruments.

For example, there are dozens of string instruments that all create music through the vibration of strings. However, although they have that trait in common, the resulting sound that each produces is vastly different. When Beethoven composed his "Ode to Joy" for the violin, he didn't assume any string instrument could represent the ethereal nature of the melody—certainly not a banjo or an electric bass. Because each string instrument offers its own unique tone, they are not interchangeable.

The same is true of minerals. They all have something important in common—they come from the earth's soil and water. Plants don't create minerals; they must extract them from the soil as they grow. However, much like the instruments we mentioned earlier, they also are not interchangeable. For example, calcium, one of the essential minerals, is required for proper bone growth, whereas zinc, another essential mineral, supports smell and taste. If your body is deficient in calcium, zinc can't just take calcium's place to ensure proper bone growth. And, conversely, if your body is short on zinc, calcium cannot aid in flavor or smell perception.

Just as all instruments in the woodwind section make music when the player blows air (wind) through a tube once made of, well, wood, all vitamins also have something in common. Vitamins are all produced by the plants and animals we consume. But just as woodwind instruments can be subcategorized by the number of reeds they have, the vitamin family can also be subdivided by characteristics. Vitamins can be either fat-soluble or water-soluble. The fat-soluble vitamins—A, D, E, and K—are absorbed with the help of bile acids and can be stored in significant amounts in your body fat and liver until they are needed. All of the other vitamins are water-soluble, which means they cannot be stored in the body in significant amounts (B12 is an exception). Instead, water-soluble vitamins travel through the bloodstream, and if the body does not use them, they are eliminated through urination; they are not readily stored for a rainy day, like fat-soluble vitamins. Again, our point here is that one vitamin cannot take the place of another vitamin. Their functions are as unique as the pitch of an instrument. Vitamin A, for example, aids in night vision, whereas vitamin B9, also called folate, helps prevent spina bifida in newborns—they are not interchangeable.

So if a piece of sheet music requires a trombone, flute, cello, and violin, and the violin and flute are missing, it does not matter how many cellos or trombones are present at the time of the performance—the music will never sound as it was intended. Additionally, it would not matter if other instruments, such as a tuba or a xylophone, were present in their stead, because only the violin and the flute can produce the correct sound required for the musical piece. Following this logic, if an essential bodily function requires calcium, magnesium, vitamin K, and zinc, and the calcium and zinc are deficient, then regardless of how much magnesium, vitamin K, or any other micronutrients are present, the bodily function will never be carried out as it should be. This can leave the door open to health conditions and diseases in the future.

However, the good news is that when all the micronutrients are available, the body can once again perform the essential function, and the health condition or disease that was manifesting itself because of the deficiency will be greatly improved or reversed completely.

In Chapter 4, we will go into great detail on the final two sections of our orchestra, the essential fatty acids and the amino acids. Both can greatly influence your ability to build bones, and we'll introduce you to all the cutting-edge research about them. However, for now, we want you to know that just like with the strings (minerals) and woodwinds (vitamins), where the instruments were not interchangeable, the same is true of the percussion (essential fatty acids) and brass (amino acids) sections. One nutrient cannot take the place of another micronutrient, as their functions are all unique.

YOUR ORCHESTRA OF MICRONUTRIENTS

THE WOODWIND SECTION OR ESSENTIAL VITAMINS

WATER-SOLUBLE	FAT-SOLUBLE
Vitamin B_1 (thiamine)	Vitamin A
Vitamin B_2 (riboflavin)	Vitamin D
Vitamin B_3 (niacin)	Vitamin E
Vitamin B_5 (pantothenic acid)	Vitamin K
Vitamin B_6 (pyridoxine)	
Vitamin B_7 (biotin)	
Vitamin B_9 (folate)	
Vitamin B_{12} (cobalamin)	
Vitamin C	
Choline	

THE STRING SECTION OR ESSENTIAL MINERALS

MACROMINERALS	TRACE MINERALS
Calcium	Boron
Chloride	Chromium
Magnesium	Copper
Phosphorus	Iodine
Potassium	Iron
Sodium	Manganese
	Molybdenum
	Selenium
	Silicon
	Zinc

THE PERCUSSION SECTION OR ESSENTIAL FATTY ACIDS (EFAs)

OMEGA-3 (ALA)	OMEGA-6 (LA)
↓	↓
EPA	GLA
↓	↓
DHA	DGLA
	↓
	AA

THE BRASS SECTION OR ESSENTIAL AMINO ACIDS

ESSENTIAL	CONDITIONALLY ESSENTIAL
Histidine	Arginine
Isoleucine	Cysteine
Leucine	Glutamine
Lysine	Tyrosine
Methionine	Glycine
Phenylalanine	Ornithine
Threonine	Proline
Tryptophan	Serine
Valine	

Your Bone-Building Micronutrients

When you think about the micronutrients needed to rebuild strong bones, you likely think of those your doctor mentioned like calcium, vitamin D, and magnesium, or if they were forward thinking, perhaps boron and vitamin K. However, simply supplementing with two or three of these key micronutrients will not do the trick. Even if your current bone-building supplement contains all five of the micronutrients we just mentioned, it still would not be enough. As the orchestra analogy shows, your body requires *all* of the essential vitamins and minerals to prevent and reverse osteoporosis. No vitamin or mineral can be deficient, and none of the micronutrients are interchangeable. There is no way around it. In fact, even if you have chosen to take the drug therapy path, becoming sufficient in your essential micronutrients is vital to help you overcome prescription-induced depletions. If bone health is your goal, then sufficiency across the board is required. Take a look at Table 2.1 to examine how each essential vitamin and mineral has been scientifically proven to aid in bone health.

TABLE 2.1 The Essential Micronutrients Required for Bone Health

Essential Micronutrient	Function in Bone Health
Vitamin A	A powerful antioxidant that protects against oxygen-based damage to cells (free radicals, inflammation). Plays an essential role in regulating osteoclast function and development of osteoblasts. A deficiency in vitamin A also limits calcium absorption and metabolism. Both low and excessively high serum vitamin A concentrations are associated with an increased risk of hip fracture.
Lutein	Although not essential, this powerful antioxidant protects against oxygen-based damage to cells (free radicals, inflammation); studies suggest that lutein can be protective in bone health because it activates Nrf2-driven antioxidant gene expression with a correlation between intake of lutein and higher BMD.

Essential Micronutrient	Function in Bone Health
Vitamin B1 (thiamine)	Required for the molecules found in carbohydrates and proteins (in the form of branched-chain amino acids) to be properly used by the body to carry out various bone-building functions. Aids in the normal endocrine function of the pancreas; helps fight off stress by maintaining proper function of the adrenal glands. Thiamine deficiency reduces stomach acid and calcium absorption, which causes increased chances for osteoporosis.
Vitamin B2 (riboflavin)	Plays a role in reducing homocysteine levels (increased homocysteine levels are a risk factor for osteoporotic bone fractures). Assists with antioxidant activity; increased dietary riboflavin has been associated with higher BMD.
Vitamin B3 (niacin and niacinimide)	Assists in calcium signaling; improves adiponectin secretion, glucose tolerance, and insulin sensitivity; required for conversion of omega-3. There is a positive significant correlation between dietary intake of vitamin B3 and BMD in premenopausal women.
Vitamin B5 (pantothenic acid)	Used in the synthesis of coenzyme A (CoA), an enzyme that participates in a variety of reactions in the body, especially the breaking down of fatty acids. A deficiency of vitamin B5 can cause an increased sensitivity to insulin. Helps fight off stress (chronic stress is a risk factor for osteoporosis) by maintaining proper function of the adrenal glands and cortisol levels.
Vitamin B6 (pyroxidan)	Plays a role in reducing homocysteine levels (increased homocysteine levels are a risk factor for osteoporotic bone fractures). Essential for the enzymatic action of lysyl oxidase in collagen cross-linking formation and bone strength. B6 deficiency causes an imbalance in the coupling between osteoblasts and osteoclasts with increased bone cavities and reduced new bone formation. Necessary for hydrochloric acid (HCl) production by the stomach, which in turn is necessary for calcium absorption; B6 may act as a regulator of the steroid hormones, including estrogen; prevents progesterone deficiency; required for mineral balance; equips you to better deal with stress by aiding in the formation of chemicals called neurotransmitters. Increased dietary B6 intake was associated with higher BMD.

Essential Micronutrient	Function in Bone Health
Vitamin B7 (biotin)	Helps metabolize carbohydrates, fats, and amino acids from dietary intake; aids in the synthesis of bone marrow. Vitamin B7 (biotin) deficiency affects IGF-1 status (insulin-like growth factor is fundamental in skeletal growth) and bone formation.
Vitamin B9 (folate)	Plays a role in reducing homocysteine levels (increased homocysteine levels are a risk factor for osteoporotic bone fractures). Equips you to better deal with stress by aiding in the formation of chemicals called neurotransmitters; in folate-deficient osteoclasts, resorption activity was found to be significantly increased. Dietary folate is a significant predictor for BMD.
Vitamin B12 (cobalamin)	Plays a role in reducing homocysteine levels (increased homocysteine levels are a risk factor for osteoporotic bone fractures). Required for osteoblasts to function; proven to have a protective role in preserving BMD and reducing fracture risk.
Vitamin C	Aids in collagen and elastin synthesis, both necessary elements in bone matrix, tooth dentin, and tendons; enhances calcium absorption; enhances vitamin D's effect on bone metabolism; protects against oxygen-based damage to cells (free radicals, anti-inflammatory); lowers cortisol. Higher vitamin C intake levels were associated with a lower risk of osteoporosis in adults over age fifty with low levels of physical activity.
Vitamin D	Mobilizes calcium and phosphorus for release from bone in the presence of parathyroid hormone; promotes intestinal absorption of calcium and phosphate; increases kidney absorption of calcium and phosphorus and carries them into the blood. Prevents muscle weakness that can promote falls and fractures. People with low levels of vitamin D in their blood have lower BMD and an increased incidence of osteoporosis. Vitamin D supplements at doses of 700–800 International Units (IU) per day reduced the incidence of hip fracture by 26 percent and other nonvertebral fractures by 23 percent.

Essential Micronutrient	Function in Bone Health
Vitamin E	A powerful antioxidant that protects against oxygen-based damage to cells (free radicals, anti-inflammatory). One of the eight forms of Vitamin E, called delta-tocotrienol, can completely prevent the erosion of the bone surface and also be effective in increasing bone formation and preventing bone resorption. Deficiency in another form of vitamin E, alpha-tocopherol, was associated with an 86 percent increase in the rate of hip fracture, whereas use of alpha-tocopherol-containing supplements was associated with a 22 percent reduction in the rate of hip fracture.
Vitamin K	Vitamin K2 is an important inducer of bone mineralization in human osteoblasts (bone-building cells); required for the synthesis of osteocalcin. Vitamin K2 has been proven in studies to be as effective as prescription drugs in reducing the incidence of bone fractures. Vitamin K2 has also been proven to induce positive changes in bone mass by allowing for proper use of calcium.
Choline	Involved in metabolism, transport of lipids, cellular reactions, and the synthesis of neurotransmitters. Subjects with the lowest dietary total choline had a higher risk of low BMD.
Boron	Enhances calcium absorption and estrogen metabolism; stabilizes and extends the half-life of Vitamin D, converting vitamin D to its most active form; reduces the excretion of magnesium; helps metabolize insulin; exhibits an estrogen-enhancing effect and reduces oxidative stress. One study found that boron supplements can increase bone formation and inhibit bone resorption.
Calcium	Acts as the primary component required for both strong and dense bone; supports tooth formation. Studies determined that increases in BMD were similar in trials of dietary sources of calcium and calcium supplements.
Chromium	Preserves bone mineral by reducing the loss of calcium in the urine, promoting collagen production, increasing adrenal DHEA levels, improving insulin regulation, and reducing the rate of bone resorption.

Essential Micronutrient	Function in Bone Health
Copper	Aids in the formation of collagen for bone and connective tissue and contributes to the mechanical strength of bone collagen fibrils (the strands of proteins that cross-link to one another in the spaces around cells); inhibits bone resorption; neutralizes superoxide radicals produced by the osteoclasts (bone-breakdown cells) during resorption. Reduced copper levels have been shown to be linked to reduced BMD.
Iodine	Iodine deficiency has been shown to result in increased oxidative stress and higher levels of oxidative damage to DNA. Increased oxidative stress has also been highlighted as one of the underlying mechanisms of osteoporosis. Iodine is an essential element for bone mineralization, and iodine deficiency is frequently observed in postmenopausal patients with osteoporosis.
Iron	Iron is a co-factor for the enzymes involved in collagen synthesis. In laboratory tests, low levels of iron may lead to lower bone strength. Essential for vitamin D metabolism. Chronic iron deficiency induces bone resorption and risk of osteoporosis.
Magnesium	A constituent of the bone matrix, required for osteoblast production, development, and activity; assists in calcium absorption; fights destructive inflammation; ensures the strength and firmness of bones; stimulates the thyroid's production of calcitonin; regulates parathyroid hormone; required for forming new calcium crystals for proper bone formation. Lower magnesium intake is associated with lower BMD of the hip and whole body.
Manganese	A co-factor in the formation of bone cartilage and bone collagen, as well as in bone mineralization. Helps with the formation of bone-regulatory hormones and enzymes involved in bone metabolism. Manganese is the preferred co-factor of enzymes called glycosyltransferases; these enzymes are required for the synthesis of proteoglycans that are needed for the formation of healthy cartilage and bone. Deficiencies in manganese have been correlated with lower bone density and bone strength.

Essential Micronutrient	Function in Bone Health
Phosphorus	Combines with calcium to form a mineral crystal that gives strength and structure to our bones and teeth. Up to 70 percent of absorbed and retained phosphorus combines with calcium to help form bone and tooth structure; the remaining 30 percent combines with nitrogen to metabolize fats and carbohydrates. High intake of phosphorus has no adverse effect on bone metabolism in populations with adequate calcium intake, and it is also associated with positive bone parameters in some age/gender groups.
Potassium	Neutralizes bone-depleting metabolic acids; potassium conserves calcium within the body and reduces urinary calcium loss. Studies show that potassium can decrease bone breakdown and stimulate new bone formation in postmenopausal women.
Silicon	Strengthens the connective tissue matrix by cross-linking collagen strands. Increases the rate of mineralization, particularly when calcium intake is low; plays an important role in initiating the calcification process, thus helping us to maintain strong, flexible bones. Stimulates osteoblasts (bone-building cells) by increasing protein collagen synthesis; inhibits osteoclasts (bone-resorbing cells) by directly discouraging bone resorption. In one study, researchers noted that at least 40 mg of daily silicon accounted for 10 percent higher BMD than lower intakes of around 14 mg of silicon per day. Another study found that individuals who supplemented with silicon enjoyed significant increases in trabecular bone volume.
Selenium	A powerful antioxidant that protects against oxygen-based damage to cells (free radicals, anti-inflammatory). Studies have shown that selenium deficiency changes bone metabolism and reduces BMD and bone volume.
Zinc	Plays a role in the activity of osteoblasts and osteoclasts; required in the production of the matrix of collagen protein threads on which the bone-forming calcium-phosphorus compound is deposited. Proper calcium absorption also depends on zinc, and a deficiency prevents full absorption of calcium. A zinc deficiency will delay bone growth, bone development, and maintenance of bone health. Low serum zinc is associated with low BMD in women.

Wow, incredible, right? Whether they play a leading role or a more supporting role, each essential micronutrient must be ready to play its unique melody if the body is to prevent and reverse bone loss. As you read the upcoming chapters, we want you to keep this table in mind so that you can see how every micronutrient we discuss can help you build strong, healthy, flexible bones. And each of the forty healing habits you'll learn increases the micronutrients in your bone-rebuilding orchestra. If creating sufficiency in just one or a few micronutrients (as they did in many of the studies highlighted in the table) can increase bone density and decrease fracture risk, imagine the benefits of creating a sustained state of micronutrient sufficiency in all of your essential micronutrients.

However, in order to see these positive benefits, you need to reach micronutrient sufficiency every day. Similarly to how your doctor may mandate that you take your drug therapy each day for it to work, with micronutrient therapy, consistency is key not only to build your bone, but to rebuild your health. We promise to do our part and deliver all the information you need to rebuild your bones in our twelve-week osteoporosis protocol. But you need to commit to it. After all, isn't getting your health back on track safely and naturally worth it?

Introducing Our Three-Step Plan

To help you meet your goal of improved bone health, we have identified three key steps to take: dietary changes, lifestyle habits, and smart supplementation. They are all equally important on your path to success, and we will cover each of the steps in the chapters to follow in great detail, identifying your forty healing habits along the way. For now, let's just learn a little bit about the incredible journey you will take and the three steps you will take in order to get there.

STEP 1: SWITCH TO RICH

We want you to switch to rich. No, we aren't talking about winning the lottery here. (Although preventing bone loss should be as exciting as winning a jackpot!) What we do mean is that eating a micronutrient-dense diet filled with "Rich Food" is our first step toward reaching micronutrient sufficiency and achieving bone health. This essential first step will fill your body with the vitamins, minerals, essential fatty acids, and amino acids it needs to function at its best. Often, the dietary doctrine you follow (Paleo, low-carb, vegan, etc.) will determine the spectrum of foods you will be choosing from. For example, vegans will not be choosing beef as their source of vitamin A, nor will a Paleo dieter be choosing dairy as their source of vitamin D; these foods do not fit into the dietary guidelines of these dietary preferences. Regardless of the dietary profile you follow, we'll show you how to choose the foods that contain the highest levels of micronutrients.

But be warned: today our food is fighting a losing battle, not only against depleted mineral levels in the soil and ever-increasing CO_2 levels, but also against genetically modified organisms (GMOs), global distribution, factory farming, and food processing and cooking methods, which all further deplete the few micronutrients that are left. And as we mentioned earlier, even some of the "healthy" foods you love may be adding to your nutrient depletion by making it so that you can't absorb your micronutrients. There is a lot to learn about finding Rich Foods that can help you reach sufficiency.

STEP 2: DRIVE DOWN DEPLETION

Although eating a Rich Food diet increases your micronutrient levels, everyday life contains many roadblocks that can stand in your way of achieving optimal health. We will show you all the ways you may unknowingly be causing your own micronutrient depletion. As mentioned in Chapter 1 during our discussion of factors that can contribute to micronutrient deficiency, some of your everyday lifestyle habits, even ones you think are healthy, may be causing you to use your vitamins and minerals faster, leaving you running low. From stress to pollution, medications to toxins, your life is filled with what we call everyday micronutrient depleters (EMDs) that reduce the amount of micronutrients in your body. In this second step, you will learn to identify these micronutrient thieves that are keeping you from thriving.

STEP 3: SMART SUPPLEMENTATION

You are already starting to learn how just how miraculous the essential micronutrients are, and how they can help you improve your bone health. In this third and final step, we will share with you the reasons that supplementation often falls short of delivering the desired outcomes. You will learn our ABCs of smart supplementation, and we'll teach you how avoiding the four major flaws common to most supplements today can guarantee that micronutrient sufficiency is met and exceptional health transformations occur.

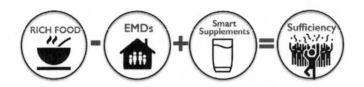

Sounds pretty simple, right? You'll recognize these steps as the path we took to reverse Mira's osteoporosis. They are the same steps we have shared with thousands before you. But remember: in order for the program to work, you have to work it! Your health depends on your willingness to make these forty small but strategic changes in your life. And you have to be in it for the long haul—your osteoporosis did not show up overnight, and neither will any reversal or prevention.

YOUR BODY, YOUR BUCKET—MAY YOUR BUCKET RUNNETH OVER!

Now before we move on, let's end this chapter with another analogy we call the bucket analogy. (You're probably noticing that we love analogies!) The purpose of *this* analogy is to create a simple, easy-to-understand mental picture of what micronutrient sufficiency and deficiency looks like.

We want you to start by picturing a bucket in your mind—think of that bucket as your body. If your body is sufficient in all of your essential micronutrients, your bucket is full. When you think about your sufficiency bucket, we want you to see a bucket that is full right up to the brim with water. However, if you are deficient in even one essential micronutrient, then we want you to picture the water level of the bucket going down. The more deficient you are, the lower the water, got it?

Your objective is to end each day with a full bucket so that your body has everything it needs to maintain your health. Every day that you do not accomplish this objective, your body is forced to allocate the available micronutrients to high-priority functions and leave other functions compromised in some way, opening the door to potential health issues. Seems pretty easy, right? Just fill up your bucket and *poof*, your body has everything it needs to keep you healthy. And although this is true, in an overly simplified way, keeping your bucket filled to the brim is not as easy as it sounds.

How Full Is Your Bucket?

As we continue together, we will show you how it is nearly impossible for you to receive even the minimum amount of essential micronutrients your body requires from today's food. Additionally, you will discover how your daily dietary and lifestyle habits create tiny holes in your bucket, causing the vital micronutrients that you have managed to put in your bucket to slowly and steadily leak out. Our goal here is not to discourage you but to offer you a stripped-down, raw view of what we are all up against. The good news is that the forty healing habits can help you plug those holes so that you can achieve your goal of a full, micronutrient-sufficient bucket. To help you identify (and then disarm) the micronutrient-depleting habits in your life, we created our Rebuild Your Bones Micronutrient Sufficiency Quiz (Table 2.2).

The first thing that we do when a client is interested in starting our Rebuild Your Bones twelve-week osteoporosis protocol is give them the quiz that we have provided here for you. It doesn't matter if that client already has had a micronutrient blood test of any kind. Our analysis is different. The quiz looks at your dietary, lifestyle, and supplementation habits along with information about your current health status to identify the areas where you most need to improve. All you have to do is answer the questions honestly. Don't worry about how you score: even if you don't score as high as you would like this time around, when you take the quiz again at the end of your twelve-week plan, after implementing all forty of our healing habits, your score is sure to improve. It may not be as scientific as blood work, but it does offer great insight into your likelihood of being sufficient or deficient in the essential micronutrients—and the more you learn about yourself and your micronutrient levels, the better equipped you will be to rebuild your bones.

TABLE 2.2 Rebuild Your Bones Micronutrient Sufficiency Quiz

	OFTEN	SOMETIMES	NEVER
1. I eat locally grown food.			
2. I eat organically grown food.			
3. Fruits, vegetables, cheese, and meats may sit in my refrigerator or the grocery store refrigerator for a few days before being used.			
4. I eat conventional eggs or those labeled as cage-free (not pasture-raised or free-range).			
5. I eat grain-fed beef (not grass-fed) and store-bought cheese (not raw cheese), eggs, and butter.			
6. I use canned or frozen vegetables.			
7. I eat potato chips, french fries, tortilla chips, nuts, or other salty snacks.			
8. I eat candy (gummy, hard, or anything else made of sugar).			
9. I use Splenda, Sweet'N Low, Equal, or any artificial sweeteners rather than stevia, xylitol, or luo han.			
10. I use products containing high-fructose corn syrup (including salad dressing and ketchup).			
11. I eat white bread, rolls, or traditional pasta.			
12. I drink carbonated sodas (Coke, Pepsi, Diet Coke, etc.).			
13. I use products containing MSG (including soy sauce).			

	OFTEN	SOMETIMES	NEVER
14. I eat dessertlike baked goods (muffins, croissants, cakes, biscuits, crepes, quiche).			
15. I eat spinach, collard greens, sweet potatoes, rhubarb, or beans.			
16. I eat whole-grain breads, corn, beans, grains (including cereal), or soy isolates.			
17. I eat nuts, apples, carrots, seeds (including flaxseeds), or oats			
18. I eat brown rice or white potatoes.			
19. I drink pasteurized (grocery store–bought) milk.			
20. I drink more than two glasses of alcohol a day (beer, wine, or spirits).			
21. I drink a lot of coffee, tea, or coffee drinks—more than 3 cups a day.			
22. I drink caffeinated sodas or energy drinks.			
23. I drink fruit juices or sports drinks sweetened with sugar or enhanced with high fructose corn syrup.			
24. I skip meals.			
25. I follow a low-carbohydrate, low-fat, intermittent-fasting, Paleo, Primal, Mediterranean, medically founded (e.g., DASH), packaged-food (Jenny Craig, Nutrisystem, or similar), vegetarian, vegan, gluten-free, or calorie-restricting diet.			
26. I limit protein intake to follow an alkaline diet.			
27. I have had surgery to help me lose weight. (Check "never" for no, "often" for yes.)			
28. I use olive oil, avocado oil, grapeseed oil, sunflower oil, corn oil, sesame oil, soybean oil, or margarine.			
29. I snack on nuts, nut butters (unsprouted), or nut milks or use nut flour.			

	OFTEN	SOMETIMES	NEVER
30. I use store-bought mayonnaise or salad dressings.			
31. I drink from plastic water bottles or store food in plastic containers.			
32. I cook with aluminum foil.			
33. I purchase conventional moisturizer, toothpaste, shampoo, or household cleaning products at the grocery store.			
34. I use nonstick Teflon pans.			
35. I have stress in my life.			
36. I sleep less than eight or nine hours a night soundly.			
37. I smoke cigarettes, cigars, or a pipe or live with (or spend a large amount of time with) someone who does.			
38. I live in a large or highly polluted city.			
39. I avoid being in the sun without wearing sunscreen.			
40. I carry my cell phone all day close to my body (in a pocket, etc.).			
41. I am physically active in a gym, at home, or outdoors and frequently sweat during workouts.			
42. I hop, jump, jog, or do osteogenic loading.			
43. I take prescription drugs for osteoporosis.			
44. I take prescription medication (including birth control and medication for erectile dysfunction).			
45. I take medication for stress, anxiety, or depression.			
46. I take aspirin or other over-the-counter pain and fever reducers (including acetaminophen and ibuprofen).			
47. I take antacids (prescription or nonprescription).			

	OFTEN	SOMETIMES	NEVER
48. I take probiotics and digestive enzymes daily.			
49. I take an omega-3 supplement that contains both EPA and DHA in two separate doses.			
50. I take a multivitamin supplement that is formulated using Anti-Competition Technology.			

Step 1: Look at statements 1 and 2. For each question, if you answered "often," give yourself a round of applause and **add 10 points**. **Add 5 points** for each time you answered "sometimes." **Don't add any points** if you answered "never."

+ _____

Step 2: For statements 3 through 41, **deduct 5 points** for every time you answered "often." **Deduct 3 points** for every time you answered "sometimes." **Don't deduct any points** if you answered "never."

- _____

Step 3: Look at statement 42. If you answered "often," **add 100 points.** If you answered "sometimes," **add 50 points.** **Don't do anything** if you answered "never."

+ _____

Step 4: For statements 43 through 47, **deduct 5 points** for every time you answered "often." **Deduct 3 points** for every time you answered "sometimes." Don't deduct any points if you answered "never."

- _____

Step 5: Look at statements 48 and 49. If you answered "often," **add 20 points**. **Add 10 points** if you answered "sometimes." **Deduct 20 points** if you answered "never."

+/- _____

Step 6: If you answered "often" to statement 50, then bravo! **Add 100 points** to your score—we'll tell you why it's so important in Chapter 6. If you answered "sometimes," **add 50 points** and try to remember to take it more often. Do nothing if you answered "never."

+ _____

Step 7: Add up all the totals from Step 1 through Step 8.

= _____

GRAND TOTAL

IF YOUR SCORE WAS NEGATIVE

A negative score indicates that you are not reaching micronutrient sufficiency. But don't worry if you have a low score, or even a *really* low score—the lower your score, the more you can improve. By reading this book, you'll learn our secrets to increase your micronutrient sufficiency level and dramatically improve your bone health.

Our goal for you is to get your score into the Optimal Zone for Bone Building, where you'll be primed to see fast, dramatic results that can last a lifetime. Don't forget to take the analysis again at the end of your twelve-week protocol. When you follow the plan exactly as we outline it, your score and sufficiency level will both greatly improve.

IF YOUR SCORE WAS POSITIVE

Bravo! You are in the Optimal Zone for Bone Building, and for that, we salute you. Your score indicates that you are making great decisions to consume high-quality micronutrient-dense foods. It is likely that you have also eliminated a few micronutrient-robbing lifestyle habits, and perhaps you supplement using a properly formulated multivitamin. (You may even be taking our patented multivitamin Nutreince already.)

Now, our goal for you is to keep your score in the Optimal Zone for Bone Building. You may not even know which things you have done right or how you scored so high. Following our Rebuild Your Bones osteoporosis protocol will reveal to you the healing habits that got you here, so you can make sure to continue them. It will also give you some important information on how to improve your score even further. This is a great starting point. Your sufficiency level means that you are primed to see fast, dramatic results that can last a lifetime.

AND OFF YOU GO!

You've analyzed your own dietary, lifestyle, and supplementation habits to get a snapshot of how likely it is that your habits are unknowingly contributing to your micronutrient deficiencies. You are now ready to start making some important changes in your life. We have already introduced you to two of the healing habits we want you to incorporate into your life—pretty sneaky of us, right? Your first healing habit is to **avoid the dangers of osteoporosis medications**, which we have shown to be potentially detrimental to your health. These drugs deplete you of the essential micronutrients that we have proven can naturally aid in bone building. Instead, we want you to incorporate our second healing habit and **choose to make micronutrient sufficiency your path to stronger bones**. Remember, if you're on osteoporosis medications, following our second healing habit and increasing your micronutrient sufficiency is just as important for you to combat the depleting effects of your medication. In the next chapter, we will move through your pantry and fridge to identify the Poor Food Perpetrators just waiting to trip you up on your path to extraordinary health.

Healing Habits Revealed in Chapter 2

1. Avoid the dangers of osteoporosis medications. However, if you decide to follow the pharmaceutical path, safeguard yourself by following all of the other healing habits in *Rebuild Your Bones*.
2. Make micronutrient sufficiency your chosen path to bone health.

Join us On the Couch for an in-depth chat about Chapter 2

OK, it's time for your next "On the Couch" chat. In this coaching video, we share important insights into your first two healing habits as well as our three-step plan. We will also talk to you about what your Rebuild Your Bones Micronutrient Sufficiency Quiz score means to you, and what you can do to improve your score to create the optimal bone-building environment in your body. Remember, this is important information regardless of whether you have chosen to take or forgo medication. Join us now at RebuildYourBones.com.

CHAPTER 3

Let Thy Food Be Thy Medicine

The journey of a thousand miles begins with one single step.
—CHINESE PROVERB

Right now, there are likely a lot of products in your kitchen that could hurt your chances of building stronger, more flexible bones. Although some are easy to spot because the micronutrient-robbing ingredients are listed right on the label, other bone blockers may be hiding in less obvious places. Get ready to take your first giant step toward creating a state of micronutrient sufficiency by Switching to Rich and becoming a nutrivore.

Becoming a Nutrivore

Do you follow a low-fat, high-protein diet? Or does the idea of eating burgers and chicken wings on a low-carb, high-fat ketogenic diet excite you? Regardless of what type of diet you choose to follow, we've got you covered. This is because being deficient in vitamins, minerals, essential fatty acids, and amino acids (the intricate family of micronutrients you learned about in Chapter 2) has negative health implications for everyone, including vegans, vegetarians, low-fat, Primal/Paleo, Mediterranean, and low-carb dieters. The bottom line is this: everyone who is on a mission to build better bones and improve their overall health should have micronutrient sufficiency as their primary goal.

Because this is such a radical new way of looking at and understanding nutrition, we created a new term to describe the person who adopts this goal. We want to personally invite you to join this group of health-conscious visionaries regardless of your dietary philosophy. By reading *Rebuild Your Bones* now and embarking on your own journey to improve your bone health, you are officially welcome to call yourself a *nutrivore*. The good news is that all you have to do to become a nutrivore is commit to taking control of your health by recognizing that regardless of your preferred dietary philosophy, micronutrient deficiency is the foundation of poor health and disease, and that micronutrient sufficiency is the foundation of optimal health. Nutrivores don't blame their poor health on genetics, or search for a cure at the bottom of a prescription bottle. Instead, they commit to retaking control of their health by achieving a state of micronutrient sufficiency.

The health-promoting, disease-preventing power of micronutrient sufficiency has the potential to prevent and reverse countless diseases, including osteoporosis, within the next century, but only if we harness it.

Throughout this chapter, our goal is help you maximize your micronutrients and identify the foods that could be blocking your path to micronutrient sufficiency and making it more difficult for your body to build healthy bones. To help you with this evaluation, we created the Rich Food, Poor Food philosophy. We define Rich Foods as foods that help increase your micronutrient sufficiency levels that are natural, unprocessed or minimally processed, high in micronutrients, and low in or devoid of problematic ingredients that can put your bone-building nutrients at risk. Poor Foods, on the other hand, are foods that reduce your likelihood of reaching micronutrient sufficiency. However, identifying them can be tricky. Poor Foods can be either highly processed foods that are low in or devoid of micronutrients or seemingly healthy foods that contain problematic ingredients, such as everyday micronutrient depleters (EMDs), that rob you of vitamins, minerals, essential fatty acids, and amino acids. Your goal, over the next twelve weeks and hopefully for the rest of your life, will be to eat as many Rich Foods as possible and to steer clear of Poor Foods. Let's get started.

Shopping Solutions—More Micronutrient Bang in Every Bite!

The following is a crash course in our top ten shopping tips from our book *Rich Food Poor Food*. These tips increase the micronutrient content of your foods so you'll have all the information you need to make your twelve-week bone-building program a resounding success. However, we highly recommend you pick up a copy of *Rich Food Poor Food* as well. It helps you identify the highest-quality foods down every aisle of the grocery store and even lists our favorite brands to make grocery-shopping super simple.

OUR TOP TEN *RICH FOOD POOR FOOD* TIPS FOR SHOPPING SMART

1. **Buy local and organic whenever possible to increase micronutrient content, reduce pesticides, and avoid GMOs.** Research published in the journal *Environmental Research* shows that when study participants switched to eating a diet of at least 80 percent organic food for just one week, urinalysis revealed a dramatic 89 percent reduction of detectable levels of pesticides. We've created a free download that can help you identify which foods are the safest to buy conventional and which are worth buying organic. It's called the Fab 14 and Terrible 20 list; grab yours now at RebuildYourBones.com.

2. **Look for raw, unpasteurized dairy products or safe milk alternatives.** Compared to conventional pasteurized milk, natural, grass-fed raw milk has as much as 60 percent more vitamin B1 (thiamine) and B6, 100 percent more B12, and 30 percent more vitamin B9 (folate). It also has an increased amount of calcium, phosphorus, and vitamin K2, and greater amounts of anti-inflammatory omega-3s. Can't find raw milk? Then opt for organic grass-fed milk in the grocery store. If you are dairy-free, leave all soy and nut milk products on the shelves and opt instead for hemp or coconut milk.

3. **Meat should be organic, grass-fed, and grass-finished.** A joint research study between the USDA and Clemson University found that compared to grain-fed beef, grass-fed beef has higher amounts of calcium, magnesium, thiamine, riboflavin, and potassium, has more than 400 percent more vitamins A and E, and is up to four times as rich in bone-building omega-3 fatty acids. Additionally, the grass-fed beef was also found to contain a healthier ratio of omega-3 to omega-6 (you'll learn the importance of omega-3 for bone health in Chapter 4).

4. **Choose organic and free-range or pasture-raised poultry and eggs.** Don't be misled by the term *cage-free*—it is not the same as free-range or pasture-raised. Eggs from hens raised on pastures (free-range) contain seven times as much beta-carotene (a form of vitamin A) and three times as much vitamin E, as well as twice the amounts of anti-inflammatory omega-3s.

5. **Always purchase wild fish that has been troll, pole, or line-caught.** Wild-caught fish can have up to 380 percent more omega-3 than factory-farmed fish, according to the USDA National Nutrient Database. Avoid canned fish unless you can confirm that it comes in BPA-free cans.

6. **Avoid unhealthy omega-6 fats when choosing oils.** Organic grass-fed/pasture-raised butter, cream, ghee, lard, tallow, and duck fat, as well as palm oil, coconut oil, and MCT oil, are recommended. Our favorite option is SKINNYFat brand, which we'll tell you more about in Chapter 7—a great-tasting cooking oil with zero omega-6.

7. **Ditch the store-bought salad dressings and condiments.** Most are loaded with sugar and unhealthy oils, so you will likely want to make your own. Chapter 9 has some great recipes.

8. **Create an alternative flour mix.** Flour alternatives, like coconut flour, almond flour, buckwheat flour, and flax meal, can produce great baked goods; however, sometimes a combination is needed for the best results. That is why you will see some of these Rich Food alternative flours used in our recipes.

9. **Choose organic stevia, xylitol, or luo han as sweeteners.** Not only are all three sweeteners low-glycemic, but stevia is currently

being researched for its ability to increase calcium metabolism, and xylitol is being researched for its ability to increase both calcium absorption and collagen production.

10. **Be smart when choosing beverages.** Ditch the sugar and caffeine-laden BPA-canned sodas as well as those sugary-sweet juices. Instead, opt for sparkling water in glass bottles. Purchase fair trade, organic coffees and teas.

Say So Long to Sugar

Although following our top ten Rich Food tips will increase your micronutrient levels, it's equally important to steer your cart away from Poor Foods that can harm you. Sugar is one of our least favorite ingredients in the grocery store—and there are so many reasons why. A recent study conducted by the Wall Street bank Credit Suisse revealed the bitter truth about global sugar consumption: the study found that sugar makes up 17 percent of the global diet. The daily average consumption for the world is 17 teaspoons (68 grams), which is 45 percent higher than thirty years ago. In the United States, which tops the list for consumption, the amount is far greater; Americans average 40 teaspoons (160 grams) a day, or 3 pounds of sugar per week.

So what gives sugar its spot on top of our list of Poor Foods? Remember, on this plan, the micronutrients come first. Sugar is one of the biggest roadblocks on your path to bone health because it can both deplete your body's essential bone-building micronutrients and block micronutrients from being absorbed. Additionally, unlike other micronutrient-leaching ingredients you will meet later on, there is not one bit of evidence of any nutritional benefit to eating refined white sugar. Although sugar's sweet flavor may be appetizing, its depletion of calcium, magnesium, chromium, and copper is not, especially when you consider the negative side effects of becoming deficient in these essential minerals. And vitamin C is also affected by sugar; because of similar chemical structures, vitamin C and glucose (a type of sugar) compete for entry into your cells. Even slightly elevated blood sugar levels can block vitamin C from getting in and can cause a weakened immune system.

Two important bone builders were on that list of nutrients depleted by sugar: calcium and magnesium. Guess what scientists discovered happens (beyond osteoporosis) when your calcium and magnesium levels fall short? You crave sugar! That's why one bite of something sweet leads to another, and you feel that you just can't put down the treat. With every bite, your levels of calcium and magnesium are further reduced, increasing your desire for more sugar—we call this the Crave Cycle. Your internal "cravings monster" calls out louder and louder, and there are only two ways to quiet him. Your first choice is to feed the cravings monster, eating more and more sugar and continuing on the path to deficiency, starving your bones of the essential nutrients they need to fight osteoporosis. Your second option, the one we hope you will take, is to break the Crave Cycle altogether by simply becoming sufficient in calcium and magnesium. It really is that easy.

There's more good news to share. Not only will you kill your sugar cravings with this one easy healing habit, but if you are a person who craves salty snacks, like pretzels or chips, research shows these cravings will be eliminated as well. Researchers at the Monell Chemical Senses Center in Philadelphia determined that salt cravings are also caused by a deficiency in calcium. They found that when you snack on something salty, the sodium temporarily increases calcium in the blood, tricking your body into thinking the calcium deficiency is over. However, although your salt craving may be temporarily satisfied, the secreted bone calcium leads to an exacerbated calcium deficiency, further salt cravings, and possibly more cravings for sugar, as well!

As you can see, when your body ingests sugar, numerous bone-strengthening vitamins and minerals are depleted. Ask yourself if that afternoon sugary snack or nightly scoop of ice cream is really worth it.

Becoming micronutrient sufficient is about to take you out of the Crave Cycle and put you and your willpower back in control. Mira got over her seemingly insatiable desire for Swedish Fish, which had plagued her in the years leading up to being diagnosed with advanced osteoporosis, and Evelyn's need for a nightly bowl of ice cream simply vanished. By eating Rich Foods and learning how to properly supplement with calcium and magnesium (warning: the two should not be taken together), you'll eliminate those deficiencies, and therefore your cravings. Additionally, by avoiding sugar, you will be avoiding any further sugar–related micronutrient depletions, which will help break the vicious Crave Cycle and quiet that cravings monster for good.

Evelyn Mann: My Success Sidestepping Sugar

It all began when I read the Caltons' book after my mother-in-law passed away from colon cancer. I'd always found reading food labels to be confusing, and to be honest, I didn't read them at all. Reading that book gave me the understanding of the importance of the micronutrients in the foods I eat. I took the first step on my own and began eating Rich Foods as well as eliminating sugar and wheat from my diet. It was a miracle. I was amazed at how my sugar cravings were wiped out within just weeks. My need for a nightly bowl of ice cream simply vanished. No more late-night runs to the store for my must-have ice cream.

However, I knew I had to do more. I suffered from intense headaches and was diagnosed with an ovarian cyst. After reading about the third step in the program, I added in supplementation with Nutreince, their multivitamin drink, and within ten days the headaches were also gone. Could it have been that I was getting headaches because of a lack of adequate vitamins and minerals? It sure seemed so. The biggest miracle of all, though, was that my cyst went away, as well. My prayers, and those of my friends and family, had been answered.

On top of having lost my cravings, my headaches, and my cyst, I realized I had lost something else. I had lost ten pounds without any additional effort. My husband was so impressed that he joined in, and immediately I noticed he had a lot more energy. (Who wouldn't want a husband with more energy?) I started teaching what I had learned from the Caltons in church, and I have personally witnessed the joy in others as they report all the numerous health benefits they have received from adopting the nutrivore lifestyle.

HIGH-FRUCTOSE CORN SYRUP: A CHEAP AND DANGEROUS SUGAR IMITATOR

Another dangerous ingredient that puts unsuspecting people on the road to micronutrient deficiency is high-fructose corn syrup (HFCS). Its popularity has skyrocketed by 1,060 percent since the 1970s because of its low cost. Today, many cereals, frozen snacks, chips, pastries, desserts, candies, and soft drinks are loaded with HFCS. As an inexpensive means of enhancing the flavor of their products, many food companies resort to using HFCS to intensify the sweetness. Although this helps their bottom line, it does not help your health.

It's bad enough that the excessive production of this monoculture crop (corn) robs the soil of its micronutrient content, but that's nothing compared to the micronutrient-depleting effects HFCS has on your bones. Fructose has been shown to have a negative effect on calcium, chromium, magnesium, zinc, and copper levels in the body, all of which are necessary for bone health. Recent animal studies have proven that chronically excessive fructose intake plays an important role in the development of osteoporosis. And because HFCS can be found abundantly in so many processed foods, it's easy to consume it unknowingly—especially for children, who need these essential micronutrients to reach peak bone mass. From a bowl of cereal in the morning to a thirst-quenching drink on a hot summer day, the ingestion of HFCS can happen anywhere, anytime, and must be avoided.

WOULD SUGAR BY ANY OTHER NAME TASTE AS SWEET?

Meryl Streep, Tom Hanks, and Jack Nicholson all seem to be able to transform themselves effortlessly from role to role in each performance on the big screen. They are capable of reinventing themselves over and over again to suit any situation and audience. Today, because so many of us are looking for different things on food labels to suit our individual dietary philosophies, food manufacturers have upped their game by using different aliases for sugar on their packaging. This marketing ploy makes it easy for anyone consuming a processed food to be fooled into thinking it's OK because the word *sugar* is nowhere to be found. But this couldn't be further from the truth! Table 3.1 lists the aliases for sugar that should be avoided at all costs.

Table 3.1 The Many Names for Sugar

Agave nectar	Evaporated cane juice
Barley malt	Fructose
Beet sugar	Fruit juice concentrate
Blackstrap molasses	Galactose
Brown sugar	Glucose
Cane juice crystals	High-fructose corn syrup (HFCS)
Cane sugar	Honey
Caramel	Invert sugar
Carob	Lactose
Castor sugar	Malt syrup
Confectioners' sugar	Maltodextrin
Corn sweeteners	Maltose
Corn syrup	Maple syrup
Crystalline fructose	Molasses
Date sugar	Raw sugar
Demerara sugar	Rice syrup
Dextrin	Sucrose
Dextrose	Syrup
Diastatic malt	Treacle
Diatase	Turbinado sugar
D-mannose	

SINISTER SUGAR SUBSTITUTES: A MENACE TO YOUR MICROBIOME

The food industry is always looking for new ways to attract customers. So it just makes sense that as sugar started to get a bad name, they've turned to food scientists at chemical companies to devise new sugar substitutes to entice you into wanting to eat their food. Although these sugar substitutes promise sweet treats without sacrifice, we know that the negative effects of these chemical concoctions extend down to our inner ecosystem of friendly and beneficial bacteria known as the *micro-biome*. Food scientists formulated these sinister sugar substitutes with the intent of having zero impact on our outsides (i.e., not causing weight gain like sugar), but their effect on our insides (i.e., our microbiome) is the real cause for concern.

Popular sugar substitutes, such as sucralose, aspartame, and saccharin (which are more commonly known by popular brand names such as Splenda, Equal, and Sweet'N Low), can all disrupt the natural balance of the microbiome, which plays an important role in the body's ability to fight disease and both absorb and manufacture essential micronutrients. In studies, when diet-induced changes improved the microbiome, researchers found a positive correlation with increases in fractional calcium absorption and increases in measures of bone density and strength.

This means that the seemingly harmless act of ingesting sugar substitutes, which has been shown to disrupt the microbiome, could negatively affect your calcium absorption and potentially lower your bone density. Additionally, scientists have discovered that ingesting aspartame (Equal) diminishes the absorption of calcium, iron, and zinc—all three of which are essential bone builders. Those sugar-free sodas are also big no-nos if your goal is to prevent or reverse your osteoporosis. (Don't worry—per our top ten Rich Food shopping tips, you can still safely sweeten your favorite foods with stevia, xylitol, and luo han.) Be on the lookout for the sinister sugar substitutes listed in Table 3.2 the next time you're at the market.

TABLE 3.2 The Many Names for Sugar Substitutes

SUGAR SUBSTITUTE	SOLD UNDER THESE NAMES
Acesulfame potassium	Acesulfame K, Sunett, Sweet One, E950 (European Union)
Advantame	The newest (2014) and sweetest addition to the aspartame/neotame family
Aspartame	NutraSweet, Equal, AminoSweet, Canderel, Spoonful, Equal-Measure, E951 (European Union)
Neotame	Newtame, E961 (European Union)
Saccharin	Sweet'N Low, Sugar Twin, and E954 (European Union)
Sucralose	Splenda, Sukrana, SucraPlus, CandyS, Cukren, Nevella, E955 (European Union)

Wheat: An All-Out Assault on Your Bones

Since our modern diet is filled with wheat-based foods like pastries, snacks, pastas, and other baked goods, exposure to wheat is common in today's society. However, as with its companions (sugar, HFCS, and sugar substitutes), wheat consumption also brings about some unfavorable bone consequences, and from this point forward, you and wheat are on the outs!

The first way that wheat works to wreck your bones is that it naturally contains oxalic acid, which binds to calcium, magnesium, and iron and blocks their absorption. Second, wheat also contains phytic acid, which binds to and blocks the absorption of calcium, magnesium, copper, manganese, chromium, iron, zinc, and niacin. It also accelerates the metabolism of vitamin D, causing the body to use up this important bone-strengthening vitamin at a faster rate. Phytate's attack on your micronutrient levels is no small matter. According to a study in the *American Journal of Clinical Nutrition*, when phytates are removed from wheat, iron absorption is increased by 1,160 percent. The consumption of wheat can even cause whole social groups to suffer. A study on Pakistani immigrants in the United Kingdom revealed that eating chapati (a Mediterranean-style bread) caused rickets and osteoporosis due to the high levels of phytates in the bread. This means that the simple act of eating too much phytate-laden bread caused vitamin D levels to be so low that rickets and osteoporosis were able to take hold.

And it doesn't end there. Wheat also contains lectins and trypsin inhibitors, which are both part of a plant's natural self-defense mechanism. Although lectins and trypsin inhibitors are good for plants, they are not good for humans to eat. Their stickiness causes them to bind to your intestinal tract. Because we require a clear intestinal tract to properly absorb vitamins and minerals, lectins and trypsin inhibitors have been shown to reduce micronutrient absorption and should be avoided. With every bite of bread, pasta, or crackers, your chances of building strong bones are being jeopardized.

These sticky antinutrients aren't done with you yet either. They also work alongside gluten, another bothersome protein in wheat. You've probably already heard of gluten, or may be among the 30 to 50 percent of the population that has a gluten sensitivity. You might even be among the one out of every 133 Americans who are diagnosed with celiac disease, a genetic condition resulting in intestinal damage whenever gluten is ingested. You probably know where we are going here—celiac disease induces micronutrient malabsorption, which means that most people who are diagnosed incur deficiencies in iron, zinc, copper, folate, calcium, and magnesium, as well vitamins E, D, B12, and B6.

The trypsin inhibitors, lectins, and gluten in wheat work in unison to cause a breach in the intestinal lining, a condition commonly known as *leaky gut*. Your gut *should* be a tightly sealed area so that the undigested food you eat stays inside, where it belongs. However, when you eat wheat, the trypsin inhibitors stimulate intestinal inflammation, and the lectins cause intestinal permeability. Then gluten induces the release of a protein called zonulin (and no, we aren't making up these intergalactic-sounding names). The villainous zonulin then damages the seals in the walls of the intestines, making an intestinal breach possible.

Once an intestinal breach exists, lectins, along with other particles, such as toxins and partially digested food, can "leak" into the bloodstream. Your body views these escapees as unwelcome foreign invaders and begins an all-out attack on these particles, leading to autoimmune mayhem and opening up the door to a wide variety of other health conditions like Crohn's disease, irritable bowel syndrome, colitis, fibromyalgia, thyroiditis, arthritis, and chronic fatigue syndrome. Additionally, leaky gut can directly affect bone loss. Because healthy bacteria in the gut produce vitamin K2, any disruption in the intestines (such as leaky gut syndrome) can result in a decreased ability to absorb or produce enough vitamin K2. Vitamin K2 is a key bone nutrient: it helps direct calcium into the bone itself. So if wheat causes you to have leaky gut and you can't create enough vitamin K2, then calcium can't be ushered into the bone, potentially causing osteoporosis.

Wheat's final strike is a one-two punch that has proven to be a real blow below the belt—actually in this case, it's a real blow to the belt line. The first punch comes from amylopectin A, which is responsible for the expansion of visceral fat (unhealthy fat that surrounds the organs) in the abdomen, often referred to as "wheat belly." Wheat's amylopectin A content and its relationship to a hormone called leptin make it far more perilous. Eating foods that contain amylopectin A makes us overexcrete leptin, which tells the brain we're full. Over time, an excess of leptin causes us to become deaf to its message. This is called leptin resistance. So not only do we eat more than we should because our body effectively can't hear leptin tell us we are full, but we are also increasing our blood levels of the hormone leptin—which carries with it some dangerous bone loss consequences of its own.

THE LEPTIN CONNECTION TO BONE LOSS (SCIENCE AND A STORY!)

New scientific research out of the College of Physicians and Surgeons at Columbia University has determined that high leptin levels decrease bone mass. Let's look at the science behind how this happens. High leptin levels inhibit a specific protein (ATF4), which effectively turns off all osteoblast (your bone-building cells) formation. This is key because your osteoblasts create osteocalcin. Therefore, increases in leptin levels directly jeopardize the production of osteocalcin. Because osteocalcin's job is to direct and carry the calcium we absorb in our gut to go to the correct tissues in our body (i.e., our bones), a halt in its production would limit bone building.

High leptin levels can also hold the benefits of your bone-building micronutrients ransom. If you have elevated leptin levels, your body will not be able to sufficiently use any ingested vitamin K2 or calcium to help build your bones. This is because in humans, osteocalcin has to be carboxylated by vitamin K2 to be made active, and thus able to do its job. This is why when vitamin K2 levels are low, and osteocalcin doesn't get carboxylated, we see calcification in places it should not be, like in your arteries. But if osteocalcin production is halted because of high leptin levels, then no matter how much vitamin K2 or calcium you ingest, via supplementation or diet, there is nothing for the vitamin K2 to carboxylate, nor is there anything to transport the calcium into your bones. This could be hugely detrimental in your fight against osteoporosis. Regardless of how hard you work or how intently you supplement, the process of building your bones will be hindered if blood levels of leptin rise too high.

Let's use another fun analogy to illustrate how high leptin can reduce your ability to build bone, even when you've spent your hard-earned money on micronutrient-rich foods and smart supplements. Think of the process of bone building like a well-run taxicab company. The taxicab's job is to take people to their desired destinations; however, as we all know, they require a payment from the passenger in order to do their jobs. When there are plenty of taxis it's easy to get a ride, but when taxis are scarce, it's difficult to get where you would like to go.

In this analogy your osteocalcin is the taxicabs. They carry passengers (calcium) to their desired location (your bone). If the passenger brings cash (vitamin K2), then the taxi brings them to their desired destination . . . your bone! However, if the passenger (calcium) has no cash (no vitamin K2) then the cabdriver is unable to take them to their desired destination (your bone) and the calcium is stuck in an undesirable location (like your arteries).

Now, let's imagine that too much leptin is like a new guy running the dispatch for the taxicabs. One day he simply doesn't dispatch enough taxis (osteocalcin) to the airport. What happens? A large number of passengers arrive at the airport (calcium you have just ingested from food or supplements), but there are too few taxis (osteocalcin) to bring them all to their desired destination (bone), even though they have plenty of money (vitamin K2) to get there. So they are stuck at the airport (i.e., your arteries), frustrated and angry (causing calcification). Can you see how this analogy illustrates how high leptin levels can both negatively impact your bone health and possibly cause dangerous arterial calcification?

The deleterious effects of high leptin levels don't stop there. The data from the labs at Columbia University made it clear that osteocalcin is also responsible for telling cells in our pancreas to produce insulin and our pituitary gland to make more testosterone—both of which, when in normal ranges, can help us form bone. Finally, when a person has high levels of leptin, it eventually drives cortisol higher, and as we covered in Chapter 2, high levels of cortisol block calcium absorption, increase bone resorption, and ultimately reduce bone density. Clearly, high leptin levels are to be avoided if bone health is your priority.

Amylopectin A is also responsible for the high blood sugar spike caused by eating wheat. Yes, wheat! Did you know that eating a slice of whole-wheat bread can spike your insulin more than a candy bar? When simple sugars react nonenzymatically with proteins and lipids (fats) in the body, it prompts something called the Maillard reaction. The sugars, proteins, and lipids combine to form nasty *advanced glycation end products*, or AGEs. Some AGEs are fine. However, if there are too many AGEs, the body may not efficiently excrete them, causing them to remain in the body. How does this affect your bones? These harmful substances damage your collagen, which is the primary substance that makes up your bone. So that lovely bread from last night's dinner, because of its amylopectin A content alone, can boost your belly fat, increase your leptin and cortisol levels, reduce your testosterone and insulin production, decrease your bone density, and damage your collagen.

The second punch to the gut comes from a protein in wheat called gliadin that, when digested by stomach acids and enzymes, becomes an exorphin, a morphinelike compound that binds to opiate receptors in your brain. Unlike other opiates that relieve pain, these exorphins cause addictive behavior and appetite stimulation that researchers have found to result in the consumption of more than four hundred additional calories every day. You know this addiction—it's the one that makes you grab that second piece of bread at the restaurant. Wheat's gliadin content is what causes this daily increase in your calories, which over time will likely lead to weight gain. Increased body weight often decreases mobility and weight-bearing movement, which is a major causative factor in osteoporosis. This is because a lack of weight-bearing movement causes

the cells that make bone (osteoblasts) to not work as well, while simultaneously causing more activity in the cells that break down bone (osteoclasts). Studies on individuals who lack weight-bearing physical exercise
have shown drastic bone loss. The one-two punch of amylopectin A and
gliadin serves up a wheat-filled recipe for insulin spikes, collagen destruction, appetite stimulation, weight gain, and expedited bone breakdown.

So between the oxalates, phytates, lectins, trypsin inhibitors, gluten, amylopectin A, and gliadin found in wheat, you should now have
plenty of reasons to ditch the dinner rolls and say bye-bye to the ba-
gels. All the various components of wheat work together to deplete
your micronutrients and fill your body with osteoporosis-causing compounds. In order to help you avoid wheat, we have made a list of the
products in which wheat and its most notable sidekick, gluten, may be
hiding (Table 3.3). Luckily, label reading for wheat has become much
easier since the Food Allergen Labeling and Consumer Protection Act
was passed in 2004. This regulation requires that the eight most common allergens be clearly identified on food labels, and wheat is one of
them. So if a food product contains a derivative of wheat, such as modified food starch, it must clearly indicate that wheat is the source. *Wheat*
may appear either in parentheses in the ingredient list or in a separate
"contains" statement, so always check thoroughly. Review the list in
Table 3.3, remove wheat from your diet, and then sit back and get ready
for a flood of bone-building micronutrients!

MSG—MAKING YOU EAT MORE . . . AND BUILD LESS

Food manufacturers just love it when you can't stop eating their products: it means that they can count on the fact that you'll be back to buy
more. So how do food scientists manipulate their products to cause you
to overeat? Three little letters: MSG. Monosodium glutamate (MSG) is
the go-to ingredient to achieve this "can't get enough" effect. Unfortunately, this frightening flavor enhancer is found in a large percentage
of packaged foods in the United States. It is frightening because out-of-
control eating can quickly lead to obesity. In fact, when scientific studies
require obese animals, MSG is the first thing they are given. Research
shows that laboratory rats given MSG increased their food intake by
40 percent.

TABLE 3.3 Where Wheat and Gluten May Be Hiding

Baked beans

Biscuits

Blue cheese

Bread and rolls

Bread crumbs

Breakfast cereals

Brown rice syrup

Bulgur wheat

Cakes

Chocolate

Chutneys (malt vinegar)

Cookies

Couscous

Crispbreads

Crumble toppings

Farina

Gravy powders

Hydrolyzed vegetable protein (HVP)

Imitation crab meat

Instant coffee

Kamut

Licorice

Lunch meat (fillers)

Malt vinegar

Malted drinks

Matzo flour/meal

Meat and fish pastes

Muesli

Muffins

Pancakes

Pasta

Pastry or pie crust

Pâtés

Pepper, white

Pickles (malt vinegar)

Pizza

Potato chips

Pretzels

Protein (HVP)

Pumpernickel

Rye bread

Salad dressings

Sauces (flour-thickened)

Sausages

Scones

Seitan (doesn't contain gluten; it *is* gluten!)

Soup stock cubes

Soups (flour-thickened)

Soy sauce

Spelt (ancient grain)

Spice mixes

Stuffing

Turkeys (self-basting)

Waffles

Yorkshire pudding

The obvious problem here is that much like wheat, MSG works by making you desire more of a tasty treat. It intensifies the flavor and potentially makes you eat greater quantities of food than you otherwise would. This can bring about weight gain and inactivity, which could result in bone loss. Additionally, MSG greatly increases your odds of becoming leptin resistant, which, as we learned earlier, has been linked through numerous processes to reduce your body's ability to build bone and increase your risk of arterial calcification.

MSG Also Messes with Micronutrient Levels

Beyond increasing leptin levels, this Poor Food ingredient also reduces our micronutrient levels because it is an *excitotoxin*. This means it can cross the blood-brain barrier and overexcite your cells to the point of damage or death, causing brain damage to varying degrees and potentially even triggering or worsening learning disabilities, Alzheimer's disease, Parkinson's disease, Lou Gehrig's disease, and more. Your micronutrient levels also pay the price because your available antioxidants are used at an accelerated rate when trying to repair MSG brain toxicity. Rather than performing other important functions in your body, available antioxidants—such as vitamins C and E and selenium—are called on to repair the damage. Additionally, magnesium, chromium, and zinc are all important protectors of neural cells, so their use is also accelerated in the presence of MSG. MSG is dangerous—take a look at Table 3.4 so you can avoid its many aliases.

TABLE 3.4 The Many Names for MSG

Autolyzed yeast	Monopotassium glutamate
Autolyzed yeast protein	Natural flavors (ask manufacturers their sources, to be safe)
Calcium glutamate	
Carrageenan	Pectin
Glutamate	Sodium caseinate
Hydrolyzed corn	Soy isolate
Ingredients listed as *hydrolyzed, protein fortified, ultra-pasteurized, fermented,* or *enzyme modified*	Soy sauce
	Textured vegetable protein (TVP)
Magnesium glutamate	Vegetable extract
Monoammonium glutamate	Yeast extract
	Yeast food

Introducing the EMDs—Your Antinutrient Thieves

Once you put everything you just learned into practice, your house will be free of sugar, HFCS, sugar substitutes, wheat, and MSG–laden products. Adopting these five healing habits will help you build an environment where your bone building can flourish. Although we identified the many ways that these Poor Foods negatively affect your health, the Everyday Micronutrient Depleters (EMDs) hiding inside them can really derail your micronutrient sufficiency and ultimately block your ability to achieve strong, flexible bones. Remember, EMDs are like stealth thieves that pop up in your foods and reduce the amount of micronutrients your body can absorb; because of this, they are often referred to as *antinutrients*. Both sugar and HFCS are EMDs in and of themselves. Their chemical structure reduces your micronutrient levels dramatically. Wheat, on the other hand, contains a quadfecta of naturally occurring EMDs. Made of phytic acid, oxalic acid, lectins, and trypsin inhibitors, wheat contains four micronutrient thieves you want to avoid.

Where else are EMDs hiding? Are there other EMDs that you need to be aware of? Should you avoid them, all of the time? These are all intelligent questions. First, it would be prohibitively difficult, if not nearly impossible, to completely eliminate all EMDs, as they're found in most foods. And since EMDs are naturally occurring in some of the "healthiest," most micronutrient-rich foods like kale, chia seeds, sweet potatoes, and berries, we are not sure we would want you to avoid all of these foods anyway. Proper preparation methods can reduce some EMDs, which makes the foods safer to consume while allowing you to enjoy them and their micronutrient benefits. Let's take a closer look at the EMDs found in our foods and drinks.

PHYTATES (PHYTIC ACID)

You've already seen that wheat contains our first EMD, phytic acid. Similarly to fiber, phytic acid works by binding to substances in our intestinal tracts. However, unlike fiber, which lowers cholesterol by binding to cholesterol-like compounds in the digestive tract, phytic acid reduces micronutrient absorption by binding to vitamin B3 (niacin), calcium, chromium, copper, iron, magnesium, manganese, and zinc. Additionally, phytic acid accelerates the metabolism of vitamin D.

Where it is found: Although wheat is the worst offender, other foods high in phytic acid include corn, beans, seeds (including flaxseeds and chia seeds), nuts, cereal grains, brown rice, and oats.

Proper preparation: Sprouting and fermenting grains, beans, flaxseeds, nuts, and chia will reduce phytic acid. According to a 2010 article that appeared in the Weston A. Price Foundation journal *Wise Traditions in Food, Farming, and the Healing Arts,* "research suggests that we will absorb approximately 20 percent more zinc and 60 percent more magnesium from our food when phytate is absent."

OXALATES (OXALIC ACID)

Green smoothies may be trendy in the wellness community, but they may also be contributing to your osteoporosis, high blood pressure, or kidney stones. As counterintuitive as it may sound, your raw greens may be to blame. As with phytic acid, oxalic acid also binds, or chelates, to specific micronutrients in the intestinal tract. Oxalates in your food bind to the calcium, magnesium, and iron in that same food (or in foods eaten with it) and block their absorption. This means no bone-building benefits for you. In the case of spinach, this results in leaving a mere 2 and 10 percent of the seemingly plentiful supply of iron and calcium, respectively. It also reduces the absorption of magnesium by 35 percent. However, the ability of oxalates to bind with calcium brings 1 out of every 1,000 Americans annually to the hospital with kidney stones. Eighty percent of all kidney stones in patients in the United States are made of calcium oxalate, which is crystalized oxalate acid bonded to calcium. Removing oxalates from the diet is essential for osteoporotic individuals who are increasing their calcium levels.

Where it is found: Foods with the highest concentration of oxalates include spinach, wheat, buckwheat, peanut butter, beets, beet greens, Swiss chard, nuts, rhubarb, and beans (green, waxed, or dried). Oxalates can be found to a lesser extent in many other foods, including collard greens, sweet potatoes, quinoa, celery, green rutabagas, soy, white potatoes, okra, tomatoes, and carrots.

Proper preparation: Make sure to cook oxalate-rich foods. According to a study in the *Journal of Agricultural and Food Chemistry,* "boiling markedly reduced soluble oxalate content by 30 to 87 percent and was more effective than steaming (5 to 53 percent) and baking (used only for potatoes, no oxalate loss)."

LECTINS

If a plant's goal is self-preservation, then lectins are its premier defense system. Lectins are sticky proteins that coat your intestinal tract, making it difficult to properly absorb micronutrients. Additionally, lectins also aid in the creation of leaky gut by binding to your intestinal walls and acting like chisels—forcing apart the cells that protect the rest of you from the undigested foods inside. As we learned earlier in this chapter, leaky gut can directly reduce your ability to produce vitamin K2. And because vitamin K2 is a key bone nutrient that directs calcium into the bone, if lectins cause you to have leaky gut and you can't create enough vitamin K2, your calcium can't get into the bone, leading to osteoporosis.

The loss of micronutrients is only one way lectins can challenge the bone-building process. They also attach to insulin receptors on fat cells. Remember, insulin is the fat-storage hormone. Once attached, lectins never detach, indefinitely telling the fat cell to store more fat. Again, weight gain can be worrisome for those with osteoporosis because increased body mass may decrease activity, which in turn can decrease bone growth. To add insult to injury, lectins also attach themselves to the receptor sites for leptin, the hormone that tells your brain when you are full, and block its effect on satiety. The result is that you become leptin resistant. Remember, excessive leptin is a double-edged sword against your bones. It causes both an increase in bone resorption (breakdown) and a decrease in bone building.

Where it is found: Lectins are present in about 30 percent of the American diet. Foods with high levels include brown rice, wheat, spelt, rye, barley, tomatoes, beans, soybeans, seeds, nuts, corn, potatoes (skin), eggplant, millet, bell peppers, and hot peppers. Lectins are also found in increased amounts in foods that have been genetically modified, as GMO scientists splice in lectins to make crops heartier.

Proper preparation: Heat destroys some lectins but not all. Pressure cooking is the only way to completely destroy lectins. Soaking, with frequent water changes, or sprouting can remove many lectins from beans, rice, and nuts.

TRYPSIN INHIBITORS

Trypsin inhibitors work by inhibiting your trypsin (an enzyme that is excreted by the pancreas) so that it cannot do its part in the digestion of food proteins and other biological processes. Trypsin inhibitors put your amino acids as well as fat-soluble vitamins A, D, E, and K and vitamin B12 in jeopardy, as they interfere with the pancreas's ability to create enzymes necessary for proper digestion.

Let's examine more closely how trypsin inhibitors in your diet can affect your vitamin B12 sufficiency. Malabsorption is the most common cause of a vitamin B12 deficiency, and vitamin B12s absorption is quite complex.

We consume B12 in our diets where it is found bound to animal proteins. Once in the stomach, the enzyme pepsin and gastric acid ensure that these proteins are digested and vitamin B12 is released. B12 then binds to endogenous transport proteins known as R-proteins, which carry the B12 to the small intestine. This is where trypsin comes in. Trypsin, a specialized pancreatic enzyme, splits the R-protein complex, releasing the vitamin B12, which then binds to intrinsic factor, a transport protein produced in the stomach, which through an even more complicated process eventually allows the B12 to enter your bloodstream. When trypsin is inhibited, then all of the B12 in your food and supplements cannot be delivered into your bloodstream—and that means you lose out on its bone benefits. In studies, a deficiency of B6, B9, and B12 has been shown to increase the resorption activity of osteoclasts.

Where it is found: Most of the USDA studies performed over the years have looked at trypsin inhibitors in soybeans, but these antinutrients are also found in other beans, as well as grains, nuts, seeds, and vegetables of the nightshade family (potatoes, tomatoes, and eggplant).

Proper preparation: Luckily, cooking deactivates most of the trypsin inhibitors. For example, when researchers heated sweet potatoes to

215°F (102°C), it led to rapid inactivation of their trypsin inhibitors. However, although trypsin inhibitors are reduced by cooking, they are not completely removed. The cooked sweet potatoes still retained between 17 and 31 percent of their trypsin-inhibitor activity. Raw foodists and vegetarians who frequently consume large amounts of soy, beans, and nuts in their raw state are most at risk from these antinutrients.

PHOSPHORIC ACID

Watch out for phosphoric acid, a chemical additive that helps keep the carbonated bubbles in soda products from going flat—it is a real calcium depleter. Your body tries to keep a 1:1 ratio of calcium to phosphorus. When you drink a beverage that contains phosphoric acid, your body steals calcium from your bones or teeth in order to keep this balance. Then, when the phosphoric acid is passed in your urine, the calcium is also lost. However, the loss of calcium does not end there. Phosphoric acid also neutralizes hydrochloric acid in your stomach, and as we have stated, hydrochloric acid is required to break down food and absorb micronutrients. Yes, you guessed it: calcium needs an acidic environment to be properly absorbed, as do both vitamin B9 (folate) and vitamin B12. Finally, phosphoric acid binds with calcium and magnesium in the stomach, creating insoluble salts and further micronutrient loss. So if you are one of the 54 million people with risk of osteoporosis, steer clear of beverages that contain phosphoric acid. The leaching of both calcium and magnesium can have detrimental effects on your bone health.

Where it is found: Follow the bubbles! Carbonated soft drinks, carbonated energy drinks, and some flavored waters contain phosphoric acid. Most sparkling waters, like San Pellegrino, are phosphoric acid–free.

Proper preparation: This EMD is simple to reduce and even eliminate—there is no need to drink these micronutrient-depleting beverages at all.

ALCOHOL

Do you remember earlier when we explained how trypsin inhibitors decrease the pancreas's secretion of digestive enzymes? Well, so does alcohol, which can cause the loss of both amino acids and fat-soluble vitamins. Excessive alcohol consumption can also damage the stomach lining and intestines. This may inhibit the absorption of any vitamins and minerals that were made available for digestion by the digestive enzymes, such as vitamin B1 (thiamine) and vitamin B9 (folate). Alcohol interferes with the pancreas and its absorption of calcium and vitamins C and D. Lastly, alcohol also affects the liver, which is important for activating vitamin D—if vitamin D is not activated, it negatively affects calcium absorption. Therefore, heavy drinking may have a very risky effect on bone health.

If we're sounding like Debbie Downers, don't worry: you don't have to let this information put a damper on your celebrations. In fact, you might even want to pop some bubbly because *moderate* alcohol consumption can actually be quite beneficial to your bones. A recent study out of the University of Oregon showed that consumption of 19 grams of alcohol—about two small glasses of wine—helped preserve bone strength just as well as bisphosphonates (and without all the negative side effects we already shared with you). Finnish researchers concur; in 2013, they determined that women who drank more than three alcoholic drinks a week had significantly higher bone density than abstainers. Additionally, two Harvard studies revealed that, compared to abstainers, the risk of death from all causes was reduced by up to 28 percent among men and women who drank alcohol moderately.

Where it is found: The main culprits are beer, wine, hard cider, mead, and hard alcohol.

Proper preparation: Alcohol is a micronutrient foe if you forget moderation! Reducing intake is the only way to enjoy it and benefit from its bone-boosting perks.

CAFFEINE

As with alcohol, caffeine has a sweet spot. Too much could be problematic, but just the right amount and you get some real benefits brewing!

Caffeine has been shown to deplete micronutrients (specifically calcium and iron), but the levels of depletion are quite minor and safe when you consume up to three cups a day. A recent study determined that the calcium loss from a 6-ounce cup of coffee could be offset by supplementing with 40 milligrams of calcium—the equivalent of 2 tablespoons of milk in your cup of coffee. Additionally, that same 6-ounce cup of joe can inhibit the absorption of nonheme iron (the main form of iron found in plants) by 24 to 73 percent. However, a Korean study on premenopausal women that was looking for the link between caffeine and osteoporosis determined that coffee consumption showed no significant association with BMD of either femoral neck or lumbar spine for those who consumed up to three cups of coffee a day. The study did find that more than four cups of coffee per day, which was considered a "high coffee intake," was associated with a very small reduction in bone density that did not translate into an increased risk of fracture. In fact, the majority of studies available fail to find any significant effects of caffeine on bone density. A review of thirty-two observational studies indicated no overall negative effect of caffeine on bone health. Potentially negative effects on BMD were recorded mainly in populations with insufficient calcium intake or very high coffee consumption (more than nine cups daily).

Although nine cups of coffee seems a tad excessive to us, caffeine-containing beverages such as coffee have been found to have some amazing bone-boosting benefits as well. Coffee, for example, is the number one source of antioxidants in the U.S. diet, containing 300 percent more free radical–fighting antioxidants than even black tea. Coffee's antioxidant content has been shown to reduce the risk of heart disease, depression, Alzheimer's, Parkinson's, type 2 diabetes, stroke, cirrhosis of the liver, gout, dementia, and certain types of cancer. All these antioxidants fight inflammation, which damages bone by increasing the activation of osteoclasts, which in turn increases the risk for osteoporosis. In fact, drinking coffee has been shown to reduce levels of CRP—a protein that is considered an indicator of systemwide inflammation and that physicians usually check as a marker of osteoporosis. Researchers have determined that high CRP levels are an indicator of poor skeletal health and an increased risk of fracture.

Additionally, coffee also lowers another hormone that promotes inflammation called leptin. (You remember leptin, right? A quick recap: chronically high leptin levels cause leptin resistance, which in turn causes both an increase in bone resorption [breakdown] and a decrease in bone building.) This means that your morning java actually helps keep your leptin level in line and is therefore bone protective. There's more good news for caffeine lovers where frail bones are considered: a 2013 study presented at the Society for Experimental Biology reported that caffeine "boosts power in older muscles, suggesting the stimulant could aid elderly people to maintain their strength, reducing the incidence of falls and injuries."

Where it is found: Caffeine can be found in caffeinated soft drinks, coffee drinks, tea, and chocolate, as well as in greater amounts in energy drinks.

Proper preparation: Reduce your intake of caffeinated beverages to three servings or less per day and offset the calcium and iron loss through food or supplementation. You can also opt for decaffeinated beverages, but then you lose all of caffeine's benefits.

TANNINS

The dry, mouth-puckering sensation you get from a breakfast tea or aged merlot tells you that tannins, our next antinutrient, are present. Like oxalates and phytates, tannins are naturally occurring molecules that bind with micronutrients—specifically vitamins B1 and B9 and the minerals calcium, magnesium, iron, and zinc—to inhibit their absorption. For this reason, UK researchers recommend that individuals wait at least one hour after eating before drinking tannin-laden tea, to lower the risk of anemia.

However, simply because a food or beverage contains tannins doesn't mean you have to avoid it altogether—again, moderation is the key here. Tea, for example, is loaded with tannins, but like coffee, the antioxidant (polyphenol) levels in tea have been shown to be bone protective. And as you already read, two small glasses of wine per day can be good for your bones. Although limiting or eliminating foods and beverages with tannins may help you achieve micronutrient sufficiency, keeping a few in your diet, in moderation, may actually help your bones.

Where it is found: In addition to coffee, tea, and red wine, tannins are also found in apples, grapes, and berries (including their juices), as well as rhubarb, beans, lentils, spices, barley (beer), nuts, and chocolate.

Proper preparation: Avoid at mealtimes if you are at risk for iron deficiency.

TIME TO TAKE INVENTORY OF YOUR EMDS

Were you surprised to learn about all the EMDs hiding in your foods? It can be upsetting to think about how some of your favorite "healthy" foods, even those suggested by diet gurus and physicians, can actually rob you of micronutrients that are essential to the health of your bones. Your current diet likely consists of at least a few of these antinutrients, and maybe a lot of them! Remember, the more antinutrients you consume, the greater the chance that they will detrimentally affect your bones.

It is now time for you to take a good, hard look at your own habits. Could your diet have unknowingly been contributing to the poor status of your bones? In Table 3.4, we list the EMDs found in foods and drink. This next part may take some calculating and perhaps fifteen to twenty minutes of your time. But take the time to do it—it's important to see how pervasive these EMDs are in your life. Remember, it is not until you can recognize that a habit is potentially hurting you that you will be motivated to change it.

Step 1: It's time to take inventory on your habits. And yes, we want you to be extremely honest with yourself here. Place a check (✓) in the Tabulations column in Table 3.5 for *each day of the week* that you might consume any EMD listed. Be honest! If, for example, for the EMD *phytates*, you determine that you currently eat wheat, beans, flaxseeds, and broccoli each once a week, but snack on nuts daily, you should give yourself one check for each of the first four foods and seven checks for nuts. That would give you a total of eleven checks for phytates.

Step 2: Now that you have identified how many EMDs you consume each week, it's time to fill in Table 3.6. This is your current Everyday Micronutrient Depleters Personal Intake Chart. Using the checks you entered in Table 3.5, calculate how many times each micronutrient might be affected. For example, if you had eleven checks next to phytates, then you will need to put 11 points next to each vitamin and mineral that phytates deplete. This means that you will write the number 11 next to B3, D, calcium, chromium, copper, iron, magnesium, manganese, and zinc. Mark down your total for each EMD in every micronutrient it depletes. You will hit some micronutrients more than once. When you do this, simply mark the second number to the right of the first. For example, you could end up with something like this:

Calcium: 11 6 27 5 3

Step 3: Total the numbers listed for each micronutrient. For example:

Calcium: 11 + 6 + 27 + 5 + 3 = 52

Step 4: It is time to analyze your data. Look at how many bone-threatening EMDs you currently have in your life. Does the sheer amount of micronutrients being depleted by your current dietary habits shock you? Are patterns emerging in the clusters of micronutrients most often lost through EMDs? Note which micronutrients are being heavily depleted because of your current dietary habits.

Remember, the intricate orchestra of micronutrients can play its bone-remodeling symphony only when every micronutrient is in attendance, and in the necessary amount. Although you may have considered your diet "healthy" in the past, is it possible that the foods you are eating are not actually delivering the micronutrient levels you think they are? Based on your EMD intake chart, does it appear that you could increase your micronutrient levels by making some simple changes to your daily diet? Remember, our goal is not to eliminate all the foods that contain these antinutrients. It is to make you aware of the micronutrient-depleting effect of the foods you have chosen to be part of your diet, so that you know which foods you can reduce or eliminate to increase your likelihood of achieving micronutrient sufficiency.

3. Choose Rich Foods and avoid Poor Foods.
4. Say so long to sugar.
5. Halt the high-fructose corn syrup (HFCS).
6. Skip the sinister sugar substitutes.
7. Whack the wheat.
8. Move away from MSG.
9. Fix the phytates (phytic acid).
10. Evade the oxalates (oxalic acid).
11. Lose the lectins through pressure cooking.
12. Take the time to cook out trypsin inhibitors.
13. Flee from phosphoric acid.
14. Escape from excessive alcohol intake.
15. Curb the caffeine.
16. Tame the tannins.

Join us On the Couch for an in-depth chat about Chapter 3

Hurry back to RebuildYourBones.com for our next "On the Couch" video chat. We know that choosing the most micronutrient Rich Foods can be difficult; in this coaching session, we will share some of our favorite tips. And don't get overwhelmed with the antinutrients—they are everywhere. Join us now to review the best ways avoid them, especially when eating out.

TABLE 3.5 Everyday Micronutrient Depleters Found in Food and Drink

Everyday Micronutrient Depleter (aka antinutrient)	Micronutrients Depleted	Found in These Foods/ Drinks (worst offenders first)	Proper Preparation and Bone-Building Guidelines	Tabulations (place one ✓ for every day of the week you consume a food)
Sugar and high-fructose corn syrup (HFCS)	C, calcium, chromium, copper, magnesium, zinc	Almost all prepackaged goods in the grocery store under all the names listed in Table 3.1	Do not consume.	
Sugar substitutes	Calcium, iron, zinc	Listed on diet foods under the names in Table 3.2	Do not consume.	
Monosodium glutamate (MSG)	C, E, chromium, magnesium, selenium, zinc	Almost all prepackaged goods in the grocery store under all the names listed in Table 3.4	Do not consume.	
Phytates (phytic acid)	B3, D, calcium, chromium, copper, iron, magnesium, manganese, zinc	Breads (any wheat product), corn, beans, seeds (including flaxseeds and chia seeds), nuts, grains (cereals), brown rice, soy products, oats, figs, artichokes, carrots, potatoes, broccoli, strawberries, rice, apples	Reduce phytates by sprouting, soaking, or fermenting grains, beans, seeds, and nuts.	
Oxalates (oxalic acid)	Calcium, iron, magnesium	Spinach, wheat, buckwheat, peanut butter, beets, beet greens, Swiss chard, nuts, rhubarb, beans (green, waxed, or dried), collard greens, sweet potatoes, quinoa, celery, green rutabagas, soy products, white potatoes, okra, tomatoes, sesame seeds (tahini), carrots	Cook oxalate-rich vegetables.	

Everyday Micronutrient Depleter (aka antinutrient)	Micronutrients Depleted	Found in These Foods/ Drinks (worst offenders first)	Proper Preparation and Bone-Building Guidelines	Tabulations (place one ✓ for every day of the week you consume a food)
Lectins	All vitamins and minerals (✓ all)	Rice, wheat, spelt, rye, barley, soy products, other beans, seeds, nuts, corn, potatoes, tomatoes, eggplant, hot peppers, bell peppers	Reduce lectin levels by soaking, sprouting, and fermenting; cooking also reduces levels, but none of these will totally eliminate lectins. (Pressure cooking is the best.)	
Trypsin inhibitors	Fat-soluble vitamins A, D, E, and K; B12; amino acids (carnitine)	Soy products, other beans, grains, nuts, seeds, vegetables of the nightshade family (potatoes, tomatoes, eggplant)	Cooking deactivates most of them.	
Phosphoric acid	B9, B12, calcium, iron, magnesium, manganese	Carbonated sodas, carbonated energy drinks, some flavored waters	Do not consume.	
Alcohol	All vitamins, minerals, and essential fatty acids (✓ all)	Beer, wine, hard alcohol	Limit to 2 drinks a day to reduce depletion while gaining bone benefits.	
Caffeine	A, B9, D, calcium, iron	Coffee, tea, soda, energy drinks, chocolate	Limit to 3 cups a day and replenish calcium to reap benefits.	

Everyday Micronutrient Depleter (aka antinutrient)	Micronutrients Depleted	Found in These Foods/ Drinks (worst offenders first)	Proper Preparation and Bone-Building Guidelines	Tabulations (place one ✓ for every day of the week you consume a food)
Tannins	B1, B9, calcium, iron, magnesium, zinc	Coffee, tea, red wine, fruit juice, rhubarb, beans (red), lentils, barley (beer), nuts, spices, chocolate, pomegranates, berries, apples, grapes	If at risk for iron deficiency, avoid consuming tannin-containing beverages at mealtimes.	

TABLE 3.6 Everyday Micronutrient Depleters Personal Intake Chart

Micronutrient	Tabulation Total
Vitamin A	
Vitamin B1 (thiamine)	
Vitamin B2 (riboflavin)	
Vitamin B3 (niacin)	
Vitamin B5 (pantothenic acid)	
Vitamin B6 (pyridoxine)	
Vitamin B7	
Vitamin B9 (folate)	
Vitamin B12 (cobalamin)	
Vitamin C	
Vitamin D	
Vitamin E	
Vitamin K	
Calcium	
Choline	
Chromium	
Copper	
Iodine	
Iron	
Magnesium	

Micronutrient	Tabulation Total
Manganese	
Phosphorus	
Potassium	
Selenium	
Zinc	
Omega-3	
Omega-6	
Amino acids (carnitine)	

CHAPTER 4

Dietary Doctrine, Alkalinity, and Omega-6 Overload . . . Oh My!

Diets, like clothes, should be tailored to you.

—JOAN RIVERS

You have seen how specific foods in your kitchen can negatively affect your micronutrient sufficiency levels, but now we are going to evaluate how your sufficiency levels are being influenced by your lifestyle habits. In Chapter 3, you took the first step to becoming a nutrivore by Switching to Rich. Now it is time to take the second step to becoming a nutrivore and focus on *driving down depletion*. It is time for you to take a good look at your life and become aware of how your lifestyle habits may be contributing to your bone loss. Unless we become aware and hold ourselves accountable for our actions, we never push ourselves to do better. Accountability forces us to take responsibility for where our health is today and make the changes that will result in success tomorrow. In this chapter, we will take a good look at how your dietary philosophy may be putting your micronutrient levels in jeopardy and review both protein and omega-6 intake—two factors that will affect your bones regardless of your chosen diet.

Your Dietary Doctrine—A Lifestyle Choice

Regardless of what city or what country we are speaking in, and regardless of the audience, be it physicians or health enthusiasts, whenever people learn that we are micronutrient specialists, they always pose one question: "Which dietary philosophy is the best at creating micronutrient sufficiency and improving bone health?" You've probably wondered this yourself. If you spend any time in the osteoporosis chat rooms on Facebook, we are sure you have read opinions that steer you in all sorts of directions. There is a constant chatter and debate over the superiority of low-carb, low-fat, Paleo, vegan, and low-acid (alkaline) diets for osteoporosis.

On the USDA website, their team of trained nutrition professionals tells you that "healthy individuals can get all of the vitamins and minerals they need from a well balanced diet." However, many other well-known and well-respected nutritional academics disagree. The late Shari Lieberman, PhD, a certified nutrition specialist, professor of human nutrition, and author of *The Real Vitamin and Mineral Book*, had a different opinion: "It is virtually impossible to meet the RDIs (Reference Daily Intakes) by eating the food available to us today." Walter Willett, MD, chairman of the Department of Nutrition at the Harvard School of Public Health, believes that even the individuals eating the healthiest diets may still be deficient in specific micronutrients. Dr. Mark Hyman, *New York Times* bestselling author and director of the Cleveland Clinic Center for Functional Medicine, believes that "even with a perfect diet, the combination of many things—including our depleted soils, the storage and transportation of our food, genetic alterations of traditional heirloom species, and the increased stress and nutritional demands resulting from a toxic environment—make it impossible for us to get the vitamins and minerals we need solely from the foods we eat."

So who is right? How can one group of nutrition professionals state that a well-balanced diet is sufficient for our micronutrient requirements, while another group tells us that our diets are virtually stripped of vitamins and minerals and that meeting the daily requirements of essential micronutrients through a balanced diet is virtually impossible? It all comes down to dietary dogmas. One of the many problems with nutrition today is that there is so much infighting between people who believe in different dietary philosophies. But it makes sense. People are very attached to their belief systems, and when you make up your mind to follow a specific dietary philosophy, it becomes a large part of your overall lifestyle and who you are. You go out of your way to find restaurants that cater to your particular preferences, and you often bond easily with others following the same dietary protocol. So when your dietary philosophy is challenged, you are bound to become a bit defensive. After all, someone is questioning your lifestyle. One's dietary doctrine really is a lifestyle choice and because of this, it is going to be the first in a long line of lifestyle choices that we'll be exploring.

During our quest to heal Mira's bones, we became confused by all of the diverse opinions on which diet would be best to achieve our goal of micronutrient sufficiency. So we decided to do something about it. We started researching each dietary philosophy to uncover the truth about exactly how many of the essential micronutrients each of these dietary profiles could deliver daily. We wanted to discover whether any diet plan would meet micronutrient sufficiency.

We started by looking to see if we could find studies showing the ability to meet micronutrient sufficiency through diet alone (any diet). It turns out that the American Dietetic Association had wondered the exact same thing. In their study published in the *Journal of the American Dietetic Association* titled "Problems Encountered in Meeting the Recommended Dietary Allowances for Menus Designed According to the Dietary Guidelines for Americans," a group of dietitians were asked to create menus that met the Recommended Dietary Allowances (RDAs) for the essential micronutrients while providing 2,200 to 2,400 *palatable* calories. Not one single dietitian was able to reach the study's objective, not even when they used software designed for creating a healthy diet. According to the researchers, "only 11 percent of the menus met the RDA for zinc. Half of the menus did not meet the RDA for vitamin B6, and one-third did not meet the RDA for iron." If these dietitians couldn't create a micronutrient-sufficient diet with that as their primary goal, then what is the likelihood that you'll happen to serve up micronutrient sufficiency for supper?

If a random diet doesn't provide micronutrient sufficiency and trained USDA dietitians couldn't create menus that meet sufficiency either, how do you think the world's best-selling diet books did at this same task? That is exactly what we wanted to know and exactly what we researched for Jayson's 2010 study published in the *Journal of the International Society of Sports Nutrition* titled "Prevalence of Micronutrient Deficiency in Popular Diet Plans."

In this study, we examined the sufficiency levels of twenty-seven essential micronutrients as recommended by the Reference Daily Intake (RDI) in four popular diet plans to see if the act of dieting itself could be creating a micronutrient-deficient state in the average American. In order to examine a variety of dietary philosophies, we included Atkins (low carbohydrate), the South Beach Diet (Mediterranean), and the Best Life Diet (low fat). The fourth diet we chose was the Dietary Approaches to Stop Hypertension (DASH) diet—rated the number one diet overall by *U.S. News & World Report* for its nutritional completeness. This medically founded diet plan was created to reverse disease, not merely lose weight, and was written by an amazing group of researchers from some of the country's most prestigious institutions. The entire concept of the DASH diet was that one could lower blood pressure through gaining sufficiency in potassium, magnesium, and calcium. Surely a diet aimed at micronutrient sufficiency as a cure for disease would perform well in our study. Later, we decided to add both the Primal and Paleo diets into the mix in order to include two of the hottest diet crazes in the bookstores.

In order to evaluate each diet plan's ability to reach micronutrient sufficiency, we measured the amount of every micronutrient in the respective menu plans, down to the last gram of salt. After all the computations were completed, not one of the popular diet plans reached micronutrient sufficiency for all twenty-seven essential micronutrients we evaluated—vitamin A, vitamin B1 (thiamine), vitamin B2 (riboflavin), vitamin B3 (niacin), vitamin B5 (pantothenic acid), vitamin B6, vitamin B7 (biotin), vitamin B9 (folate), vitamin B12, vitamin C, vitamin D, vitamin E, vitamin K, calcium, choline, chromium, copper, iodine, iron, magnesium, manganese, molybdenum, phosphorus, potassium, selenium, sodium, and zinc. See Table 4.1 for our findings.

The study determined that a typical dieter using one of these six popular diet plans would be, on average, 48 percent sufficient at reaching RDI requirements and would meet sufficiency in only thirteen out of the twenty-seven essential micronutrients required every day to prevent diseases from micronutrient deficiency. These diet plans were literally starving their followers of more than half of the micronutrients they needed to prevent disease, even when requiring them to eat up to six meals a day. Furthermore, these diet plans weren't limiting calories either. Their average caloric intake was over 1,844 calories per day. Curious as to how many calories one would have to eat on each program in order to create micronutrient sufficiency, we increased the amount of each ingredient in each meal proportionally until RDI sufficiency for all twenty-seven essential micronutrients was met. The shocking truth is that the world's leading diets, if followed perfectly to plan, would require you to eat—on average—an excessively large and unhealthy 23,566 calories a day in order to reach micronutrient sufficiency.

TABLE 4.1 Independent Research on Six Popular Diet Plans

Name of Diet Plan	% RDI Sufficient	Number of Micronutrients out of 27 That Met RDI
Atkins for Life	44%	12
Best Life	56%	15
DASH	52%	14
Practical Paleo	56%	15
Primal Blueprint	56%	15
South Beach	22%	6
Average	**48%**	**13**

Our point in sharing these studies with you is to show you that no matter how much we all want to believe that a balanced diet can provide all the essential micronutrients we need, the idea of any diet delivering micronutrient sufficiency each and every day is a myth. In fact, to our knowledge (and, believe us, we have searched), no study has ever been published proving that this is possible for any dietary philosophy. The American Dietetic Association could not create a micronutrient-sufficient meal plan, even when using computer software designed to do so. And America's most popular diet books, written by some of the most trusted doctors and nutritionists, haven't been able to do it either—regardless of which dietary philosophy they were following. This does not mean, however, that micronutrient sufficiency is impossible to achieve; it just means we have to work a little harder to get there. Understanding the shortcomings of your dietary philosophy is a good place to start on your mission to prevent bone loss.

The Pros and Cons of Your Dietary Doctrine

Remember, as a nutrivore, you can follow whatever dietary philosophy you believe in on your quest for better bones as long as you make micronutrient sufficiency your main goal. But what exactly makes a dietary philosophy a dietary philosophy? In other words, what makes the Paleo diet the Paleo diet or a vegan diet a vegan diet? When you start to look at how a dietary philosophy is designed, you realize it basically comes down to one thing—elimination. The Paleo diet eliminates dairy and legumes, whereas a vegan diet eliminates food sourced from animals. Each dietary philosophy is designed to eliminate specific foods or food groups that don't fit into their protocol's philosophy. What do you think happens when foods get eliminated? Well, the vitamins and minerals that are abundant in those eliminated foods are also eliminated, and this can lead to certain dietary philosophies falling short in specific groups of micronutrients.

Being aware that your diet may fall short at supplying enough of the essential bone-building micronutrients is important. Once you are aware of these shortcomings, you can focus on either eating foods that contain these missing micronutrients or supplementing them instead. Let's look at today's most popular dietary philosophies more closely to identify their problematic pitfalls when it comes to micronutrient sufficiency.

LOW-CALORIE, FASTING, PREPACKAGED, AND GASTRIC BYPASS DIETS

Low-calorie diets are a popular method of losing weight by simply cutting back on the total number of calories consumed each day by eating less food. This not only supplies the dieter with fewer calories, it also supplies them with fewer vitamins, minerals, and essential fatty acids to build their bone, as well as amino acids to build muscle, which may result in increased falling and fracture risk. Research published by the National Institute of Hygiene in Poland evaluated the effects of a low-calorie diet and found participants with insufficient intakes of vitamins A, B1, B2, B3, C, and E.

Fasting or skipping meals (via the new and wildly popular trend called intermittent fasting) is becoming more common but may not be a wise solution if micronutrient sufficiency is your goal. Although this style of diet can reduce overall daily caloric intake and likely reduce weight, what are the chances that a dieter following these starvation-style weight-loss strategies can achieve micronutrient sufficiency in only two meals a day (or less)—especially when studies show no chance of reaching sufficiency even when eating as many as six meals a day?

Following a diet that makes things easy with prepackaged prepared foods and shakes such as Jenny Craig and Weight Watchers also puts you at risk of micronutrient deficiency. A study published in *Nutrition Journal* evaluated dieters following the Weight Watchers protocol and found "significant declines" in vitamin B2 (riboflavin), vitamin B3 (niacin), potassium, calcium, magnesium, iron, and zinc. This could be from the quality of the foods (highly processed, nonorganic), the fact that they had been frozen (freezing can lower micronutrient content), or perhaps because of the antinutrient content in some of their prepackaged platters, such as breakfast quesadillas or "diet lasagna," which supply you with high levels of phytates, oxalates, lectins, trypsin inhibitors, sugar, and gut-wrenching gluten.

Finally, when all else fails and weight loss is seemingly out of reach, many frustrated dieters turn to surgical procedures such as laparoscopic banding (lap band) and gastric bypass surgery. These procedures cut out or "band off" a portion of patients' stomachs so they cannot eat large portions, which in turn ensures that they will not be able to fully absorb their micronutrients. Although this can result in significant weight loss of 50 to 75 percent of excess body weight, due to the malabsorption created by virtue of the bypassed surface area, more than calories are lost. Deficiencies in vitamins B1, B9, B12, and D, along with copper and calcium, are common postsurgery. The resulting deficiencies may leave the patient thinner but much more vulnerable to osteoporosis. One recent study by investigators at Massachusetts General Hospital in Boston found that not only do patients who have had gastric bypass surgery have a high rate of bone loss in the first year after surgery, but their bone loss persists two years after surgery, even after the patient's weight stabilizes.

VEGAN AND VEGETARIAN DIETS

If you follow a vegan or vegetarian diet, you have chosen to eliminate or restrict animal products from your diet. These dietary doctrines have been shown to fall short in supplying adequate amounts of vitamins B12, D, and K2 as well as iron, calcium, zinc, and omega-3 fatty acids. Did you notice a few of the important bone builders in there? Studies show that the vegan diet only provides one quarter the amount of vitamin D that the omnivore diet provides. This lack of vitamin D directly complicates bone growth, because activated vitamin D (calcitriol) regulates blood calcium levels in concert with parathyroid hormone. In the absence of an adequate intake of vitamin D, less than 15 percent of calcium is absorbed from foods or supplements. Vegans as well as vegetarians who exclude dairy products should consider supplementation of vitamin D, because milk is the primary source of vitamin D in the United States.

Vitamin K2, the micronutrient responsible for ushering calcium into the bone and not allowing it to form plaque in the arteries, has also been shown to be deficient in a vegan diet. This is because vitamin K2 is primarily found in meat, cheese (highest in Gouda), and eggs. Vegans can get K2 from a fermented soy product called natto. However, natto may not be the best option since 94 percent of all U.S. soy is genetically modified and because soy contains an abundance of antinutrients (phytates, oxalates, lectins, trypsin inhibitors), which deplete many of the micronutrients in which you are trying to become sufficient.

Many advocates of the vegan/vegetarian lifestyle point out that beneficial bacteria in the intestinal tract can produce vitamin K2, and this is true. But research is not conclusive as to whether the quantity would be enough to prevent or reverse osteoporosis, or how the high lectin and trypsin inhibitor content of the vegan diet (which can cause leaky gut and diminish K2) affects production. Additionally, since the body can also convert vitamin K1 (from green leafy vegetables) into K2, one could assume that increasing vitamin K1 consumption could help meet K2 requirements. However, here the evidence is conclusive and shows that the body does not convert enough K1 into K2 to prevent osteoporosis and heart disease. In one study published in the *Journal of Nutrition*, for example, it was found that taking vitamin K2 reduced heart disease, but intake of K1 had no beneficial effect. This shows that although K2 is capable of driving calcium into the bones and out of the arteries (where it can cause heart disease), vitamin K1 could not perform this task. Therefore, the idea that simply eating an abundance of K1 in your diet and relying on it converting to K2 is not scientifically sound. Another study from the Netherlands found that vitamin K2 is three times as effective at carboxylating osteocalcin (a chemical that controls bone formation) as K1.

Additionally, in a study published in the *American Journal of Clinical Nutrition*, 73 percent of lacto-ovo vegetarians (vegetarians who do not consume animal flesh but do consume eggs and dairy) and vegans were found to be deficient in vitamin B12, an essential vitamin that cannot be found naturally in any plant-based sources and is only found naturally in animal products. This B12 deficiency puts the vegetarian and vegan populations at risk for elevated homocysteine levels—a risk factor for osteoporotic bone fractures, as well as cardiovascular disease, disorientation, dementia, and mood and motor disturbances. Finally, because vegan diets do not include fish or eggs, they generally lack the essential fatty acids EPA and DHA (from omega-3) and have high levels of omega-6 fatty acids, which, later in this chapter, we will show are detrimental for bone health.

As we learned in Chapter 3, achieving micronutrient sufficiency is not as easy as simply eating foods high in specific micronutrients. We have to take into account those nasty EMDs hiding in foods as well. Individuals following a vegetarian or vegan diet often increase their intake of foods like legumes, soy, nuts and seeds, spinach, and grains, which contain phytic acid, oxalic acid, trypsin inhibitors, lectins, and tannins, antinutrients that can cause further micronutrient depletion. The fact that vegan and vegetarian diets are both low in specific micronutrients and high in antinutrients may help explain the findings of researchers who examined the effects of vegetarian diets on BMD. In a study published in the *American Journal of Clinical Nutrition*, researchers identified "all relevant articles on the association between vegetarian diets and BMD" and determined that BMD was approximately 4 percent lower in vegetarians than in omnivores at both the femoral neck and the lumbar spine. Compared with omnivores, vegans had a significantly lower lumbar spine BMD, which was more pronounced than in lacto-ovo-vegetarians (vegetarians who also eat egg and dairy). Although many studies differ on how significant bone loss is on a vegan or vegetarian diet, we feel that the take-home message here is the same. If this is your chosen dietary philosophy you must do two things: you must be extremely vigilant in supplementing with these key bone-remodeling micronutrients, and you must properly prepare as many of the foods containing antinutrients as possible.

PALEO AND PRIMAL DIETS

The Paleo and Primal diets are ancestral-style diets that encourage their followers to achieve better health by focusing on eating foods that would have been available to our Paleolithic ancestors. You would expect that a diet like this, which focuses on eating fresh, high-quality meat, fish, eggs, nuts, seeds, and vegetables, would be successful at providing a wide range of essential micronutrients, but again, both the Paleo and Primal diets fall short. Although these ancestral-style diets are among the most micronutrient-rich dietary philosophies we have examined, because of key food group eliminations—including wheat (gluten), legumes, and dairy (for Paleo)—both diets were shown to be deficient in key micronutrients. The deepest deficiencies were found in calcium (one of the heroes in bone remodeling), chromium (which promotes production of collagen by our bone-building osteoblasts while moderating bone breakdown), and vitamin B7 (aka biotin, a nutrient that aids in the synthesis of bone marrow). Two recent Australian studies found that the Paleo program also fell short in the intake of numerous B vitamins—including thiamine (B1), riboflavin (B2), and folate (B9)—as well as iodine and iron.

Both the Paleo and Primal diets eliminate gluten. Although we don't define ourselves as "pure Paleo" dieters, we too eliminate gluten and suggest that you follow suit. After reading Chapter 3 (and seeing how gluten negatively affects your gut and your nutrient levels), you should be on the road to being gluten free too, if you weren't already. However, as we stated earlier, every time you eliminate specific foods you decrease the likelihood that you will be sufficient in the micronutrients normally found in those foods. However, the benefits of removing wheat from your diet greatly outweigh the benefits of the micronutrients that can be found there. Gluten-free diets are often low in vitamin A, the B vitamins, vitamin D, calcium, iron, magnesium, phosphorus, and zinc. Since we encourage you to eliminate gluten, we'll also show you how to increase your intake of those bone-enhancing micronutrients that are reduced on a gluten-free diet. We want you to pay special attention to vitamin B6 and vitamin B9 (folate) because in studies, more than half of the individuals following a gluten-fee diet were found to be deficient in both, and deficiencies in both have been linked to osteoporosis.

Just as in the vegan and vegetarian diets, many common Paleo and Primal foods further increase the likelihood of deficiencies due to their antinutrient content. You can't read a Paleo plan without noticing that they rely heavily on nuts and seeds to create bread recipes and numerous other treats. Remember that nuts and seeds contain five micronutrient-thieving EMDs. Replacing grains is a great idea, but replacing them with excessive amounts of nut flours is not the answer. Nuts and most seeds, as well as nut flours, nut milks, and nut butters, are high in inflammation-causing omega-6 fatty acids. Additionally, although the Paleo and Primal diets recognize the importance of replacing cheap, oxidized vegetable oils (like canola) with healthy saturated fat, they don't spend a lot of time discussing how to choose fat and oil sources that don't add to an omega-6 overload. (You will learn all about the omega-6 crisis causing inflammation and bone loss, and how to reverse it, later in this chapter.)

For now, just recognize that both of these ancestral diets have been shown to cause deficiencies in specific micronutrients, so make sure you supplement appropriately to fill in the gaps.

LOW-FAT DIETS

Following a low-fat diet means you are simply eliminating foods that are high in fat. Although it may now be obvious that low-fat dieters greatly decrease their chances of reaching sufficiency in essential fatty acids (think omega-3), the reduced-fat philosophy also brings about likely deficiencies in the fat-soluble vitamins A, D, E, and K, as well as calcium. Remember, the fat-soluble vitamins are just what their name implies: fat-soluble. Therefore, they require fat to transport them in the body. No fat in the diet means no transport system, and no transport system leads to a high likelihood of deficiencies in these important nutrients. But a low-fat diet can also put your calcium at risk. According to calcium researcher Randi Wolf of Columbia University, low-fat diets have a 19 percent lower mean fractional calcium absorption value than high-fat diets. This is because fat intake increases calcium absorption by slowing transit time and increasing the duration of contact with the absorptive surface. It makes sense, then, that low-fat diets would be deficient at delivering the fat-soluble vitamins, omega-3, and calcium needed to build strong bones. Like all the diets before them, low-fat diets are also high in antinutrients and put their followers at an increased risk of micronutrient deficiency without proper supplementation.

LOW-CARB OR KETOGENIC DIETS

Just as low-fat diets restrict fat from the diet, following a low-carbohydrate diet means nearly cutting out one of the three macronutrient groups (carbohydrates, fats, and proteins) altogether. It generally also means increasing fat and protein consumption compared to a standard American diet (SAD). When the Atkins diet (a popular low-carb, high-fat diet) was studied by researchers at the Children's Nutrition Research Centre of the Royal Children's Hospital in Australia, they found it to be significantly deficient in vitamin B2 (riboflavin), vitamin B9 (folate), calcium, magnesium, and iron. One possible advantage to a low-carb, high-fat diet is that it naturally contains less wheat, beans, rice, and sugar than high-carbohydrate diets, which greatly reduces the number of antinutrients followers have to deal with. It also typically contains some of the best dietary sources of vitamins D and K2, key bone-building micronutrients—such as butter, cream, fish, and eggs.

Possible disadvantages include the fact that many studies have shown low-carbohydrate diets to increase calcium urine excretion, which may lead some to link a low-carbohydrate, high-fat diet with potential bone loss. However, these studies do not show a reduction in calcium absorption. With calcium absorption dependent on fat-soluble vitamin D, it makes sense that a low-carb, high-fat diet would support calcium absorption. This leads us to the question, could a higher level of calcium absorption balance the increased calcium excretion? Interestingly, when researchers looked at high-fat diets and their effects on bone health, they found that high-fat diets with sufficient levels of vitamin D3, phosphorus, and calcium increased bone strength and increased bone mineral content, whereas the same high-fat diet that was deficient in these bone-building micronutrients aggravated bone loss and decreased bone strength.

Individuals making a low-carb, high-fat diet part of their lifestyle need to understand that by greatly reducing carbohydrates in their diet, they are increasing their likelihood of becoming micronutrient deficient. Make sure to supplement properly to fill those gaps if bone health is your goal.

What about Fiber in Your Diet?

Unlike fat that increases calcium absorption, studies indicate that high fiber intakes may "inhibit calcium absorption by increasing the bulk of intestinal contents, speeding the transit time of the stool, and in theory allowing less time for absorption to occur." Any diet that includes large amounts of high-fiber foods, be it low-fat, low-calorie, intermittent fasting, vegan, or vegetarian, may be deficient at delivering the calcium needed to build strong bones.

Beyond Micronutrient Deficiency

It should be becoming clear that *all* the dietary doctrines cause depletions in numerous micronutrients to some extent. You should now be aware that from the perspective of achieving micronutrient sufficiency, there is no perfect diet! All diets have their pros and cons. Your diet alone will not bring you to micronutrient sufficiency—proper supplementation will be necessary. Remember, as a nutrivore, the dietary philosophy you choose is up to you. As you move forward, remember that your dietary philosophy may have micronutrient gaps, caused by either eliminated foods or antinutrients. So pay special attention to filling in these gaps on a daily basis. Now let's shift our focus to two dietary factors that must be considered regardless of dietary philosophy. In this next section we'll examine how both an alkaline diet (low-protein) and your omega-6 to omega-3 ratio can directly impact your bone.

THE ALKALINE DIET: MIRACLE OR MYTH?

If you have osteoporosis, it won't be long before someone tells you to increase your intake of alkaline foods and decrease acidic foods if you want to protect your bones. It's called the alkaline diet and it is being preached like the gospel all over the Internet. Let's look at this controversial theory and see if this advice benefits or harms your bone health.

The position of the alkaline diet is that your body gets energy by *burning* foods for fuel. The remaining by-product (called *ash*) is either acidic or alkaline. Choosing more alkaline foods than acidic foods (about a 3:1 ratio) "alkalizes" your body and helps promote a balanced internal environment that will improve your health. The alkaline diet focuses on eating alkalizing foods, including nearly all vegetables and fruits, many nuts and seeds, and spices. The acid-forming foods include most high-protein foods, such as meat, fish, eggs, dairy, and most legumes (peas and some beans). The goal of the alkaline diet is to try to keep your body's pH between 6.5 (slightly acidic) and 7.5 (slightly alkaline). According to this theory, your food intake, whether alkaline or acidic, is reflected in your urine pH, as well as the pH of other fluids, such as blood and extracellular fluid. Proponents of the alkaline diet believe that if you don't eat enough alkaline foods, the minerals in your bones will be used to buffer acid to support pH balance, which will wear down your bones. But extraordinary claims require extraordinary evidence, and in the case of the alkaline diet theory, the evidence is less than extraordinary.

LET'S EXAMINE THE EVIDENCE

Alkaline Diet Claim 1: Changes in urine pH are evidence that different foods have different effects on pH in the body overall, and that those changes matter to the pH of the environment your cells are in.

Examination: Yes, the foods that you eat change the pH of your urine. But what does that actually tell you? It tells you what you ate recently—which you already knew. But here's the key flaw in the logic of the alkaline diet: your urine pH changes so that your blood pH doesn't have to. Your blood pH is kept in a tight range and will not change much based on your food consumption. Extracellular fluids (outside your cells) and intracellular fluids (inside your cells) cannot drastically alter their pH, or cells won't function properly. Other factors change your urine pH as well, such as fasting, exercise, and medications. Finally, there are cultures all over the world, both modern and historical, that do not have higher rates of osteoporosis and consume a mainly acid diet.

Besides, your body isn't all about that base. Acids are actually essential building blocks of life . . . think essential fatty *acids*, amino *acids*, and even your DNA (deoxyribonucleic *acid*). You actually have a range of pH in different tissues. Your saliva is slightly alkaline to protect your esophagus from the acid in your stomach. Your stomach contains strong acid to start digesting protein, kill invading pathogens, and boost your absorption of several key micronutrients, including B vitamins and minerals like iron, calcium, and zinc. (This is why drinking high-alkaline waters could have a negative effect. By diluting your stomach acid with high-alkaline water, you could be reducing your body's ability to digest food and absorb micronutrients.) Your blood is almost a neutral pH—it is just a tad alkaline—whereas urine pH varies day to day.

MAKE NO BONES ABOUT IT

Alkaline Diet Claim 2: Choosing more acid than alkaline foods (such as protein) will make your blood acidic. To buffer this acidity, your body uses the minerals in bone (such as calcium), which can lead to osteoporosis.

Examination: Sort of, but not really. This claim misunderstands what your kidneys, lungs, and parathyroid gland *do*. Mostly, your kidneys use bicarbonate to support your pH balance. Also, phosphate, found in bone, is used to make phosphoric acid, found in urine. But you have an entire parathyroid gland to tightly regulate your blood calcium and phosphorus. This gland produces hormones that control making and breaking bone. Moreover, your blood passes through your lungs, which help regulate blood pH by exhaling carbon dioxide produced in your kidneys. You exhale more carbon dioxide to remove excess acidity (e.g., yawning); carbon dioxide is also used internally to make bicarbonate to buffer your blood. You also have a protein (albumin) that helps buffer your blood. In short, calcium bone loss is not correlated with a high-protein (acid) diet.

The bottom line is that although the human body can benefit in many ways from eating high-quality, properly prepared plant-based (alkaline) foods, high-quality, properly prepared animal-based (acid) foods are equally beneficial. Whether a food is acid or alkaline is *not* what you should be focusing on to improve your bone health. Instead, focus on food quality and becoming sufficient in your essential micronutrients (vitamins, minerals, fatty acids, and amino acids) and leave the myth of the alkaline diet where it belongs—in storybooks.

HIGH TIME FOR HIGHER PROTEIN

Although claims that high protein intake has detrimental effects on bone health continue to circulate in the osteoporosis communities, you may be surprised to learn that science now points to just the opposite conclusion. According to research published in the *European Journal of Clinical Nutrition*, "no clinical data supports the hypothesis of a detrimental effect of HP [high-protein] diet (acid) on bone health, except in a context of inadequate calcium supply." It's already a well-established fact that long-term inadequate calcium intake causes osteoporosis. So if scientists have debunked the myth that high-protein diets cause bone loss, what new data do we have about protein intake? New research shows the complete opposite of these claims to be true. Scientists have determined that low-protein, fruit-and-vegetable-based (alkaline) diets may actually discourage your production of stomach acid and compromise calcium absorption and that high-protein (acid) intake increases intestinal calcium absorption, effectively offsetting its effect on calcium excretion, so whole-body calcium retention remains unchanged. Not only have multiple studies confirmed that high protein intake provides collagen, phosphate, and other bone-building nutrition that is correlated with better bone health, but a 2018 study endorsed by the International

Osteoporosis Foundation found that "in older people with osteoporosis, higher protein intake (above the current RDA) is associated with higher BMD, slower rate of bone loss, and reduced hip fracture risk, provided that there is also adequate dietary calcium intake. Researchers concluded, "There is no evidence that diet-derived acid load is deleterious for bone health . . . Insufficient dietary protein intakes may be a much more severe problem than protein excess."

You may be one of the thousands of people who have been told to avoid protein because it will cause bone loss, but research clearly points us in the opposite direction. So if protein (animal or plant based) is not the enemy, then just how important is it to our overall success at rebuilding bone? As it turns out protein is really important, and it affects you regardless of which dietary profile you follow. Although it may at first seem controversial, the research is backed by one of the giants in the field of osteoporosis research. Dr. Robert P. Heaney, a renowned clinical endocrinologist who spent nearly fifty years researching bone biology, osteoporosis, and human calcium and vitamin D physiology, believed that protein might be an important key to bone health.

To better understand the link between protein requirements and bone health, we first must understand bone itself. Bone is made up of a protein matrix within which the calcium salts are embedded. According to Dr. Heaney, "While bone is the body's reservoir of calcium, that calcium is tied up as part of a structure, the largest component of which is protein. When the body needs calcium and has to make withdrawals from the skeletal reserves, it does so not by leaching the calcium from this protein-mineral complex, but by physically tearing down microscopic units of bone and scavenging the calcium that is released in the process. Inevitably, therefore, the protein matrix—the structure—goes as well."

Dr. Heaney explains that in order to profit fully from a high calcium intake, a patient who has lost bone would need to consume enough protein to allow the body to rebuild the lost structure. Without enough protein, the extra calcium might reduce further bone loss, but it would be ineffective at building new bone. A few years ago, a study at the Tufts Nutrition Research Center on Aging in Boston proved just that. Researchers led by Bess Dawson-Hughes noticed that a high calcium intake led to increased bone gain if the patient's intake of protein was high. The Tufts research study first proved that supplementation of both calcium and vitamin D produced a better than 50 percent reduction in fracture risk in healthy elderly Bostonians with those two nutrients alone.

But, like other researchers before her, Dawson–Hughes noted that although high calcium intakes reduced or stopped bone loss in treated subjects, the two nutrients didn't lead to bone gain. They didn't, that is, in individuals consuming usual protein intakes. However, in a subset of treated patients, who, it turns out, had protein intakes above 1.5 times the RDA (0.8 g/kg body weight), bone gain was dramatic! To figure out your ideal bone-building protein intake, you can multiply your weight in pounds by 0.545. For example, if you weigh 130 pounds, then the amount of protein you need daily is at least 71 grams per day (130 × 0.545), or 18 grams (71 ÷ 4) per meal over four meals. Take a look at the figure below, which shows the three-year change in BMD at the hip in the calcium- and vitamin-D-supplemented participants in the Tufts study. Dramatic bone gains were seen only in participants with the highest protein intakes.

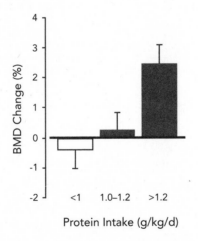

Protein Intake (g/kg/d)

This study was groundbreaking, even for Dr. Heaney, who was in bone research for half a decade. Dr. Heaney writes, "For me, it was an 'Aha!'" moment. Why hadn't we thought of that? It was known that bone is 50 percent protein by volume (but only about 20 percent calcium by weight). And it was known that when bone is torn down (as with estrogen or calcium deficiency), its protein is degraded in the process. So it made sense that, to rebuild the lost bone, you would need not just calcium but fresh protein as well."

In another study, researchers found that participants with protein intakes below the median for the group could not retain calcium, no matter what their calcium intake. This means they couldn't build bone. By contrast, those with protein intakes above the median for the group retained extra calcium reasonably well.

So there you have it! Two distinct studies exhibited the same interdependence of calcium and protein. According to Dr. Heaney, most clinical nutritionists had failed to recognize that the adult RDA for protein is just barely enough to prevent muscle loss, and is not enough to support tissue building or rebuilding. When calcium deficiency leads to bone loss, the bone protein is lost as well, and that has to be rebuilt to restore the lost bone. Although the alkaline diet theory told us to reduce protein, scientific studies prove that we cannot build new bone without adequate and even higher levels than normal of protein. Now that you know the importance of getting enough protein, let's take a more in-depth look at protein and how it can benefit our bones in three distinct ways.

#1: PROTEIN HELPS SUPPORT THE BONES AND PREVENT FALLS

Sarcopenia, which is a gradual loss of muscle mass as one ages, has been credited with causing a slew of health problems, including low BMD and fractures. Studies have shown that muscle quality is critical for balance control in elderly individuals. People with osteoporosis often have muscle weakness leading to fractures, poor balance, and even falling. Therefore, improving muscle quality and strengthening weak muscles are essential elements for the prevention of falls and fractures in older adults with osteoporosis. In Chapter 5, you will learn how to best work your muscles safely to fight sarcopenia.

#2: YOUR ESSENTIAL AMINO ACIDS ARE ESSENTIAL FOR BONE BUILDING

We have been talking a lot about protein, but don't forget that quality protein delivers more than just help building strong muscles. Protein is also the delivery system for another class of essential micronutrients called amino acids, which act as building blocks of protein. Just as certain foods contain different vitamins and minerals, protein-based foods (both plant and animal) contain your amino acids. If you don't eat enough protein, you will become deficient in these essential micronutrients.

There are twenty-two standard amino acids, nine of which are essential amino acids (histidine, isoleucine, leucine, lysine, methionine, phenylalanine, threonine, tryptophan, and valine), and eight of which are conditionally essential amino acids (arginine, cysteine, glutamine, tyrosine, glycine, ornithine, proline and serine). They are called essential or conditionally essential amino acids because our bodies cannot manufacture them or need certain conditions to manufacture them. Subsequently, we need to get a sufficient amount of each one from the food we eat or supplements we take daily. Failure to get enough of even one of the essential amino acids can have serious health implications.

Here are some studies showing just how essential amino acids are for bone health:

- Arginine, lysine, alanine, proline, leucine, and glutamine have been shown to promote osteoblast growth and differentiation.
- Arginine has also been shown to stimulate growth hormone (GH) secretion, thereby promoting production of insulinlike growth factor (IGF–1), which are both fundamental in skeletal growth and bone health throughout life.
- Arginine, lysine, and glycine have been associated with an improvement in collagen formation or synthesis. We've previously discussed how crucial collagen is to bone health, so you know that these three amino acids play a huge role in your battle against osteoporosis.
- Leucine has a direct effect on the initiation of mRNA translation (the second imperative biological process of gene expression) and

is thought to be the most efficient of the branched-chain amino acids at increasing muscle protein synthesis, which is critical for the maintenance of adequate bone strength and density.

- Supplementation with L-arginine (2 g/day) for 2 years increased BMD by 11.6 percent in 150 osteoporotic postmenopausal women.
- A study published in the *Journal of Bone and Mineral Research* proved that higher intakes of six of the bone-protective amino acids (alanine, arginine, glutamic acid, leucine, lysine, and pro-line) were significantly associated with higher BMD at the spine and forearm.

#3: LACTOFERRIN—WHEY PROTEIN'S SECRET BONE-BUILDING AGENT

Milk: it really does do your body (and your bones) good! Actually, it is a natural bioactive glycoprotein found in milk, called lactoferrin, that science has determined is excellent for bone health. Lactoferrin works in two distinct ways. First, it reduces inflammation, which causes a reduction in the destructive actions of the osteoclasts, the cells responsible for bone loss that lead to osteoporosis. Second, new studies suggest that lactoferrin also enhances bone-building activity. Lactoferrin's anabolic (building) effect on bone stems from its ability to increase the number of osteoblasts capable of creating (synthesizing) new bone—through both stimulation of proliferation and inhibition of cell death. It also enhances the ability of the osteoblasts to synthesize and mineralize bone matrix. Lactoferrin is one of those few molecules that has been proven to affect both osteoclasts and osteoblasts in the remodeling activity of bone. Drinking a whey protein shake (there is no lactoferrin in plant protein) is a great way to increase your intake of lactoferrin.

In the end, protein (and the amino acids it delivers) has been shown to have a multitude of incredible, scientifically proven health benefits such as lowered stress and improved mood, protection against cognitive decline, weight loss, decreased risk of cardiovascular disease, lowered risk of type 2 diabetes, increased lean body mass, boosted beneficial gut bacteria, and even inhibited growth of cancer cells. Now, we can confidently add bone building to this list. Getting enough protein (animal or plant) in your diet, thereby creating a positive protein balance in your body, is extremely important on your journey to bone health. In Chapter 7, you will learn how to purchase the healthiest protein powder that fits into your dietary doctrine.

Your Omega-6 to Omega-3 Ratio

This next factor has been shown to have a direct effect on both bone loss and your ability to rebuild bone. If you have been reading about nutrition for a while, you have probably heard about the omega-6 to omega-3 ratio. Getting this ratio right is vital for not only your bone health but for your overall health in general. Omega-6 and omega-3 make up the essential fatty acids, which are of course part of the essential micronutrients. (Remember, micronutrients are vitamins, minerals, amino acids, and essential fatty acids.) And just as the amino acids that we covered in the last section are found in protein-based foods, essential fatty acids are found in foods that contain fat.

Our Paleolithic ancestors, who were free of modern diseases like heart disease, cancer, autoimmune conditions, diabetes, and of course osteoporosis, ate a diet that was naturally lower in omega-6 and higher in omega-3 than our modern diets. Their diets were roughly a 1:1 ratio of omega-6 to omega-3. Today, our diets have skewed to a reported average someplace around a 16:1 ratio (and as high as 25:1 in some people). This is the foundation of a really big problem: all research shows that a lower ratio of omega-6 to omega-3 is more desirable in reducing the risk of many of the chronic diseases of high prevalence in Western societies—including osteoporosis. In fact, a study published in the *American Journal of Clinical Nutrition* concluded, "A higher ratio of omega-6 to omega-3 fatty acids is associated with lower BMD (bone mineral density) at the hip in both sexes."

So why is omega-6 so bad and omega-3 so good? Well, in reality, both omega-6 and omega-3 are good. They are both essential fatty acids, and we need both to survive. The real problem is in the ratio of the two in our diets. This is because, for the most part, omega-6 is pro-inflammatory, meaning it causes inflammation in the body, and omega-3 is anti-inflammatory. So to prevent or reduce diseases linked to inflammation, like osteoporosis, it is essential to attempt to create a 1:1 ratio (or at least below a 4:1 ratio) between your omega-6 and omega-3 intake every day.

OK, this sounds relatively simple to do—right? Just eat foods or take supplements that help increase your omega-3 levels and that should improve your ratio. Well, unfortunately, it's not that simple. The problem is that although a 16:1 ratio of omega-6 to omega-3 might not sound so bad, when we look at how much omega-6 and omega-3 that ratio really delivers in an average daily diet, a problem becomes immediately apparent.

ARE YOU OVERLOADED BY OMEGA-6?

Let's look at an average day's menu for Wilma, a typical Paleo dieter (a diet that is praised for its healthy amount of omega-3). For breakfast, Wilma starts her day eating three eggs with four slices of bacon. She follows this with a Cobb salad for lunch, which is topped with an egg, two slices of bacon, $2/3$ cup avocado, $2^{1}/_{2}$ ounces chopped chicken thigh, and 4 tablespoons of her favorite avocado-oil-based salad dressing. Wilma enjoys a small 1.75-ounce snack pack of almonds in the afternoon, and then for dinner she eats 6 ounces dark meat chicken and sautéed vegetables with garlic cooked in 4 tablespoons olive oil.

Now, you may not follow a Paleo diet (or ever even consider eating any of the foods included in this sample menu), and that's OK. Our point is that Wilma's menu would be considered an almost perfect daily menu by most Paleo dieters, and yet what you're about to see is just how far from perfect it is when we take into account the omega-6 to omega-3 ratio. Wilma's "healthy" daily menu delivers a 15:1 ratio of omega-6 to omega-3 (37,308 mg/2,481 mg). And although this is just below the average 16:1 ratio most people eat, what is really disturbing is that it leaves Wilma with a deficit of 34,827 mg of omega-3. This means that in order to get to a 1:1 ratio, which is recommended for optimal health, Wilma would have to ingest 34,827 mg of pure omega-3 through either food or an omega-3 supplement.

So what are Wilma's options? Let's crunch the numbers to find out. She could choose any number of foods to try to equalize the ratio, but the problem is that most foods that contain omega-3 also deliver more omega-6. For example, they may provide 1,000 mg of omega-3, but they also contain that much or more omega-6—so you never actually improve your ratio. Her best options would be to choose either omega-3-rich wild-caught salmon or to opt for a fish oil or flaxseed oil supplement. If she chooses wild-caught sockeye salmon, then she would have to eat between 6.5 and 8.75 *pounds* of salmon *on top* of her daily menu. Obviously, this is completely unrealistic. Her next option would be to supplement with approximately *thirty-five* (1,000 mg) fish oil or flaxseed oil pills—also entirely unrealistic! The fact is, no one ever has or will do either of these options; this is why we are making such a big deal about this issue.

Even if Wilma *did* take 2,000 mg of fish oil or flaxseed oil daily and increased her omega-3s to 4,481 mg per day (2,481 mg through diet plus 2,000 mg through supplements), she would still have a ratio of approximately 8:1 (37,308/4481)—nowhere near where it needs to be. You should notice something else about this example. Wilma was sufficient in her omega-3s. Her diet delivered 2,481 mg of omega-3, and the RDI is 1,600 mg per day. In fact, she exceeded the RDI by 55 percent. However, because her omega-6 was so high, even a very high omega-3 intake will not save her from the total body inflammation and low bone mineral effects that an unbalanced ratio of omega-6 to omega-3 will cause.

We have another bit of bad news for you: scientists have determined that omega-6 and omega-3 compete in the body. High quantities of omega-6 will greatly diminish the chances that your ingested omega-3 can convert to the EPA and DHA that you need to build bone. In short, the more omega-6 you take in, the lower your chances that any ingested omega-3 will actually benefit you. However, the opposite is also true. If you can create a positive omega-3 to omega-6 ratio, then omega-3 will block the inflammation-causing bone-loss effect of the omega-6. Pretty cool, right?

OMEGA-3 BUILDS BONE!

Let's take a deeper dive and explore how omega-3 and omega-6 contribute to and undermine our bone health specifically. Omega-3 (ALA) elongates into two fatty acids called EPA and DHA that defend our bones against osteoporosis. They do this by reducing inflammation through a large number of mechanisms, and reducing inflammation is essential for those with bone loss because research shows that inflammation activates osteoclasts, the cells that break down bone. Since it takes more time to build bone than to break it down, chronic inflammation from too much omega-6 results in a loss of BMD and, ultimately, in osteoporosis.

So EPA and DHA inhibit osteoclast production and activity, preventing excessive bone loss, but they do something else too: they help us build healthy bones by signaling to special cells that live in our bone marrow called mesenchymal stem cells (MSCs) to become osteoblasts rather than fat cells. Yes, you read that right. You have cells in your bone that can choose to become fat cells or osteoblasts (bone-building cells). When more osteoblasts are produced, more of these bone-building cells are available and bone mineral loss is reduced or reversed. But there is more good news! Mature osteoblasts also produce an important anti-inflammatory compound called osteoprotegerin (OPG).

To understand OPG we have to think back to Chapter 2, where we discussed osteoporosis medications—specifically RANK ligand (RANKL) inhibitors. If you remember, when RANK binds with RANKL, a series of inflammatory events results in the production of osteoclasts and bone removal. These RANKL inhibitors work to prevent RANK from binding with RANKL, thus reducing the formation and activity of osteoclasts. Well, guess what? OPG does the same thing. When OPG binds to RANKL, no inflammatory response takes place and no osteoclasts are produced. This makes it crystal clear that drug companies are trying to mimic the natural, easy-to-achieve effects of omega-3 supplementation with their prescription RANKL inhibitors.

This is really exciting, especially when you realize that the only thing you have to do to get your body to inhibit osteoclasts and increase osteoblasts and OPG production is even out your omega-6 to omega-3 ratio. Remember only EPA and DHA omega-3 fatty acids can do this, not ALA. If you have too many omega-6 fatty acids, you get a completely different outcome.

So next, let's look at this whole thing from the omega-6 perspective. Just as omega-3 creates two elongated fatty acids called EPA and DHA, omega-6 creates an elongated fatty acid called AA, which is pro-inflammatory. Remember, inflammation activates osteoclasts, the cells that break down bone. Too much AA means chronic inflammation, which results in a loss of BMD and, finally, in osteoporosis.

And remember how EPA and DHA signal to our MSCs to become osteoblasts rather than fat cells? Well, AA does the exact opposite and signals for them to become fat cells, greatly reducing the number of bone-building osteoblasts. And, as if that weren't enough, AA also inhibits the osteoblasts you *do* have from producing that amazing, anti-inflammatory compound OPG.

Can you now see why we are really trying to drive home the importance of this often overlooked ratio between omega-6 and omega-3? Above and beyond bone health, don't forget that your omega-6 to omega-3 ratio is important to your health in general. According to research published in the prestigious medical journal *The Lancet*, a diet with an omega-6 to omega-3 ratio of 4:1 or less may reduce total mortality by up to 70 percent over two years.

But there is still more to this story. If we need to get our omega-6 to omega-3 levels to as close to a 1:1 ratio as possible, and we know that the average healthy diet delivers a ratio of 16:1 or higher, and even eating over six pounds of salmon per day or taking more than thirty fish oil or flaxseed oil pills will not achieve this desired ratio, then how in the world are you going to do it? Well, it really comes down to a two-part plan. You must increase your intake of omega-3 through food and proper supplementation *and* drive down your omega-6 intake by avoiding or eliminating high-omega-6 foods. In order to do this you must become acutely aware of the foods that contain high amounts of omega-6. But the problem with this is that many of these foods are the exact foods millions of people around the world consider to be some of the healthiest foods on the planet—foods like nuts, seeds, vegetable oils, olive oils, grapeseed oil, avocados, salad dressings, bacon, dark meat chicken, nut milks, rice bran, wheat germ, and oat bran. Of course, it is also found in higher quantities in snack foods, fast foods, and baked goods such as cookies, cakes, pastries, and muffins—you are really going to have to limit these foods in your chosen dietary profile. Look at Table 4.2 for a list of foods that can have the largest impact on your daily omega-6 intake. Also, if you don't see a particular food on this list that appears frequently in your menu—google it and find out how much omega-6 and omega-3 it has per serving so you can calculate your daily intake properly. Don't brush this ratio under the rug—if you do not get your omega-6 to omega-3 ratio right, you will be setting yourself up not just for poor bone health but for poor health in general. Before you run off and purchase an omega-3 supplement, make sure to read our purchasing guidelines in Chapter 7. There are additional micronutrient competitions (between EPA and DHA) and safety hazards you need to be aware of.

TABLE 4.2 Omega-6 to Omega-3 Ratios in Popular Foods

Foods are listed in order from least to most amount of omega-3 necessary for counterbalancing omega-6.

Foods per 100-g serving (3.5 oz or 7 Tbsp)	Omega-6	Omega-3	Omega-6 to Omega-3 Ratio	Omega-3 mg Needed to Equalize
Avocados ($^2/_3$ cup cubed)	1,673 mg	126 mg	13:1	1,547 mg (2 fish oil caps)
Whole scrambled eggs ($1^1/_2$ eggs)	1,916 mg	154 mg	12:1	1,762 mg (2 fish oil caps)
Dark meat chicken w/skin ($3^1/_2$ oz)	3,040 mg	220 mg	14:1	2,820 mg (3 fish oil caps)
Egg yolks (5–6 yolks)	3,538 mg	282 mg	13:1	3,256 mg (3 fish oil caps)
Pork belly/ bacon (5–7 slices)	5,020 mg	480 mg	10:1	4,540 mg (5 fish oil caps)
Cashews ($3^1/_2$ oz)	7,782 mg	161 mg	48:1	7,621 mg (8 fish oil caps)
Olive oil (7 Tbsp)	9,763 mg	761 mg	13:1	9,002 mg (9 fish oil caps)
Avocado oil (7 Tbsp)	12,531 mg	957 mg	13:1	11,574 mg (12 fish oil caps)
Almonds ($3^1/_2$ oz)	12,053 mg	6 mg	2,008:1	12,047 mg (12 fish oil caps)
Brazil nuts ($3^1/_2$ oz)	20,564 mg	18 mg	1,142:1	20,546 mg (21 fish oil caps)
Sunflower seeds ($3^1/_2$ oz)	37,389 mg	79 mg	473:1	37,310 mg (37 fish oil caps)

I was athletic and eating an extremely healthy diet, so I was shocked when I was diagnosed with osteoporosis. To make matters worse, my bone density didn't improve, even when I was following a whole-food diet suggested by countless doctors and healthcare professionals. It wasn't until I spoke to a Calton Nutrition specialist that I saw some real changes. The specialist pointed out that I was using way too much olive oil on my salads. In addition, I was snacking on nuts and nut butters. Both my Calton Nutrition coach and the functional medicine practitioner that I was seeing stressed that inflammation might be to blame for my weakening bones. They suggested I lower my omega-6 intake by removing nuts from my diet and replacing my regular olive oil with SKINNYFat, a special olive oil with 85 percent less omega-6. I also increased my omega-3 intake with a triple strength omega-3 supplement (four capsules a day of Origin Omega).

Within just a few months, these changes started proving to have exceptional results. My omega-6 to omega-3 ratio went from 8:1 to a 2.4:1 in just seven months! Additionally, my AA to EPA ratio (AA is the bad omega-6 and EPA is the good omega-3 that can help me improve my bone health) went from 20:1 to only 2.6:1 in that same amount of time.

My doctor was thrilled when my markers of bone resorption went from elevated bone loss to normal and my urinary lipid peroxides score (which is an indicator of oxidative stress) went from extremely elevated at 11.3 (>4 is elevated) to really amazing at 1.55! There is no doubt in my mind that making these changes and improving my omega-3 to omega-6 ratio is helping to make strides in my fight against osteoporosis. Following the Caltons osteoporosis protocol this past year has allowed me to stop losing bone for the very first time. Every DEXA prior to this last one showed bone loss, and finally, utilizing the Caltons amazing products and advice I have had my first DEXA in ten years that proved my bones were no longer deteriorating. My doctors were amazed, and I couldn't be more excited.

You can see that many of these foods have some pretty high omega-6 to omega-3 ratios. To up your ratio of omega-3s, eat plenty of low-mercury fatty fish like sockeye salmon, go for grass-fed butter and meat, swap omega-6 oils for those higher in omega-3s, and always check the ingredients when you buy packaged food to make sure there aren't any unwanted omega-6 sources hiding inside. In our experience, as you will see in Denise's story, making just one or two simple changes (or healing habits) can bring about great rewards even for those who believe they are following healthy diet plans.

Healing Habits Revealed in Chapter 4

17. Overcome the deficiencies of your chosen dietary doctrine.
18. Pick up the protein.
19. Increase your omega-3 intake.
20. Eliminate omega-6-rich foods.

Join us On the Couch for an in-depth chat about Chapter 4

As always, don't forget to come to our "On the Couch" video coaching session at RebuildYourBones.com, where we will talk about the main points of this chapter and reveal our favorite tips for getting enough protein and how to avoid high omega-6 foods at restaurants.

CHAPTER 5

It's Time to Play the Game of Life

Make no mistake about it. Bad habits are called *bad* for a reason. They kill our productivity and creativity. They slow us down. They hold us back from achieving our goals. And they're detrimental to our health.

—JOHN RAMPTON (AMERICAN ENTREPRENEUR)

In Chapters 3 and 4, we helped guide you toward eating the most micronutrient-rich diet possible to greatly increase your chances of micronutrient sufficiency. Your first lifestyle habit, your personal dietary philosophy, is the first step to filling your "micronutrient bucket." Each dietary doctrine will differ in the quantity and diversity of the nutrients delivered. But now, we must account for everyday life. Your daily habits act as EMDs, subtracting the vitamins, minerals, essential fatty acids, and amino acids you've worked so hard to build through your diet—often unexpectedly leaving you further away from meeting your goal of micronutrient sufficiency. As we mentioned before, EMDs create tiny holes in our sufficiency buckets, causing the vital micronutrients we do manage to get in there to slowly and steadily leak out. Now it's time to learn about how lifestyle habits are putting holes in your bucket and, more importantly, how to plug the holes before it's too late.

Toxic Load

Look around: this is not the world of our ancestors. In fact, it isn't even the same world that our grandparents lived in. Not only are our soil and our food supplies becoming more and more micronutrient-depleted by the day, but the world around us, including the foods we eat and the everyday items we surround ourselves with, are being filled with potentially dangerous toxins. How did this happen? To put it plainly—industrialization. In an attempt to make our lives easier, we have destroyed the natural environment of our ancestors and replaced it with an unhealthy human-made environment filled with industrialized chemical runoff, animals forced to live in unnatural environments, and products sold globally with little to no testing and regulation for safety. Although we can't jump into a time machine and return to simpler times, we can learn how to avoid many of today's micronutrient pitfalls. Let's get to lightening your toxic load. It's time to pitch the plastics, mind the metals, and clean up your casa!

PITCH THE PLASTICS

This first set of micronutrient thieves we are going to discuss will not be listed on labels, but chances are you have recently ingested these plastics. Odds are that you're among the 93 percent of Americans with detectable levels of bisphenol A (BPA) in their bodies, and also among the 75-plus percent of Americans with phthalates in their urine. Statistics seem to show us that we are not only what we eat, but also what we touch *and* what touches what we eat.

Both BPA and phthalates are synthetic chemicals that mimic estrogen in the body. BPA can be found in reusable drink containers, toilet paper, DVDs, cell phones, eyeglass lenses, and automobile parts. In the grocery store, you are most likely to come in contact with it in its polycarbonate plastic form in water bottles and in its epoxy form in the linings of food cans. It is even in the thermal paper used for cash register receipts. Phthalates can be found in food packaging, plastic wraps, pesticides, children's toys, PVC pipes, air fresheners, laundry products, personal care products, and even in medical supplies.

All of this plastic is playing with your hormones. In a 2012 study published in the journal *PLoS ONE*, research indicated that BPA triggers the release of almost double the insulin actually needed to break down food. Although normal insulin secretion has been shown to benefit bone, high insulin levels can desensitize the body to this hormone over time, causing insulin resistance. Recent studies have also determined that several prevalent phthalate metabolites showed statistically significant correlations with insulin resistance in American men. Insulin resistance has been proven to negatively influence bone remodeling and leads to reduced bone strength.

Plastic also affects two other hormones, estrogen and testosterone. Research published in the *Journal of Clinical Endocrinology and Metabolism* in 2014 proved that men, women, and children exposed to high levels of endocrine-disrupting phthalates tended to have reduced levels of testosterone in their blood compared to those with lower chemical exposure. Recent research suggests that testosterone may increase the bone's ability to retain calcium. Women who experience rapid bone loss are typically deficient in both estrogen and testosterone, and up to 30 percent of men with osteoporotic fractures have low testosterone levels. Studies also reveal that women with high levels of phthalates are likely to go through menopause earlier and have estrogen disruption, which can then have an unhealthy effect on bone formation. The research on both BPA and phthalates is clear. Both affect calcium absorption at the cellular level by blocking calcium channels. Individuals with bone loss should be keenly aware of eliminating all BPA and phthalates from their lives.

Each year about six billion pounds of BPA and eighteen billion pounds of phthalate esters are created worldwide—that's a lot of problematic plastics! Here are our top five recommendations to help you avoid them, which can greatly reduce the risk of osteoporosis:

1. Stop microwaving food in plastic containers. In fact, stop buying plastic food storage units altogether. Use porcelain, glass, or stainless steel containers instead.
2. Look on the bottoms of plastic containers for recycle codes (products with codes 3 or 7 may contain BPA).
3. Reduce the use of canned foods or, at the very least, switch to cans that are labeled as BPA free; preferably, opt for products in glass jars.
4. Ask your butcher to wrap your meat or fish in paper, which helps keep the conventional PVC plastic wrap that most markets use out of your cart.
5. Try not to touch cash register receipts unless it is absolutely necessary.

HEAVY METALS

The next thing that adds to your overall toxic load is heavy metals. These toxins may be hiding in plain sight in your refrigerator and pantry, or perhaps you come into contact with them in your daily hygiene regimen. Regardless of where you find them, you have to learn to mind them.

As it turns out, micronutrients work as the body's natural detoxifiers, affecting both the absorption and excretion of these toxic contaminants. This is both good and bad news. It is good news because even if you are exposed to toxic heavy metals, your mighty micronutrients can help you detoxify them. The bad news is that the more micronutrients used up in the detoxification process, the higher the likelihood that you will become deficient. In Table 5.1, we outline a few examples of heavy metal toxins. How many of these products do you buy at the grocery store and possibly feed to your family that contain these four toxins? Could their micronutrient-depleting effects be putting holes in your sufficiency bucket?

TABLE 5.1 Heavy Metals That Cause Toxic Load

Heavy Metal	Where Is It Found? How to Avoid It?	Concerns	Micronutrient Interactions
Lead	Found in rice, protein powder, juice, imported canned goods, and foods containing synthetic nitrates (like bacon) Avoid by choosing meat products without synthetic nitrates and reducing rice and juice consumption; make sure the manufacturer of your protein powder can show you a heavy metal third-party lab analysis.	Fatigue, headaches, irritability, uneasy stomach, reduced IQ and attention span, impaired growth, reading and learning disabilities, osteoporosis, hearing loss, mental retardation, coma, convulsions, death	Vitamins B1, B6, C, and E; calcium; iron; phosphorus; selenium; zinc; alpha-lipoic acid; and quercetin have the ability to scavenge free radicals and chelate lead ions. Although vitamin D usually increases the absorption of calcium, magnesium, and zinc, if those minerals are deficient, it may work to increase intestinal absorption of lead instead. Because lead and iron share a common absorptive mechanism, lead uptake is enhanced in iron deficiency.

Heavy Metal	Where Is It Found? How to Avoid It?	Concerns	Micronutrient Interactions
Mercury	Found in fish, usually the largest predatory ones, like swordfish and shark, that have eaten the greatest majority of toxin-containing smaller fish for the longest period of time Avoid by choosing smaller fish.	Sensory impairment (vision, hearing, speech); disturbed sensation; lack of coordination; profuse sweating; faster-than-normal heartbeat; increased salivation; high blood pressure; damage to brain, lungs, and kidneys	Selenium and vitamins C and E help detoxify mercury. N-acetylcysteine enhanced excretion of mercury by 400 percent in comparison to control animals.
Arsenic	Found in rice, juice, protein powder, foods containing synthetic nitrates, poultry from conventional farms Avoid by choosing meats without nitrates and organic poultry; make sure the manufacturer of your protein powder can show you a heavy metal third-party lab analysis.	Nerve damage; scaling skin; skin pigment changes; circulatory problems; increased risk of lung, bladder, kidney, skin, and liver cancer	Phosphorus, selenium, and vitamins A and E help detoxify arsenic.
Aluminum	Found in aluminum foil, cookware, beverage containers, preservatives, fillers, coloring agents, anticaking agents, emulsifiers, baking powders, soy-based infant formula, cigarette smoke, cosmetics, antiperspirants, sunscreen, antacids, and some vaccines Avoid by making sure not to heat food in aluminum foil; choose personal sundries and hygiene products that are aluminum free.	Increased risk of breast cancer, cognitive impairment, dementia, and Alzheimer's; linked to autism, diabetes, neuropathy, and cancer; reduces intestinal activity	Silica and L-theanine help detoxify aluminum; high aluminum levels in the bloodstream compete with calcium and ultimately weaken bone. Other chelators and antagonists include magnesium, zinc, and vitamin C.

TOXINS IN HOUSEHOLD ITEMS

Just because you don't eat something doesn't mean that you aren't ingesting it—all of the things you come into contact with are being absorbed by your skin, and the average person sure is giving it a lot to drink in. Women take in the most toxins, with the average woman using twelve beauty and skin products containing 168 different ingredients daily. Men don't fare too much better, using six products daily with 85 unique ingredients. But who is at the highest risk? It might surprise you, but teen girls (whose smaller bodies are still developing bones) actually use an average of seventeen personal care products each day— 40 percent more than an adult woman.

And these numbers reflect only beauty and skin products. Think about the dish detergent, stain-resistant chemically coated carpeting and furniture, cleaning products, Teflon-coated pans, laundry cleaners, dryer sheets, and air fresheners you come into contact with daily. It really adds up. According to the United Nations Environment Programme, approximately seventy thousand chemicals are commonly used across the world, with one thousand new chemicals being introduced every year. Many of these new industrialized chemicals disrupt your endocrine system, which has been scientifically proven to cause bone loss. In fact, a 2019 study discovered that the use of one single chemical called triclosan may double women's chances of osteoporosis. The good news is that the US government has banned its use from antiseptic soaps. However, the bad news is that is still commonly found in toothpaste, deodorants, and shampoos. While all toxic add-ins may not be directly linked to osteoporosis, all of them increase your toxic load.

Your body only has two ways of handling this toxic load: either the toxins wreak havoc in your body—causing hormonal changes, neurological damage, or even cancer—or, preferably, you have enough essential micronutrients around for natural detoxification to occur. As with the heavy metals you just encountered, micronutrients work as the body's natural detoxifiers, affecting both the absorption and excretion of these toxic contaminants. So you may not be able to tell your boss that the air freshener has to go, but you can reduce its endocrine-disrupting effect by making sure you are sufficient in your essential micronutrients, specifically the antioxidants (vitamins A, C, E, and alpha-lipoic acid) as well as magnesium, selenium, and zinc. Any reduction in these bone-building micronutrients puts your bones at risk.

Our Top Ten Tricks to Reduce Household Toxins

Remember, our plan is all about driving down your micronutrient depletion by making changes in your diet and lifestyle. This is to ensure that you don't poke too many holes in your micronutrient bucket. As you will discover later, in Chapter 8, our program is designed for you to make changes in your diet and supplementation first. Changes to your lifestyle and environment will come second. However, if you already shop using our Rich Food, Poor Food philosophy and are ready for the next step, then jump right in and change out your household and beauty products for safer nontoxic ones. Make changes at your own pace; remember, you can always add another healing habit tomorrow! Here are our top ten tricks to get you started no matter where you are on your journey to micronutrient sufficiency.

1. Forgo the fragrances. Whether it is the air freshener in your car or home or your favorite perfume, lotion, or body spray, it is important to eliminate endocrine disruptors in these products. You can eliminate these hidden toxins by avoiding any products that say *perfume* or *fragrance* on the label. Don't fret, there are a ton of great-smelling, safer alternatives. Organic essential oils are safe substitutes for perfume, and diffusing them through your home can cover up food and pet odors easily. *Safe alternatives include* In Essence organic essential oils and Mrs. Meyer's Clean Day air fresheners. You can also try a lotion like Face Naturals Organic Creamy Coconut and Key Lime Body Butter to keep your skin smelling delicious all day or rejuvenate your skin with Annmarie Gianni's Wild Fruit Serum Brightening Facial Complex.

2. What's hiding in shampoos and conditioners is shameful. Watch out for triclosan, parabens, fragrances, sodium lauryl sulfate, and polyethylene glycol (often listed as PEG) in your shampoos and conditioners. As an added bonus, the alternative healthy products are so gentle that you can save money by using them on both your hair and body. *Safe alternatives include* products by Beauty Without Cruelty (BWC), Maia's, Annmarie Gianni Skin Care, Face Naturals, and The Honest Company.

3. Put your best face forward. Plenty of responsible brands these days have removed lead from lipstick and mercury from mascara. Also, give your skin time to breathe and detox naturally when at home or out with loved ones. When you do want to doll up, choose from brands that keep you healthy on the inside while making you beautiful on the outside. *Safe alternatives include* products by Maia's, Beauty Without Cruelty (BWC), Au Naturale, W3LL PEOPLE, Beautycounter, and Jane Iredale. Some drugstore products like Revlon Colorburst lipstick and Almay Intense I-Color Volumizing Mascara also hit the mark.

4. Take time for your teeth. Think of how much your body (especially your bones) will thank you for searching out a product that does not contain fluoride, artificial flavors and colors, triclosan, polysorbate-80, ethanol, titanium dioxide, benzoate or benzoic acid, or sodium lauryl sulfate. Fluoride accumulates in your bones, creates weaker bones, and may increase your risk of fractures. There are a plethora of options for your pearly whites. *Safe alternatives include* toothpaste by Redmond Clay, JĀSÖN, Jack N' Jill (for the little ones), Just the Goods, and Tom's of Maine.

5. Deodorants can be a stinky mess. Ditch those deodorants that mimic estrogen, as well as any antiperspirants that contain aluminum, which has been linked to cancer. Search labels for unwanted parabens, triclosan, steareth, propylene glycol, and talc, which are all possible allergens—not to mention that unwanted mystery "fragrance" again. *Safe alternatives include* Lume seventy-two-hour odor shield deodorant, Pure & Natural Crystal Deoderant Mist body spray, Schmidt's Bergamot + Lime natural deodorant, and unscented Arm & Hammer.

6. Clean your clothes without poisons. The clothes you put on your body likely stay on it all day, so you want them to be clean, not coated with a film of irritants and potential carcinogens, right? Always avoid products with labels that say "warning," "danger," or "poison." Forgo fabric softener and instead add 2 cups organic vinegar to the wash. *Safe alternatives include* detergent by GreenShield Organic, Dr. Bronner's, Seventh Generation, and Mrs. Meyer's Clean Day.

7. Ditch the dryer sheets. These fluffing and perfumed pads are filled with camphor, chloroform, or ethyl acetate, all of which are on the Environmental Protection Agency's (EPA's) hazardous waste list, or with alpha-terpineol, benzyl alcohol, or linalool, all of which are known to cause nervous system disorders. *Safe alternatives include* adding in.essence organic essential oils to a wet cloth before starting the dryer, purchasing wool balls, or using Mrs. Meyer's Clean Day dryer sheets.

8. Clean up your dish soaps. To begin, toss out any product that says *antibacterial*. Thankfully, the USDA has now banned the commonly added ingredient triclosan from antibacterial soaps because it has been shown to interrupt the endocrine system, even in very low doses. As always, avoid artificially fragranced products, and it is always a good idea to follow the rule that the products with the fewest and least unpronounceable chemicals listed on the back are preferred. *Safe alternatives include* Mrs. Meyer's Clean Day, GreenShield Organic, Seventh Generation, and The Honest Company.

9. Toss the Tupperware. Pass on the plastic wrap and plastic food storage containers. Instead, purchase glass storage containers in a variety of sizes with covers to match in lieu of aluminum foil and BPA-laden plastics. Find BPA-free, lead-free, PVC-free, and phthalate-free lids as well. You will be excited, because not only will you have less toxic exposure, but your food will last longer in your fridge as well. *Safe alternatives include* glass storage containers with BPA-free lids (we use Pyrex, MightyNest, and Martha Stewart).

10. Toss Teflon and Gore-Tex. Teflon nonstick coating can help make cleanup a cinch, but there is no easy way to clean its toxins out of your system. The repelling action comes from a class of toxins called perfluorinated compounds (PFCs), and they are found not only on your favorite frying pan but also on your raincoats, your boots (think Gore-Tex), and popcorn bags and buckets to keep the grease from seeping through onto your lap in the movie theater. The harmful PFCs in Gore-Tex and Teflon, which can be found in the blood of 98 percent of the population, can remain in your body for five to eight years! High levels of PFCs in the blood have been linked to early onset of menopause. Early menopause can bring about lowered estrogen levels and bone decline. PFCs have also been shown to increase the risk of cancer, ADHD, heart disease, infertility, and obesity. *Safe alternatives include* cookware made of glass, enamel, stainless steel, or "Made in the USA" cast iron. We love Xtrema Ceramic cookware. Look for clothes treated with Nikwax.

Introducing the Seven Sinister S's

Although reducing your toxic load is important, you are not through dealing with life's micronutrient-depleting curveballs yet. We will now shift our focus to the Seven Sinister S's to uncover how stress, sleep, smoking, smog, sunscreen, smartphones, and sweat can cause micro-nutrient depletions and threaten your bone density.

STRESS

From traffic jams to business meetings, stress is hiding everywhere— and our modern world is making it happen. Time seems to be moving faster, and the stress to get everything done seems to be ever-increasing. Stress and anxiety plague 80 percent of Americans. And the problem is a global one: according to WHO, more than 15 percent of the world population has a stress-related disorder. In fact, it is hard to imagine that anyone today isn't affected by stress in some way. Have you ever considered whether stress may be at least partly responsible for your osteoporosis?

Although studies have shown that the cumulative impact of stress has been linked to a host of age-accelerating conditions and degen-erative diseases, including cardiovascular disease, diabetes, and various cancers, there has been little research until recently on the effects that stress might have on fracture rates. In a 2018 study published in the journal *Menopause*, lead scientist Dr. Antonino Catalano determined that women who had the most anxiety and stress in their lives faced a noticeably higher fracture risk, compared with women with the low-est degree of anxiety. Higher anxiety was linked to a 4 percent greater risk for a major fracture over a ten-year period, as well as lower BMD scores in both the lower back area (known as the lumbar spine) and the femoral neck area (just below the ball of the hip joint). In the study, researchers determined that this decline in bone was caused by three distinct factors: micronutrient depletion, hormone disruption, and poor health behaviors.

Let's start with the first link between stress and bone loss: our dear friend micronutrient deficiency. In times of stress, certain metabolic reactions occur, and this causes certain micronutrients to be used up at a faster rate by the body. The water-soluble micronutrients—such as the B vitamins, vitamin C, and all of the minerals—are generally excreted at a faster rate during stress, and because these micronutrients are not stored to any great extent in the body, deficiencies can develop rather quickly. In fact, the B vitamins have come to be known as anti-stress nutrients because they are often the first deficiencies to develop during times of stress.

Although vitamins B1 and B5 help fight off stress by maintaining proper function of the adrenal glands (the most important glands in the fight against stress), vitamins B6 and B9 help equip you to better deal with the stress that you do experience by aiding in the formation of chemicals called neurotransmitters, which are necessary for balancing emotions. According to a study conducted by the Mayo Clinic and published in the *Archives of Internal Medicine* (now *JAMA Internal Medicine*), you don't need a great deficiency in the B vitamins to set in before you really start to feel it. The study revealed that subjects who were given just half the daily requirement of vitamin B1 (thiamine) became "irritable, depressed, quarrelsome, uncooperative, and fearful that some misfortune awaited them."

Similarly, the demand for vitamin C, which assists in the formation of collagen, increases tenfold during stressful periods, which can cause this water-soluble vitamin to become depleted relatively quickly. And much like with the B vitamins, when you deplete vitamin C, you are depleting the same micronutrient that can help eliminate the stress in the first place. Research shows that people with high levels of vitamin C do not show the expected mental and physical signs of stress when subjected to acute psychological challenges. What's more, they bounce back from stressful situations faster than people with low levels of vitamin C in their blood. Finally, stress causes all of the minerals to be used quickly, resulting in rapid depletion. With all of these depletions occurring, you can see that stress can really take its toll on your bone-building micronutrient levels.

The final way that stress reduces micronutrients is by harming your friendly gut bacteria. A reduction in the beneficial organisms in your digestive tract can lead to both digestive upset and malabsorption of the micronutrients taken in through your food.

However, a 2013 study published in *Psychosomatic Medicine* concluded that individuals taking a multivitamin supplement for at least twenty-eight days enjoyed a 65 percent and a 68 percent reduction in stress and anxiety, respectively, so instead of getting stressed, rest assured that your Rebuild Your Bones osteoporosis protocol has you covered.

The second link that researchers identified between osteoporotic fractures and stress was changes in hormone levels. Pregnenolone, a multitasking hormone manufactured in your adrenal glands, is a pre-cursor to both stress hormones and sex hormones, and it will go wher-ever the demand is. When everything is fine and you're feeling relaxed, pregnenolone helps make progesterone and just enough of the stress hormone cortisol. However, when you're stressed, your body snaps up the pregnenolone that it would otherwise use to make the sex hor-mone progesterone, and instead creates substantially more cortisol. That means your progesterone comes up short and can't do its job. Progester-one contributes to bone-forming activity by binding to receptors on the osteoblasts. In the Michigan Bone Health Study, premenopausal women with the lowest bone mass had the highest rates of progesterone defi-ciency. So when stress levels rise, your progesterone falls, which causes decreases in bone mass.

While all that bone loss is occurring, the other side of the hormone story is occurring at the same time. Cortisol, often called the stress hormone, is produced by your adrenal glands during stressful episodes. It is responsible for the fight-or-flight response to stress that allows us to spring into action when we sense danger. As the body experiences stress, it not only diminishes progesterone production but also increases cortisol levels in the bloodstream. Cortisol indirectly acts on your bones by blocking your calcium absorption, which decreases your bone cell growth. The disruption increases bone resorption and can ultimately reduce BMD. Even a short bout of elevated cortisol secretion may cause a decrease in BMD.

Luckily, certain micronutrients can clobber cortisol. According to *Psychology Today*, vitamin C can "abolish the secretion of cortisol." Conversely, according to researchers at the University of Maryland, even slight deficiencies of vitamin C can increase cortisol output. So although stressful situations cause the adrenal glands to release cortisol, which relays the news of stress to all parts of the body and mind, they also release vitamin C, which fervently attempts to squash the physiological and psychological stress you're experiencing. However, if you don't have enough vitamin C in your body, then cortisol sends the message of stress throughout your body. This is another way that stress can further reduce micronutrients, because when too much cortisol is present in the body for an extended period of time, your immune system is weakened. This causes your body to use your immune-boosting micronutrients, including your antioxidants, at a more feverish pace.

Your ever-important omega-3s will also come to your aid in times of stress. Recent research shows that omega-3 fatty acids can play a key role in keeping stress at bay. DHA, part of the omega-3 family, has been shown to affect aggressive behavior in young adults. Researchers proved that DHA prevented the study's forty-one participants from becoming more frustrated, even when put under mental stress. Scientists believe that omega-3 supplementation "inhibits the adrenal activation elicited by a mental stress," leaving cortisol levels "significantly blunted" when omega-3 levels are high. In fact, omega-3 supplementation can reduce the body's stress-induced production of cortisol by 22 percent. Studies have also shown that omega-3 can cause fat loss and increased muscle mass.

This is great news—by adding the omega-3 fatty acids EPA and DHA into either your diet or your supplementation regimen, you can quiet cortisol, reduce stress, and eliminate much of the micronutrient depletion that stress may have cost you (all while perhaps losing a few pounds of fat and adding a few pounds of body-stabilizing muscle while you are at it!).

Finally, let's discuss the third link between stress and bone fracture rates, something the researchers called "poor health behaviors." The study determined that just as stress caused micronutrient depletion and hormonal changes, it also caused unhealthy habits, like making poor dietary choices for sweet and salty treats. The researchers determined that high stress levels brought on "stress eating" of micronutrient-poor foods. These foods delivered fewer nutrients, which caused weaker bones and, in the end, a greater number of fractures.

However, although stressed individuals may think they are eating to stifle their emotions or anxiety, it is stress and anxiety themselves that may be physically responsible for the snacking. Remember in our earlier discussion of the Crave Cycle when we identified how magnesium and calcium deficiencies can cause cravings for both sweet and salty foods? Well, stress causes both of these water-soluble minerals to be used quickly, resulting in rapid depletion. It is because of these mineral deficiencies that you begin stress eating. So if you are a stress eater, know that you're not mentally weak, just mineral deficient. Make sure to supplement smart, and the stress, the cravings, and the bone loss will all be things of the past.

Stop Stressing . . . Here Are a Few Tips!

Let's be honest: your life isn't going to magically become less stressful. However, it is still really important for you to de-stress, so you need to find a stress-reduction technique that works for you. We've listed five top techniques here—choose one or more that match both your personality and your situation. It's worth taking this special time to center and de-stress yourself, and your bones will thank you for it!

1. Meditate with a mantra. A mantra is a word or phrase repeated to aid in your concentration while meditating. Choose a mantra for yourself that expresses what you desire from life. Perhaps try "I welcome healing, happiness, and balance to my life." Reciting your mantra in rhythm with your breathing can help calm you in times of stress. This is a great technique when you are in your office, as well as both in the morning to center you and in the evening to prepare you for a night of bone-building sleep.

2. Perform a "full body scan." This is our personal choice to perform before bed. Begin with the tips of your toes and move up your body to the crown of your head. Pay attention to any pains, aches, and stress being held throughout your body. You'll quite literally release tension one muscle at a time. This is great tool for self-awareness and de-stressing.

3. Dance away your stress. You simply can't be anxious when you are listening to one of our favorite tunes, right? This technique may not be suitable when panic rears its head in public, but letting loose and grooving to the music allows you to turn off your tension—with the added bonus of boosting your metabolism.

4. Focus on your breathing. Listen to your body breathing. After all, breathing is your body's natural relaxation response. Take time to focus on deep breaths in and out; this will elicit a physical state of deep rest that decreases heart rate, blood pressure, respiratory rate, and muscle tension. Practice focused breathing when you are in public and faced with frightening or stressful circumstances.

5. Get moving! When you exercise, you de-stress your body while helping it achieve the strength, weight regulation, and bone health you deserve. Exercise reduces levels of the body's stress hormones, such as adrenaline and cortisol. It also stimulates the production of endorphins, chemicals in the brain that act as natural painkillers and mood elevators.

These are just a few of our favorites. Luckily, today, there are tons of ways to de-stress, including listening to relaxation tapes, adult stress-relieving coloring books, yoga, gardening, knitting, or just simply spending time with friends. We don't care what you choose—we just want you to choose to de-stress daily!

SLEEP

The next nutrient thief that you need to be aware of is lack of sleep. Studies have shown that sleep deprivation causes deregulation of two hormones, leptin and ghrelin. As both low leptin (the hormone that tells you that you are full) and high ghrelin (the hormone that tells you that you are hungry) stimulate hunger and appetite, individuals who didn't sleep reported higher overall hunger ratings, especially cravings for energy-dense, micronutrient-poor processed foods like sweets, baked goods, and bread. Thus, scientists speculate that sleep deprivation causes deregulation of appetite hormones, which then ultimately leads to micronutrient deficiencies. So obviously the advice to sleep a good eight to nine hours a night makes sense if our goal is micronutrient sufficiency. But following this advice is even more important when we look at other ways that sleep influences bone growth.

In 2017, Christine Swanson, MD, an assistant professor at the University of Colorado, spoke at the Endocrine Society's ninety-ninth annual meeting in Orlando, Florida, urging that insufficient sleep might also be an unrecognized risk factor for bone loss.

Not getting enough sleep at night can definitely affect your bone health. During sleep, your body works to repair itself and cortisol levels decrease. Remember that cortisol, the stress hormone, can be detrimental to bone health by blocking your calcium absorption and increasing your bone resorption, which can ultimately reduce your BMD. Lowered levels of cortisol during sleep are beneficial—studies have shown that sleep restriction reduced levels of a marker of bone formation, whereas a biological marker of bone resorption, or breakdown, was unchanged, indicating that old bone was breaking down without new bone being formed. Decreased sleep duration has also been closely associated with lower BMD, especially in middle-aged and elderly women. The study concluded, "These findings may lead to the development of better preventive approaches to osteoporosis in women." Other recent studies have shown that patients with sleep apnea or insomnia have a much higher risk of osteoporosis, at 270 percent and 52 percent, respectively.

SMOKING

Hey, there are some habits that are simply bad for you—no sugarcoating this one. Smoking cigarettes has no benefits to your health. And although you have probably heard that smoking causes osteoporosis, cancer, and accelerated aging, and wrecks your teeth and skin, you might never have considered the micronutrient-depleting aspects of cigarette smoke. Cigarette smoke causes a rapid depletion of vitamins A, C, and E. Smoke itself is an oxidant that creates free radicals, and your antioxidants play a protective role, trying to repair the damage that this oxidant (smoke) is causing. Smoking reduces the amount of calcium your bones can absorb—we know that vitamin D helps bones absorb calcium, and smoking interferes with how your body uses vitamin D. Less calcium is then available to build strong bones. As a result, your bones start to get brittle. Again, and we hope you see a pattern here: the micronutrients that may be able to repair the damage from smoking are the same ones you are using and depleting with every puff. If you live with a smoker or work in a smoke-filled environment, you need to know that the secondhand smoke you are being forced to inhale is having a detrimental effect on your health. Research out of Johns Hopkins revealed that exposure to passive smoking (secondhand smoke) may also result in decreased concentrations of selected micronutrients, primarily antioxidants.

Now that we recognize the micronutrient-depleting effects of smoking, let's look at how it directly affects bone health as well. As we stated earlier, cigarette smoke generates huge amounts of free radicals—molecules that attack and overwhelm the body's natural defenses. The result is a chain reaction of damage throughout the body—including cells, organs, and hormones involved in keeping bones healthy.

The nicotine and toxins in cigarettes affect bone health from many angles. The toxins upset the balance of hormones (like estrogen) that bones need to stay strong. Smoking also triggers other bone-damaging changes, such as increased cortisol levels, which leads to bone breakdown. Research also suggests that smoking impedes the hormone calcitonin, which helps build bones. Furthermore, nicotine and free radicals kill the osteoblasts—the bone-making cells. When you consider all of smoking's deleterious effects on bone, it proves that it's time to put down your pack!

SMOG

Exposure to poor air quality is another daily habit that can negatively affect those living in large cities. According to WHO, at least twenty thousand premature deaths occur every year in the United States because of air pollution. Globally, this number may exceed five hundred thousand per year. The polluted air you inhale—which can be caused by high ozone levels, smog, and car exhaust—is also acting as an oxidant. Luckily, the surface of the lungs is covered with a thin layer of fluid containing a range of antioxidants that appear to provide the first line of defense against oxidant pollutants. Studies show that supplementation of antioxidants, as well as vitamins B6, B9, and B12, also helps prevent damage from air pollution, and the EPA suggests antioxidant supplementation for those living in large, polluted cities.

Beyond the effect that smog has on your micronutrient levels, smog also has a direct effect on your bones by reducing levels of the parathyroid hormone, a key hormone that strengthens bones by boosting calcium levels. A recent study in *The Lancet Planetary Health* determined that exposure to higher levels of PM2.5 (fine particles that can come from power plants, motor vehicles, airplanes, and agricultural burning), and black carbon (which is a component of air pollution from automotive emissions) caused lower levels of parathyroid hormone. U.S. researchers have found that even a small increase in the concentration of tiny particulates contained in vehicle exhaust and other smoke can reduce a bone's density, making it more likely to break.

Obviously, if smog is a factor in your life then we aren't going to suggest that you move to a new city while you are rebuilding your bone. However, because your environment is not going to change, you need to recognize the inevitable micronutrient depletion and bone-hindering effects that your habitat invokes. You might want to consider purchasing a high-efficiency particulate air (HEPA) filter for your urban home, which can capture ultrafine particles, or check the air quality forecast in your area on days when you know you'll be spending a lot of time outside.

SUNSCREEN

As we mentioned in Chapter 1, you have likely been conditioned to believe that it's essential to use gobs of sunscreen to keep you from burning up in the sun and developing skin cancer. We've all heard the risks of getting too much sun. An estimated 9,320 people will die of melanoma in 2018, according to the Skin Cancer Foundation, with every year bringing in more new cases of skin cancer than the combined diagnoses of cancers of the breast, prostate, lung, and colon. Obviously, there's definite cause for concern when it comes to stepping out into the sun, which is why our first instinct is to hide away in the shade and cover ourselves from head to toe in sunscreen. But in doing so, we actually rob ourselves of vitamin D, an essential micronutrient that we just cannot afford to lose. If deficient, we could actually give osteoporosis the upper hand if we decide to become vampires and stay out of the sun completely.

Vitamin D reduces the risk of osteoporosis, cancer, Alzheimer's disease, diabetes, and multiple sclerosis; supports our immune system; acts as an anti-inflammatory; and has been scientifically linked to maintaining a healthy body weight. After getting direct exposure to sunlight, your body will naturally generate ample amounts of bioavailable Vitamin D (calciferol). Pretty cool, right? Yet according to the USDA, only 7 percent of the entire U.S. population over age two has an adequate intake of Vitamin D.

The people who are most at risk for developing a Vitamin D deficiency include those who live at latitudes north of Atlanta (approximately 33 degrees north), people with dark skin, the elderly (who produce Vitamin D less efficiently than they did when they were younger), those who spend too much time indoors, those who are overweight or obese, and anyone who continuously uses sunscreen.

Did you get that last part? *Anyone who continuously uses sunscreen.* And the scariest part is the effects that start to unfold in the wake of this micronutrient deficiency. Remember, vitamin D is essential in the complex interplay between magnesium, calcium, and your bones. So if bone growth is your goal, then depleting your body of vitamin D from the sunshine by wearing a huge brimmed hat and chemically laden sunscreen should be avoided.

Burning isn't the answer either. So be smart about your time in the sun and follow these three rules. First, load up on these superheroes—your antioxidants! According to Dr. Elizabeth Plourde, Clinical Laboratory Scientist (CLS) and specialist in the research of cancer and DNA, when it comes to protecting ourselves from the sunlight-induced free radical exposure, "antioxidants are the exact answer. [They] act exactly the same as the sunscreens . . . antioxidants have been proven to be protective . . . to act just like a sunscreen. And there's many of them, there really are. Our skin is so well-designed that when the solar rays hit it, the antioxidants that are in the body actually move up and form a protective shield and act just like sunscreen."

Second, allow your skin to be exposed to the sun (vitamin D time!), but stop or apply sunscreen before burning. Depending on your skin tone and how quickly you burn, this could mean starting with as little as five to ten minutes in the sun before applying sunscreen, or for those with darker skin or who don't burn quickly, thirty minutes to one hour. Finally, choose a safe, healthy mineral sunscreen such as zinc oxide or titanium dioxide so you don't add to your toxic load. (You can learn more about these on our website!) Now get outside, get some sunshine, and boost those bones!

SMARTPHONES

Can you remember back when there was a phone booth on the corner in case you had to make a call? Times were tough. If your car broke down, you were in trouble. Luckily, the invention of the cell phone has made our lives a bit easier. You can order food on the go, check in on loved ones, and work from anyplace you might find yourself. However, although all of this progress has made things better, where your bones are concerned, it has also made things worse.

Whether you love them or hate them, cell phones emit potentially harmful electromagnetic fields (EMFs), which are areas of energy that surround electronic devices. According to WHO, EMFs affect us because our bodies have their own electric and biochemical responses (e.g., nervous system, digestion, brain function, heart function). So exposure to EMFs can interact with your body in adverse ways. Possible side effects include disrupted sleep patterns and changes in DNA. These days, most people cannot function without their cell phone, so understanding how cell phones affect our micronutrient levels and our bones is essential.

Martin Pall, PhD, professor emeritus at Washington State University, has identified and published several papers describing the molecular mechanisms of how EMFs from cell phones and wireless technologies damage humans, animals, and plants. Many studies indicate that your intracellular calcium (calcium in the cells) increases with exposure to EMFs. The problem here is that when intracellular calcium is elevated, so are your levels of free radicals—molecules that attack and overwhelm the body's natural defenses. Remember, the more free radicals there are, the more cellular damage is done. So antioxidants—like vitamins A, C, and E; alpha-lipoic acid; and selenium—are extremely important because they are fabulous free-radical scavengers and can help reduce this cellular damage. But keep in mind that these antioxidants will be depleted more quickly because they are used in the fight against your cell phone rather than for bone-building tasks. Also, being sufficient in magnesium has been shown to be extremely important in counteracting EMFs. This is because studies have revealed that high magnesium levels can block the elevated intracellular calcium, thus reducing the EMF-induced creation of free radicals.

Here again, there is a lot of evidence, beyond micronutrient depletion, that EMFs also directly affect bone mass. Several studies have shown that keeping your smartphone in your pocket on one side may modestly accelerate hip and pelvic bone loss on that side. We aren't going to ask you to give up your smartphone, don't worry—we aren't about to give up ours either. We will, however, make the point that sufficiency in antioxidants and magnesium will help you curtail any side effects caused by your cell phone. Try to keep your phone out of your pockets and in a purse or drawer across the room whenever possible.

SWEAT

The faster and harder you work out, the more micronutrients you lose through sweat (yes, electrolytes are micronutrients too!). And the amount of micronutrients you lose directly correlates with the intensity and the duration of the activity you perform. Studies show that because these micronutrients play key roles in energy metabolism, their utilization rate may be increased by up to 20 to 100 times the resting rate during intense physical activity.

Iron is a great example of this "intensity equals loss" principle. Strenuous exercise stimulates an increase in red blood cell and blood vessel production, which creates an increased demand for iron. Individuals who work out less than four hours a week don't need to be concerned with this depletion; however, those exerting themselves for over six hours a week need to be cautious of iron-deficiency anemia. Calcium, another essential mineral/electrolyte, is also at risk for exercise-induced depletion. This should be of particular interest to the cardio kings and queens out there, who, like Mira back when she lived in New York City, love to spend hours sweating in the gym or dance studio. As an individual perspires, calcium is released, but the body leaches calcium from the bone to replace it. This means that as you increase intensity, you could be causing your own bones to weaken because of the large amounts of calcium that escape via your sweat. The great news is that findings presented at the 2013 meeting of the Endocrine Society found that fitness enthusiasts may be able to offset some of this bone loss by simply supplementing with calcium. We know that calcium is of critical concern for those suffering from osteoporosis, so here's a tip for you. Always take your calcium supplements before your workout. (For those taking Nutreince, our patented multivitamin, calcium is in the a.m. dose, so you are all set as long as you drink it before beginning your morning workout.) Research has shown that those who take calcium supplements thirty minutes before a workout can offset some of the bone leaching caused by exercise.

However, iron and calcium aren't the only minerals affected—zinc and magnesium can also be depleted through strenuous exercise. USDA research shows that marginal magnesium deficiency can both impair exercise performance and amplify the oxidative stress that exercise can cause. When you perform aerobic activities such as cardio, your body undergoes oxidative cell damage, and this causes the formation of free radicals. The more free radicals there are, the more cellular damage is done. So antioxidants—like vitamins A, C, and E; alpha-lipoic acid; and selenium—are extremely important for individuals who choose to sweat at the gym because they are fabulous free-radical scavengers and can help reduce this cellular damage. Reduced oxidative stress not only results in a lower likelihood of bone loss but also shortens recovery time and improves athletic performance.

OSTEOGENIC LOADING IS ESSENTIAL FOR BUILDING BONE

Don't be misled. Although exercise is an EMD, draining you of a wide variety of essential vitamins and minerals, we are in no way saying that it should be avoided. In fact, the opposite is true—we are huge advocates of exercise. We are not giving you permission to be a couch potato in the name of micronutrient sufficiency! As we said earlier, some EMDs—coffee and alcohol, for example—have been shown to have some really healthy side effects. Where bone building is concerned, exercise is absolutely essential. In fact, individuals who don't exercise, or don't do the correct form of exercise, will have a much harder time improving their bones. Although you might feel like bed rest is the safest thing for your diminished bone density, the exact opposite is true. In fact, after only one week of complete bed rest, your muscle strength can decrease as much as 20 to 30 percent, and bone loss can be seen in as little as 3 weeks. This is why astronauts, who can't perform weight-bearing activities while floating in space, lose (on average) 1 to 2 percent of bone mass each month of their mission. Prolonged bed rest (or space travel) causes the bones to "unload," which results in lost bone density.

Do you remember in Chapter 4 when we told you that calcium supplementation didn't build bone without adequate protein intake? Well, even with adequate calcium and protein intakes, your body can't build bone without weight-bearing activity. Exercises such as running, jumping, and weight lifting put stress on the bones, and this stress stimulates bone building. The weight that you put on your bones compresses the bone matrix, telling the matrix to gather more essential minerals in order to increase bone density. The amount of weight or "load" that is required for bone building is called *osteogenic load*, and inducing osteogenic load has been shown to be an extremely effective tool against osteoporosis. A 2015 study published in the *Journal of Osteoporosis and Physical Activity* found that when women with osteoporosis or low BMD did osteogenic loading for only twenty-four weeks, they were able to increase BMD by nearly 15 percent in the hip and nearly 17 percent in the spine. It is so effective that in the spring of 2015, the World Congress on Osteoporosis announced its official recommendation of osteogenic loading as a viable, drug-free method of treating osteoporosis.

Scientists in the UK have determined that the amount of loading required to stimulate the bone-building process equals 4.2 times body weight. So a 120-pound person would need to load 504 pounds to build bone. Simply standing is loading because of our helpful friend gravity. You can nearly double this load by walking briskly, and triple it by jogging or running, but you can only reach the 4.2 times body weight necessary for osteogenic load through higher-impact activities like jumping or through specific strength training.

So should you start jumping rope right away? Maybe not—it all depends on what's safe for your stage of osteoporosis and your fitness level.

The great news is that there is some form of exercise for any situation. Those at high fracture risk may want to start with brisk walking, but as your fitness level increases, there are a lot of ways to reach the higher levels of osteogenic load. Climbing stairs, dancing, hiking, jogging, jumping rope, tennis, and even pushing your lawn mower are all great exercises to consider. Although yoga and Pilates may help with your balance, they do not create an osteogenic load and cannot help build bone. Additionally, some of their movements may actually put you at a higher risk of fracture.

Hitting the traditional weight room can also be a little tricky. Remember, you need 4.2 times your body weight to stimulate bone growth. For that 120-pound person, that would mean lifting 504 pounds. This is not recommended—especially with osteoporosis. Although you will likely not hit optimal osteogenic load using free weights in a gym, we do recommend that you still lift weights. Working with a trainer to learn safe weight-lifting strategies is important for muscle building, and your muscles will keep you strong and steady on your feet as you age. Getting in the habit of a weight-bearing routine is essential as you age. But for optimal osteogenic loading in the gym, you will need to work on equipment that is specially designed to help you achieve load safely. Look for OsteoStrong facilities in your area. You only need to visit once a week, and the benefits are big, strong, beautiful bones. We are thrilled to partner with OsteoStrong. Visit us at RebuildYourBones.com to claim your free gift!

Commercials Call for Osteogenic Loading!

One of Mira's favorite ways to get in extra osteogenic loading is hopping. During TV commercials, simply stand up and hop on one foot five times, then on the other foot five times (if you can do this safely). Continue doing this through the commercials on your favorite TV show or news program. Feel free to hold on to the back of a chair or sofa till you get the hang of it. You don't have to hit the gym to rebuild your bones! Come to RebuildYourBones.com to learn more about osteogenic loading at home.

Medications: Prescriptions and OTC Drugs

The Centers for Disease Control and Prevention (CDC) reports that one out of every five children and nine out of ten older Americans have used at least one prescription drug in the past month. Although many of these prescriptions can be lifesaving, their use in this country has increased steadily over the past decade, and what's more, overdoses involving prescription drugs are at new, epidemic levels, now killing more Americans than heroin and cocaine combined. Prescription drug use is soaring worldwide—the average person in the UK takes eighteen prescriptions a year, and approximately two-thirds of Australians over age sixty are reported to take four or more drugs. Although many of these prescription drugs may make you feel better, they likely will not fix the underlying problem. In fact, on a micronutrient level, they may be making matters quite a bit worse—they may be greatly affecting your bone loss.

Although most Americans take prescription meds, the number who pop over-the-counter (OTC) drugs is much higher. These nonprescription medications—such as aspirin, acetaminophen, nonsteroidal anti-inflammatory drugs (NSAIDs), antacids, laxatives, and H2 blockers (found in heartburn medications)—may seem harmless, but they also work to deplete your vital micronutrients, threatening bone loss with every single dose.

Although we don't have time to review all of the numerous drugs that initiate bone loss through promoting micronutrient deficiencies, we will focus on three of the worst culprits: corticosteroids, antidepressants, and antacids. Later in this chapter, you will have an opportunity to review hundreds of prescription medications and over-the-counter drugs to identify which micronutrients your personal prescriptions may be depleting.

CORTICOSTEROIDS

The first class of drugs we will discuss is called corticosteroids. They are often prescribed to treat allergies, asthma, severe inflammation, and autoimmune diseases. You have likely heard of these drugs (or taken these prescriptions) under the names cortisone or hydrocortisone, or the nasal spray Flonase. Although taking this prescription may have relieved your asthma symptoms or inflammation, you may not know that it also robbed your bones of essential micronutrients including vitamins A, B6, B9, B12, C, D, and K, as well as calcium, magnesium, phosphorus, potassium, selenium, zinc, and amino acids.

Making matters worse is that corticosteroids also have a direct, twofold negative effect on your bones. They interfere with bone formation while simultaneously stimulating bone resorption, thus accelerating bone loss significantly. It shouldn't surprise you to learn that studies have shown that within the first year of corticosteroid use, BMD drops 6 to 12 percent and approximately 3 percent the following year. Even more startling is that the risk of fracture escalates by as much as 75 percent within the first three months. On a brighter note, there is also a remarkable decrease in the risk of fracture within the first three months after the medication is discontinued.

ANTIDEPRESSANTS

As if being diagnosed with osteoporosis isn't depressing enough, you may become even more depressed when you hear what your antidepressant prescriptions are doing to your bones. We will examine two classes of antidepressants: tricyclic antidepressants (TCAs) and selective serotonin reuptake inhibitors (SSRIs).

These days, TCAs are less frequently prescribed for managing depression than in the past, but their use has been linked to deficiencies in vitamin B2 and CoQ10. More popular today are the SSRIs, such as Prozac and Paxil, that bring about many more micronutrient depletions including vitamins B6, B9, B12, C, and D, as well as omega-3, CoQ10, and amino acids. Remember that B6, B9, and B12 work in unison to reduce homocysteine levels, which reduces bone loss, whereas a deficiency of omega-3, which you just learned all about in Chapter 4, also puts your bones at risk. These prescription-drug-induced micronutrient deficiencies cannot be ignored.

Here again, these antidepressants also directly attack your bone health as well. All of these drugs do two things that threaten your bone. First, they inhibit dopamine production, and second, they cause chronic elevation of the hormone prolactin. Let's examine that first part. Dopamine is a "feel-good" signaling molecule that acts as a messenger and produces feelings of relaxation and calm in the body. And when you're feeling calm, you don't feel stress. This is because less of the hormone cortisol is released from the adrenal glands. Remember, less cortisol means less calcium extracted from the bones, which results in less bone loss. So in order to maintain bone, we don't want to take a medication that inhibits a cortisol blocker. Second, antidepressants elevate the hormone prolactin because dopamine is responsible for regulating the prolactin production in the pituitary gland. Lower levels of dopamine in the body cause increased production of prolactin, which in turn can lead to reduced estrogen production, further compromising bone health.

Researchers have proven, time and time again, that these drugs (as well as different classes of antidepressants) can affect your bone loss. Studies have shown that SSRIs increased risk for osteoporosis by as much as 46 percent and osteoporotic fractures by 45 percent. Two other antidepressants, atypical antipsychotics and benzodiazepines, increased risk of osteoporosis by as much as 55 percent and 17 percent, respectively, and those taking benzodiazepines increased risk of fracture by 10 percent. Those using TCAs lost more than three times as much bone as women not taking antidepressants. SSRIs also increased the rate of bone loss, and the higher the dose, the more significant amount of bone was lost. If you are currently taking an antidepressant, talk to your doctor about how to choose one that might have a less antagonizing effect on dopamine receptors in the brain.

ANTACIDS: PROTON PUMP INHIBITORS AND H2S

Let's examine how a simple case of heartburn may cause depletions leading to osteoporosis. Two classes of medications are commonly used to treat heartburn: prescription drugs called proton pump inhibitors (PPIs), which include Nexium and Prevacid, and OTC drugs called H2 blockers, which include Axid, Pepcid, Tagamet, and Zantac. Both types work by reducing the production of hydrochloric acid in the stomach and thus likely weakening micronutrient absorption. Research indicates that these medications can deplete vitamins A, B1, B9, B12, C, and D, as well as calcium, copper, iron, magnesium, phosphorus, potassium, and zinc. PPIs are the most potent of the acid blockers; just one PPI pill can reduce stomach acid secretion by 90 to 95 percent for twenty-four hours. Many studies evaluating PPI use for more than one year have consistently demonstrated an increased risk of hip fracture (20 to 62 percent) and an increased risk of vertebral fracture (40 to 60 percent). Short-term PPI use is not associated with an increased fracture risk, whereas long-term use for more than one year increases the risk by approximately 44 percent, and with more than seven years of exposure, the odds increase by approximately 355 percent. Thus, fracture risk is greatly dependent on the duration of therapy. But the great news is that fracture risk is lowered when an individual stops taking these antacids and allows their body to absorb essential micronutrients.

So if you can't take antacids, what should you do to treat acid reflux or gastroesophageal reflux disease (GERD)? Simply take digestive enzymes (more on how to choose them in Chapter 7) before meals until the situation is under control. Heartburn is almost always a case of too little acid for proper digestion, not too much. Antacids not only deplete you of your essential micronutrients, but they also don't address the real problem at all.

Accounting for Your Actions

It is now time to review your lifestyle habits to discover how they may be contributing to your current state of micronutrient deficiency. To reiterate, we don't want you to just up and quit all of your micronutrient-depleting habits; some habits, like exercising, are encouraged. Other lifestyle EMDs, like living in a big city, you will not likely be able to change. This exercise is simply to help you realize which micronutrients you are unknowingly putting at risk so you can fully understand the need for more quality, micronutrient-dense foods, along with proper supplementation to fill in these gaps. Take your time and be as accurate as you can. Once you complete the charts, you will be able to quickly identify which micronutrients your current lifestyle is putting at serious risk of deficiency.

Step 1: To see just how many lifestyle habits may be affecting your micronutrient sufficiency levels, place a check (✓) in the Tabulations column of Table 5.2 for every day of the week that you might take part in one of these lifestyle EMDs. If, for example, you determine that you exercise three days a week, then you should give yourself three checks. Make sure to follow the directions at the top of the category. You need to tabulate your usage of each EMD in the chart.

Step 2: Fill in Table 5.3. This is your current Everyday Micronutrient Depleters Lifestyle Habits Chart. Using the checks you entered in Table 5.2, calculate how many times each micronutrient might be affected. For example, if you had three checks next to exercise, then you will need to put three points next to each vitamin and mineral that exercise depletes. This means that you will write the number 3 next to vitamins A, B2, C, and E; iron; magnesium; manganese; potassium; selenium; zinc; alpha–lipoic acid; and CoQ10. Mark down your total for each EMD in every micronutrient it depletes. You will hit some micronutrients more than once. When you do this, simply mark the second number to the right of the first. For example, you could end up with something like this:

Calcium: 11 6 27 5 3

Step 3: Total the numbers listed for each micronutrient.

For example: Calcium: 11 + 6 + 27 + 5 + 3 = 52

Step 4: It's time to analyze your data. Are you a bit surprised at how micronutrient-depleting your lifestyle actually is? Even your healthy habits, such as exercise, may unknowingly be putting you at risk of depletions that could lead to further health issues later on. Our goal is to make you aware of your deficiency so that you can hold yourself accountable for your actions and incorporate healing habits in your life that will lead to micronutrient sufficiency, improved bone density, and, ultimately, optimal health. The most important thing is that between your diet analysis (completed at the end of Chapter 3) and your dietary doctrine and lifestyle analysis (both completed in this chapter as they both relate to lifestyle), you are now aware of the micronutrients you will want to focus on becoming sufficient in during your Rebuild Your Bones twelve-week osteoporosis protocol.

You have just been introduced to thirteen more healing habits that you will be able to incorporate into your new Rebuild Your Bones lifestyle. By honestly evaluating your personal dietary philosophy and making the necessary changes to your lifestyle habits, you will be well on your way to improving your bone health We have now covered two of our three steps to better bone health. In Chapter 6, we examine smart supplementation, the third and final step of our plan. Although supplementation is likely something you are already doing to improve your bone density, the information you are about to learn is some of the most cutting-edge in the field of supplemental science and could save you years in your fight against osteoporosis. We'll teach you how to supplement to avoid competing nutrients, as well as which supplements we consider essential to build bone. So turn the page and let's get started!

Healing Habits Revealed in Chapter 5

21. Pitch the plastics.
22. Mind the heavy metals.
23. Toss toxic household products.
24. Stave off stress with de-stressing exercises.
25. Sleep eight to nine hours a day.
26. Stop smoking or exposing yourself to secondhand smoke.
27. Combat the negative effects of smog.
28. Use sunscreen sparingly.
29. Be smart about your smartphone.
30. Minimize micronutrient loss due to excessive cardio and sweating.
31. Perform a weight-bearing, osteogenic-loading exercise routine.
32. Minimize your prescription medications (if possible).
33. Reduce the use of OTC medications.

Life sure can leave you depleted! But don't worry, because it's time for your next "On the Couch" chat, where we will give you some easy ways to accomplish osteogenic loading and share some of our favorite tips to reduce toxins and heavy metals in your home. There is so much information we want to share in this next video coaching session. Join us now at RebuildYourBones.com.

TABLE 5.2 Everyday Micronutrient Depleters Due to Lifestyle Habits

Lifestyle Habit	Micronutrients Depleted	Tabulations (place one ✓ for each day in a week you come into contact with any of these EMDs)
Lead (see suspected sources on page 121)	B1, B6, C, E, calcium, iron, phosphorus, selenium, zinc, alpha-lipoic acid	
Mercury (see suspected sources on page 122)	C, E, selenium	
Arsenic (see suspected sources on page 122)	A, E, phosphorus, selenium	
Aluminum (see suspected sources on page 122)	C, calcium, magnesium, zinc	
Stress	A, B1, B2, B3, B5, B6, B7, B9, B12, choline, C, D, E, calcium, chromium, copper, iodine, iron, magnesium, potassium, selenium, zinc, omega-3, amino acids	
Lack of sleep	A, D, E, K, calcium, iodine, magnesium, potassium, zinc, omega-3	

Lifestyle Habit	Micronutrients Depleted	Tabulations (place one ✓ for each day in a week you come into contact with any of these EMDs)
Smog	A, C, D, E, copper, manganese, selenium, zinc, alpha-lipoic acid	
Smoking	A, B1, B6, B9, C, E, selenium, zinc, alpha-lipoic acid	
Sunscreen	D, calcium	
Smartphones (EMF)	A, C, E, magnesium, selenium, alpha-lipoic acid	
Sweat (exercise)	A, B2, C, E, iron, magnesium, manganese, potassium, selenium, zinc, alpha-lipoic acid, CoQ10	

Toxins	Micronutrients Depleted	Tabulations (place one ✓ for each day you come into contact with any of these household toxins)
BPA and phthalate	Calcium	
Household toxins (refer to "Our Top Ten Tricks to Reduce Household Toxins" on page 124)	A, C, E, selenium, zinc, alpha-lipoic acid	

OTC Drugs	Micronutrients	Tabulations (place one ✓ for each time taken in a week)
NSAIDs: ibuprofen (Advil, Motrin), naproxen (Aleve, Midol)	B9, C, iron, zinc	
Aspirin: Bufferin, St. Joseph, Bayer, Excedrin	B9, C, K, iron, potassium, zinc	
Acetaminophen: Tylenol	B9, C, iron, potassium, CoQ10	

OTC Drugs	Micronutrients	Tabulations (place one ✓ for each time taken in a week)
Antacids: Gaviscon, Gelusil, Maalox, Mylanta	B1, B9, D, calcium, chromium, copper, iron, magnesium, manganese, phosphorus, zinc	
Laxatives: Carter's Little Pills, Correctol, Dulcolax, Feen-a-mint	A, B12, E, calcium, potassium	
H2 inhibitors/ blockers: Axid, Pepcid, Mylanta, Tagamet, Zantac	B1, B9, B12, D, calcium, copper, iron, magnesium, phosphorus, potassium, zinc	
Alli diet aid (orlistat)	A, D, E, K, omega-3, omega-6	

Prescription Medications	Indications for Usage	Micronutrients Depleted	Tabulations (place one ✓ for each time taken in a week)
Opiates: hydrocodone/ acetaminophen (Vicodin)	Pain relief	B9, C, iron, potassium	
Statins: atorvastatin (Lipitor), ezetimibe (Zetia), fluvastatin (Lescol), lovastatin (Mevacor), pravastatin (Pravachol), rosuvastatin (Crestor), simvastatin (Zocor)	Lowering cholesterol	A, B9, B12, D, E, K, calcium, iron, magnesium, phosphorus, CoQ10	
Bile acid sequestrants: (Questran, Colestid)	Lowering cholesterol	A, B9, B12, D, E, K, iron, phosphorus	

Prescription Medications	Indications for Usage	Micronutrients Depleted	Tabulations (place one ✓ for each time taken in a week)
ACE inhibitors: lisinopril (Prinivil, Zestril), ramipril (Altace), quinapril (Accupril), enalapril (Vasotec)	High blood pressure	Phosphorus, zinc	
Thiazide diuretics: hydrochlorothiazide (Esidrix, Hydrodiuril, Oretic)	High blood pressure	D, calcium, magnesium, phosphorus, potassium, zinc, CoQ10	
Beta blockers: atenolol (Tenormin, Senorman), carvedilol (Coreg), nadolol (Corgard), metoprolol (Lopressor, Toprol XL)	High blood pressure; congestive heart failure	B1, chromium, CoQ10	
Calcium channel blockers: amlodipine (Norvasc), felodipine (Plendil), nifedipine (Procardia, Adalat), nimodipine (Nimotop), nisoldipine (Sular)	High blood pressure	D	
Vasodilators: hydralazine (Apresoline)	High blood pressure	B6, magnesium, CoQ10	
Antihypertensives: methyldopa (Aldomet)	High blood pressure	B12	

Prescription Medications	Indications for Usage	Micronutrients Depleted	Tabulations (place one ✓ for each time taken in a week)
Loop diuretics: bumetanide (Bumex, Burinex), ethacrynic acid (Edecrin), furosemide (Lasix), torsemide (Demadex)	High blood pressure; heart failure	B1, B6, B9, C, calcium, chromium, iron, magnesium, phosphorus, potassium, zinc	
Potassium-sparing diuretics: amiloride (Midamor), spironolactone (Aldactone), triamterene (Maxzide, Dyazide, Dyrenium)	High blood pressure; heart failure	B9, calcium, magnesium, phosphorus, potassium, zinc	
Cardiac glycosides: digoxin (Lanoxicaps, Lanoxin)	Heart failure; arrhythmias	B1, calcium, magnesium, phosphorus, potassium	
Anticoagulants: warfarin (Coumadin)	Blood clots	K, iron	
Bisphosphonates: alendronate (Fosamax), risedronate (Actonel), ibandronate (Boniva), tiludronate (Skelid)	Osteoporosis	C, E, calcium, magnesium, phosphorus, CoQ10	
RANK ligand inhibitors: Denosumab (Prolia, Xgeva), teriparatide (Forteo)	Osteoporosis	Magnesium	

Prescription Medications	Indications for Usage	Micronutrients Depleted	Tabulations (place one ✓ for each time taken in a week)
Proton-pump inhibitors: lansoprazole (Prevacid), omeprazole (Losec, Prilosec), rabeprazole (Aciphex), pantoprazole (Pantoloc, Protonix), Nexium	Gastroesophageal reflux disease (GERD); severe gastric ulceration	A, B1, B9, B12, C, calcium, iron, magnesium, zinc	
Methylxanthines: theophylline (Accubron, Theobid, Elixicon)	Asthma; chronic obstructive pulmonary disease (COPD)	B6	
Beta-2 adrenergic receptor agonists: albuterol (Salbutamol, Proventil, Ventolin), bitolterol (Tornalate), fluticasone/salmeterol (Advair), isoetharine (Bronkosol, Bronkometer), levalbuterol (Xopenex), metaproterenol (Alupent), pirbuterol (Maxair), salmeterol (Serevent), terbutaline (Brethine)	Asthma; COPD	Calcium, magnesium, phosphorus, potassium	

Prescription Medications	Indications for Usage	Micronutrients Depleted	Tabulations (place one ✓ for each time taken in a week)
Corticosteroids: cortisone (Cortone), hydrocortisone (Cortef, Hydrocortone), prednisone (Deltasone, Meticorten, Orasone, Panasol-S), prednisolone (Delta-Cortef, Prelone, Pediapred), triamcinolone (Aristocort, Atolone, Kenacort), methylprednisolone (Medrol), fluticasone (Flonase, Cutivate, Veramyst), beclomethasone (Beconase, Qvar, Vancenase, Vanceril)	Severe inflammation; auto-immune disease; immune system suppression; asthma; allergic rhinitis	A, B6, B9, B12, C, D, K, calcium, magnesium, phosphorus, potassium, selenium, zinc, amino acids (carnitine)	
Sulfonylureas: glyburide (Diabeta, Glynase, Micronase), glipizide (Glucotrol), glimepiride (Amaryl), chlorpropamide (Diabinese, Insulase)	Diabetes	CoQ10	
Biguanides: metformin (Glucophage)	Diabetes; prediabetes	B1, B9, B12, CoQ10	
Colchicine: (Colcrys)	Gout	A, B9, B12, D, iron, potassium	
Probenecid:	Gout	B2	

Prescription Medications	Indications for Usage	Micronutrients Depleted	Tabulations (place one ✓ for each time taken in a week)
Progestin: medroxyprogesterone (Depo-Provera, Provera, Amen, Curretab, Cycrin, Prodroxy)	Birth control	B2	
Conjugated estrogens: estrogen replacement therapies (Alora, Cenestin, Climara, Estinyl, Estrace, Estraderm, Estratab, FemPatch, Menest, Ogen, Premarin, Premphase, Prempro, Vivelle); estrogen and progesterone–containing oral contraceptives (Ovral, Lo/Ovral, Low-Ogestrel)	Hormone replacement therapy; birth control	B1, B2, B3, B5, B6, B9, C, D, calcium, magnesium, manganese, zinc, amino acids (carnitine)	
Antimalarial medications: chloroquine, Primaquine	Malaria	B2	
Antimycobacterials: isoniazid, ethambutol, pyrazinamide	Tuberculosis	B3, B6, D, K, zinc	
Nucleoside metabolic inhibitors: 5-fluoracil (Efudex, Adrucil, Carac, Fluoroplex)	Cancer	B1	
Anticonvulsant barbiturates: carbamazepine (Carbatrol, Epitol, Equetro, Tegretol), primidone (Mysoline), phenytoin (Di-Phen, Dilantin, Phenytek)	Seizure medication	B1, B3, B6, B7, B9, B12, C, D, E, K, calcium	

Prescription Medications	Indications for Usage	Micronutrients Depleted	Tabulations (place one ✓ for each time taken in a week)
Levothyroxine (Synthroid, Levoxyl, Levothroid, Unithroid)	Hypothyroidism	Calcium	
Human immunodeficiency virus (HIV) nucleoside analog reverse-transcriptase inhibitors: azidothymidine (AZT), zidovudine (Retrovir)	HIV	Copper, zinc	
Tricyclic antidepressants: amitriptyline (Elavil), doxepin (Silenor, Zonalon, Prudoxin), desipramine (Norpramin), imipramine (Tofranil, Tofranil-PM), amoxapine (Asendin), protriptyline (Vivactil)	Depression	B2, CoQ10	
Psychoactive drugs: benzodiazepines (Valium, Xanax, Ativan, Klonopin); SSRIs (Celexa, Luvox, Lexapro, Prozac, Paxil)	Anxiety, depression	B6, B9, B12, C, D, omega-3, omega-6, CoQ10, amino acids	
Atypical antipsychotics: clozapine (Clozaril, Fazaclo), aripiprazole (Abilify)	Schizophrenia	Selenium	

Prescription Medications	Indications for Usage	Micronutrients Depleted	Tabulations (place one ✓ for each time taken in a week)
Phenothiazines: chlorpromazine, promethazine, thioridazine	Antipsychotic	B2, CoQ10	
Sulfonamides, sulphonamides, or sulfa drugs: sulfadiazine, sulfamethizole (Thiosulfil Forte), sulfamethoxazole (Gantanol), sulfasalazine (Azulfidine), sulfisoxazole (Gantrisin)	Bacterial infection	B1, B2, B7, B9, B12, C	
Macrolide antibiotics: amoxicillin (Amoxil, Trimox), erythromycin (Robimycin), azithromycin (Zithromax), clarithromycin (Biaxin)	Bacterial infection	B1, B2, B3, B6, B7, B9, B12, K	
Aminoglycoside antibiotics: gentamicin (Geromycin), neomycin (Mycifradin, Neo-Fradin, Neo-Tab)	Bacterial infection	A, B6, B12, K, calcium, iron, magnesium, potassium	

Prescription Medications	Indications for Usage	Micronutrients Depleted	Tabulations (place one ✓ for each time taken in a week)
Fluoroquinolone antibiotics: ciprofloxacin (Cipro), enoxacin (Penetrex), gatifloxacin (Tequin), levofloxacin (Levaquin), lomefloxacin (Maxaquin), moxifloxacin (Avelox), norfloxacin (Noroxin), ofloxacin (Floxin), sparfloxacin (Zagam), trovafloxacin (Trovan)	Bacterial infection	B1, B2, B3, B6, B7, B9, B12, K, calcium, iron, magnesium, zinc	

TABLE 5.3 Everyday Micronutrient Depleters Lifestyle Habits Chart

Micronutrient	Tabulation Total
Vitamin A	
Vitamin B1 (thiamine)	
Vitamin B2 (riboflavin)	
Vitamin B3 (niacin)	
Vitamin B5 (pantothenic acid)	
Vitamin B6 (pyridoxine)	
Vitamin B7	
Vitamin B9 (folate)	
Vitamin B12 (cobalamin)	
Vitamin C	
Vitamin D	
Vitamin E	
Vitamin K	
Calcium	
Choline	
Chromium	
Copper	
Iodine	
Iron	
Magnesium	
Manganese	
Phosphorus	
Potassium	
Selenium	
Zinc	
Omega-3	
Omega-6	
Amino acids (carnitine)	

CHAPTER 6

Smart Supplementation

When spiderwebs unite they can tie up a lion.
—AFRICAN PROVERB

L et's review what we've learned so far:

1. We have seen that statistically speaking there is nearly a 100 percent chance you are micronutrient deficient and that micronutrient deficiency is the root cause of osteoporosis (as well as other health conditions and diseases).
2. We have analyzed peer-reviewed studies on popular diet plans and found that regardless of dietary philosophy, no diet adequately supplies the essential micronutrients required to meet minimum Reference Daily Intake (RDI) levels.
3. We have proven that our micronutrient levels are reduced by a multitude of Everyday Micronutrient Depleters (EMDs). Some, such as phytic acid, tannins, and lectins, are found in our foods and drinks, whereas others are hidden in the habits and products that make up our everyday lives, such as stress, medications, and toxins from household and personal care products.

We'd understand if at this point you're feeling a bit disheartened about your chances of achieving micronutrient sufficiency and rebuilding your lost bone, even with all the healing habits you've learned so far. But remember: the darker the night, the brighter the stars, and the star in our story is the third and final step to living the nutrivore lifestyle: smart supplementation. This last step will help you fill in the gaps between where your rich-food diet and lifestyle habits left off and where micronutrient sufficiency is finally realized.

Supplementation Takes You to the Finish Line

Let's go back to that bucket analogy we used earlier. If you remember, your goal is to fill your bucket to the brim with essential micronutrients in order to achieve micronutrient sufficiency. However, we learned that no dietary philosophy has been shown to provide an adequate amount of essential micronutrients to accomplish this goal, which means your diet alone can't fill the bucket. Next, we learned that EMDs in the foods you eat and numerous lifestyle habits, some avoidable and others unavoidable, poke "holes" in your bucket. These holes cause the micronutrients you worked so hard to get into your bucket to slowly drain out, making it even more difficult to achieve micronutrient sufficiency. And remember, without actually achieving and maintaining a state of micronutrient sufficiency, your body will not have what it needs to heal your bones. So what should you do when you see the level of water in your bucket getting low? The answer is, fill it back up. That is where smart supplementation comes in. In this chapter, we will show you how a smart supplementation program can help you achieve micronutrient sufficiency, even if you still have a few of those pesky holes in your bucket.

Do you remember Table 2.1 back in Chapter 2 (page 40), where we outlined each essential vitamin and mineral and the role they played in bone health? We created that table because we wanted you to understand that your body requires *all* of the essential micronutrients to build healthy bones. We know what you may be thinking: you already take a multivitamin and, although you might be getting some benefits, it hasn't produced any magic bone-building results so far, right? We totally agree with you. The fact is, *most* of the multivitamins on the market are, for the most part, a waste of money. In fact, even major magazines and newspapers like *Forbes* and the *New York Times* have published stories highlighting research showing no benefits to taking a multivitamin and even going so far as saying multivitamins should not be used. It took us years of studying the multivitamin to figure out why.

If you consider a multivitamin to be the sum of all its ingredients, then it should be the most powerful bone-building and health-enhancing tool available. After all, as we have learned, each micronutrient has been shown to be beneficial to our bone health in some unique way. Thousands of high-quality, peer-reviewed research papers published around the world have confirmed that individual micronutrients like vitamin D and calcium really are superstars at preventing cancer and building strong bones, and others like zinc and vitamin C really do help support a properly functioning immune system. In fact, no one in the nutrition or medical communities disputes the fact that micronutrients are absolutely essential for optimal health. However, when all of these amazing individual micronutrients are combined into a single multivitamin, their benefits all but disappear. Why? This was the question that we wanted to answer, the riddle we needed to solve. We had a hunch that the negative results researchers were finding with the multivitamin were not the fault of the individual micronutrients themselves but rather an issue of how the multivitamin had been formulated.

Would you be surprised to learn that it has been only about eighty years since the multivitamin was first created and that many of the individual vitamins we take for granted today were not identified until the mid-1930s? It's true; it has only been just over a century since the first vitamin (vitamin A) was discovered. So it shouldn't surprise us, then, that we are still learning so much about them. However, with all advancements in micronutrient science, the multivitamin still remains pretty much the same as that first prototype—a mix of vitamins and minerals haphazardly thrown together into a tablet with almost no thought concerning absorption, their quantity or form, or how the individual micronutrients may affect each other. Can you think of anything in your life that still uses technology from the 1930s, without a redesign? Probably not.

IDENTIFYING THE FOUR FLAWS
IN THE MULTIVITAMIN

So it's really not hard to imagine that a multivitamin that has not been updated and reformulated using the latest advances in supplemental science may not be living up to its ultimate potential. But this is great news because if this is true, it means that by simply identifying the outdated design flaws and updating the way we formulate the multivitamin, we should be able to greatly improve its ability to enhance our health.

After years of reviewing research conducted by scientists around the world, we were able to identify four distinct areas where multivitamins don't make the grade. In this chapter, we will explore each of these areas to learn how to unlock the full power and potential of the multivitamin. In order to keep it simple, we created an easy acronym. We call it the ABCs of Optimal Supplementation Guidelines, and the *A*, *B*, *C*, and *s* stand for the four flaws we identified in a typical multivitamin: **A**bsorption, **B**eneficial quantities and forms, and micronutrient **C**ompetition and **s**ynergy.

The ABCs of Optimal Supplementation Guidelines

A STANDS FOR ABSORPTION

Have you ever wondered why your doctor might tell you that taking a multivitamin is no better than flushing money down the toilet? Well, most of the time they are right—because of poor disintegration, many of the multivitamins we ingest end up in septic tanks, sewers, or bedpans. Absorbing micronutrients is more difficult than you might think, and if your body isn't absorbing the vitamins and minerals found in your daily multivitamin capsule or tablet, then they cannot help you build your bones. This makes absorption a huge issue for most multivitamins and the first of the four flaws we will examine.

When it comes to micronutrient absorption, the form by which the vitamins and minerals are delivered greatly affects their absorption rates. For example, if the vitamins and minerals are delivered via a multivitamin pill or capsule, the pill or capsule itself must first break down or disintegrate before the vitamins and minerals it contains become available for absorption. According to Raimar Löbenberg, PhD, lead researcher in a study published in the *Journal of Pharmacy and Pharmaceutical Sciences*, "active ingredients [micronutrients] can only be absorbed if they are released into solution from the dosage form. Disintegration is the first step in this process. . . . If a mineral has to be absorbed within an absorption window, but the dosage form does not release its content in a timely manner, the therapy might be compromised or fail." To determine if poor disintegration might be a problem with multivitamins, Dr. Löbenberg conducted a research study. In it, he tested forty-nine well-known, commercially available multivitamins in both capsule and tablet forms to find out if they would disintegrate and release their contained vitamins and minerals within the twenty-minute time period necessary for potential absorption. The researcher found that out of the forty-nine multivitamins studied, only twenty-four (49 percent) disintegrated within the allotted twenty-minute window, leaving more than half of the multivitamins (51 percent) unable to perform this essential action. The worst performers were Kirkland Signature formula (Costco brand), Nu-Life The Ultimate One for Men, Trophic, SISU Only One, Swiss One, and GNC Mega Men—all of which failed to disintegrate at all!

Surprising, right? And since disintegration is the first step in absorption, if you happen to be one of the 51 percent of people who were taking one of these popular multivitamin brands, your ability to absorb the essential vitamins and minerals contained within these multivitamins would be compromised at best and possibly completely inhibited. So based on Dr. Löbenberg's research, your physician is right, you have slightly less than a 50/50 shot at choosing a multivitamin capsule or tablet that will properly disintegrate and deliver the vitamins and minerals you need to protect your bone health. So how did your physician know this? They know it because the *Physicians' Desk Reference (PDR)*, a pharmaceutical guide to all things prescribed, indicates that the contents of both capsules and pills, which make up the majority of multivitamin sales, are only 10 to 20 percent absorbed by the body, due to poor disintegration. No wonder so many people in the medical community feel that there is little value to most multivitamins; they know that most of them do not properly disintegrate.

However, that same *PDR* recognizes one delivery system for having nearly perfect absorption. It states that liquid formulas have an absorption rate of up to 98 percent, the highest rate of absorption of any delivery system. This is great news, because it means that in order to easily avoid this first formulation flaw, all you have to do is simply drink your multivitamin. Not only will taking your multivitamins in a liquid form rather than pills or capsules increase the potential of absorption, as there is no need for disintegration to occur, but it is also easier and more enjoyable for most people. According to a nationwide survey conducted by Harris Interactive, the global market research firm that conducts the Harris poll, 40 percent of all adults surveyed have difficulty taking pills. Additionally, bariatric patients (who are at greater risk for osteoporosis) and individuals with irritable bowel syndrome, diverticulitis, and hiatal hernias have particular difficulty when taking their supplements in pill or capsule form. This makes a liquid multivitamin the best way to ensure complete disintegration and increase the absorption potential of each essential vitamin and mineral.

The Potential Problems with Liquid Delivery Systems

Although you have just learned that a multivitamin delivered as a liquid does increase the absorption potential of each of its micronutrients, we still want you to be aware of several pitfalls. First, just because you *take* your multivitamin in a liquid form doesn't mean you necessarily *purchased* it as a liquid. It could be a powdered drink mix as well. Either way, it is important to know that the potency of micronutrients is degraded when they come into contact with heat, air, and light. So you want to minimize this exposure as much as possible. If your liquid multivitamin has been exposed to high heat during its long journey to the store in the back of a container truck and has been sitting in a clear bottle on the store shelf exposed to fluorescent lighting, there is a good chance the micronutrients have been degraded to some extent. To make matters worse, as certain micronutrients degrade, they release competitive (or antagonistic) elements that further degrade other micronutrients in the same formula. For example, in a liquid solution, vitamin B12 can break down and release a cobalt ion, which in turn can then contribute to the destruction of vitamins B1 and B6.

Powdered multivitamins sold in large canisters or tubs may not be the best delivery system either. Not only can the powder become oxidized each time the tub is opened and exposed to air and light, but it's nearly impossible to guarantee which micronutrients you will be getting in each daily serving. This is because most vitamins are light and fluffy, whereas most minerals are dense and heavy. Over time, if stored in a large tub, the heavier micronutrients will naturally sink to the bottom, making it difficult to know which ones you are scooping into your daily multivitamin drink. This could become problematic, as some of your heavy, bone-building minerals such as calcium and magnesium may remain at the bottom of your tub rather than in your daily drink. Not only could this cause stomach upset and put your bone health at risk, but the imbalance in micronutrients will also leave your micronutrient orchestra playing a very off-key musical concerto.

Unwanted Ingredients Can Hinder Absorption

Another issue with most multivitamins, whether liquid, powdered, pills, or capsules, is unwanted add-ins. For example, is it really necessary for a multivitamin designed for women to be pink and a multivitamin for men to be blue? Unscrupulous manufacturers also use potentially carcinogenic artificial colors—such as Blue #1, Blue #2, Yellow #5, Yellow #6, and Red #40—to make their chewable gummy vitamins more attractive to our children. These potentially dangerous artificial colors have no place in any product, and neither do flavor-enhancing sugar, HFCS, and other artificial sweeteners and flavors (often containing MSG). As you learned in Chapter 3, these EMDs reduce your body's ability to absorb the micronutrients that your multivitamin is supposed to deliver. So, when focusing on *A* for *absorption*, avoid these potential roadblocks.

We should note that not all multivitamin capsules have poor disintegration rates (remember that 49 percent of the multivitamins tested did pass Dr. Löbenberg's disintegration test), and not all flavors, sweeteners, and colors are artificial. For example, the Vcaps Plus capsule by Capsugel (which we use with our Nutreince capsule product) is vegetarian, non-GMO-project verified, and kosher and halal certified, and clinically proven to have a high disintegration rate (even when stomach acid is low). Additionally, natural flavors (without MSG), natural sweeteners (such as stevia, luo han, and xylitol) and natural colors (from riboflavin or quercitin) are completely safe and will not reduce your ability to absorb essential micronutrients. However, you do have to do your due diligence to make sure that the manufacturer of your supplements is using these healthy and natural ingredients.

Table 6.1 identifies many of the absorption-inhibiting ingredients that act as binders, fillers, excipients, sweeteners, flow agents, flavors, and preservatives in multivitamins. Check to make sure these do not appear on the labels of your supplements.

TABLE 6.1 Ingredients That Inhibit Proper Absorption

All artificial sweeteners	Maltodextrine
Artificial flavors	Polyvinyl alcohol
BHA or BHT	Red #40
Black iron oxide	Red iron oxide
Blue #1 or #2	Shellac
Cane sugar	Sodium benzoate
Caramel color	Sodium starch glycolate
Corn syrup, cornstarch, or solids	Stearic acid
Croscarmellose sodium	Sucrose
Crospovidone	Sugar
Disodium hydrogen phosphate	Talc
Fructose	Tapioca syrup
Fruit juices	Titanium oxide
Gellan gum	Wax
High-fructose corn syrup	Yellow #5 or #6
Magnesium or calcium stearate	Yellow iron oxide

Fixing Flaw 1: Absorption

We identified disintegration as a key problem in the absorption of micronutrients and have proven that most tablets and capsules just don't cut it if you want to make sure your multivitamin is able to do its important job. To help you avoid all of the aforementioned absorption issues, we've included a quick checklist in Table 6.2 that you can use when purchasing your supplements. By using the *A* part of our ABCs of Optimal Supplementation Guidelines, you will be able to overcome the multivitamin's first flaw—inhibited absorption.

TABLE 6.2 Identifying Whether Your Supplement Follows the Rules of Absorption

Make Sure Your Multivitamin . . .	✓ if Yes
Is delivered in powdered form in single-serving packets or in a capsule proven to disintegrate in twenty minutes or less	
Does not contain sugar under any name, such as sucrose, maltodextrin, fructose, fruit juice, corn syrup solids, high-fructose corn syrup, cane sugar, tapioca syrup, or corn syrup, to name but a few	
Does not contain the preservatives sodium benzoate, BHA, or BHT	
Does not contain any binders, fillers, or flow agents, such as magnesium or calcium stearate, disodium hydrogen phosphate, talc, polyvinyl alcohol, cornstarch, sodium starch glycolate, crospovidone, croscarmellose sodium, or gellan gum	
Is not coated with shellac or wax	
Does not contain artificial colors, sweeteners, or flavors	

B STANDS FOR BENEFICIAL QUANTITIES AND FORMS

The letter *B* in our ABCs of Optimal Supplementation Guidelines has two equally important parts: beneficial quantities and beneficial forms. Both allow us to harness the miraculous healing power of the multivitamin's individual micronutrients. Unfortunately, you will find that most products on the market fall short in both categories.

Luckily, you don't have to figure out how much of each micronutrient is beneficial: the RDI is the amount of each micronutrient that will keep you from getting a micronutrient deficiency disease. But is that the same amount necessary to keep you thriving and increase bone density? Probably not. However, because you will already be eating a micronutrient-rich diet during your twelve-week Rebuild Your Bones osteoporosis protocol, you will be receiving a good portion of your essential vitamins, minerals, essential fatty acids, and amino acids through your food. Even after you take into account the stress, pollution, alcohol, and any other micronutrient-leaching EMDs you may have identified in your life, your smart supplementation will get you above the sufficiency line every time, *if* the supplement you choose supplies both the beneficial quantities and forms of the all of the individual micro-nutrients your body needs. Mathematically speaking:

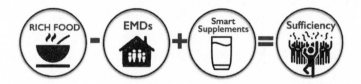

Now, when we say *beneficial quantities*, we are not implying that you should take a supplement that delivers megadoses. Sometimes too much of a good thing can be a really bad thing. For example, back in Chapter 2, you learned that vitamin A plays an essential role in bone health. However, scientists have determined that too much vitamin A can result in bone loss and an increased risk of hip fracture. According to the NIH Osteoporosis and Related Bone Diseases National Resource Center, "excessive amounts of vitamin A trigger an increase in osteo-clasts, the cells that break down bone. They also believe that too much vitamin A may negatively interfere with vitamin D, which plays an important role in preserving bone." In science, this is what we refer to as the Goldilocks Principle. Finding the "beneficial quantity" or the amount that is "just right" is the key!

However, there is one vitamin that most health professionals agree should be taken at levels higher than RDI, especially if you are work-ing to prevent or reverse osteoporosis. We are talking about vitamin D. To be fair, let's consider our ancestors. They trekked and labored for hours in the sun, and that sunshine kept them replete with vitamin D. We currently recommend 2,000 IU of vitamin D in your multivitamin, which is 500 percent of the Daily Value (DV). (The RDI is used to determine the DV of foods, which is printed on Nutrition Facts labels in the United States. The DV tells you what percentage of the RDI is delivered.) Although 500 percent may at first sound high, imagine how much more the human body is acclimated to receiving. For ex-ample, a fair-skinned individual in Miami would make 10,000 IU of vitamin D in only about six minutes of exposure to the sun in summer and fifteen minutes in winter. It is more than likely that generations of men, women, and children have been outside for more than six minutes at a time per day, thus manufacturing far greater amounts than even 10,000 IU of vitamin D. And don't worry because although 2,000 IU is 500 percent of the RDI, it is definitely *not* "too much" and should not raise safety concerns in your mind.

Although many multivitamin manufacturers often add megadoses of some micronutrients, such as inexpensive B vitamins, more often than not, the problem is one of insufficient quantities. Calcium and magnesium are two important bone-building minerals that manufacturers skimp on most. Both are bulky and expensive and don't fit neatly into just a few capsules or tablets. Manufacturers actually leave out essential micronutrients from their formulas so they can keep the number of pills you have to take each day as low as possible. They simply don't want to deter you from taking their products.

You can see the problem here, right? In order for Mira to rebuild her bones, we needed a multivitamin that contained beneficial quantities of each essential vitamin and mineral. Unfortunately, we couldn't find a single multivitamin that was formulated to include this basic requirement. Leaving out beneficial quantities of each specific micronutrient is a flaw that can lead to potentially dangerous micronutrient deficiencies, even in individuals who are purchasing supplements to protect themselves.

TIME IS OF THE ESSENCE

What would happen if you ate only one meal a day? Well, you would probably feel pretty exhausted and drained by midafternoon. This is because your body requires fuel all day long to help it with the myriad of functions it performs throughout the day. These bodily functions require both adequate amounts of macronutrients (carbohydrates, protein, and fat) for energy, as well as essential micronutrients to be there at the exact time the biological function needs to be performed. Do you remember in the orchestra analogy how we told you there are two families of vitamins—water-soluble and fat-soluble? The water-soluble vitamins move through your system very quickly and are often absorbed by the body and excreted within a twelve-hour window. So if you take your multivitamin at seven a.m., your water-soluble vitamins, such as

B vitamins and vitamin C, may not be there to perform the functions necessary at nine p.m. This is why many leading health professionals, including Dr. Oz, suggest taking several water-soluble micronutrients in multiple doses.

"You want to give your body the right amount of fuel for when you need it," says Dr. Oz. "Vitamins have water-soluble elements to them, so they are quickly moved through your system." He recommends splitting your multivitamin into morning and evening doses because "by taking half your multivitamin in the morning and half in the evening, you're guaranteeing that your body can absorb all the nutrients it can."

An additional justification for taking micronutrients multiple times a day is their limited absorption capacity. For example, and this is key for those with osteoporosis, although the RDI recommends that all adults take in 1,300 milligrams of calcium a day, scientists have determined that calcium can be absorbed only in increments of no more than 500 to 600 milligrams at one time. In order to meet the RDI, one would have to take calcium multiple times during the day, through either food or supplement. So the "beneficial quantities" part of the equation makes it clear that if we are to reach the health-promoting state of micronutrient sufficiency, we must opt for supplements that are taken multiple times during the day and that deliver the RDI levels (or, in the case of calcium, only 500–600 milligrams) without megadosing or omitting essential vitamins and minerals.

B ALSO STANDS FOR BENEFICIAL FORMS

What most consumers don't know is that each micronutrient has numerous forms that a manufacturer can choose from to include in its formula. Some offer high performance at a higher cost to the manufacturer; others are less expensive and less effective. However, unless you can distinguish the high-performance form from the lesser form, you may be paying a Bentley price tag but receiving the multivitamin equivalent of the Yugo.

For many individuals today, finding the most bioavailable form of each micronutrient is of the utmost importance. Research published in the *American Journal of Epidemiology* shows that more than 34 percent of the U.S. population may have a genetic enzyme defect known as the MTHFR mutation. This mutation makes it difficult to convert vitamin B9 (both folate and folic acid) into biologically active 5-MTHF, and new estimates suggest that up to 60 percent of the population may be affected. These individuals cannot metabolize the unmethylated forms of specific B vitamins, namely the forms of vitamins B9 and B12 that are commonly added to most multivitamins. The active forms of these B vitamins are referred to as the *methylated* form. This is the form that your body can actually use.

Above and beyond those B vitamins, approximately twenty to thirty additional vitamins and minerals are included in the formulation of a typical multivitamin. Table 6.3 lists many of these essential micronutrients and their beneficial forms, along with brief explanations of why we prefer these forms in your smart supplementation.

TABLE 6.3 **Beneficial Quantities and Forms of Specific Micronutrients**

Essential Micronutrient	Beneficial Quantities (DV) and Forms	Why Is This Superior?
Vitamin A	3,000 IU, or 100% DV, of mixed vitamin A from both retinyl acetate and beta-carotene	Some multivitamins contain only beta-carotene, an inactive form of vitamin A (provitamin A), which must be converted in the body to retinyl (preformed), an active form (conversion rate of 21:1). Because of the poor conversion rate of beta-carotene, a supplement should be formulated to include at least 2,500 IU of preformed vitamin A in the natural form, retinyl acetate (preferred), or in the synthetic form, retinyl palmitate.

Essential Micronutrient	Beneficial Quantities (DV) and Forms	Why Is This Superior?
Lutein (not essential)	6 mg lutein	Most multivitamins do not contain lutein at all, but we recommend 6 mg of lutein because this is the amount that is recommended to prevent/reverse age-related macular degeneration and combat oxidative damage.
Vitamin B1 (thiamine)	1.2 mg thiamine pyrophosphate	Thiamine pyrophosphate is the metabolically active form of thiamine and does not require conversion by the body.
Vitamin B2 (riboflavin)	1.3 mg riboflavin-5-phosphate	Although many products contain riboflavin HCL, it is inferior to riboflavin-5-phosphate because it is not the bioactive form of vitamin B2. Riboflavin HCL needs to be converted in the liver to the active form.
Vitamin B3 (niacin)	16 mg niacin and niacinamide	Most multivitamins contain only niacinamide. However, the two forms of vitamin B3 perform different functions in your body. Niacinamide controls blood sugar, but only niacin has been shown to lower LDL (bad cholesterol) and raise HDL (good cholesterol). It is best to include both forms to cover all bases.
Vitamin B5 (pantothenic acid)	5 mg pantethine	Pantethine is the bioactive form of B5, making it readily used by the body.

Essential Micronutrient	Beneficial Quantities (DV) and Forms	Why Is This Superior?
Vitamin B6 (pyroxidan)	1.7 mg pyridoxal-5-phosphate	Pyridoxal-5-phosphate is the bioactive form of B6. However, many inferior products use pyridoxine HCL, which is not the active form of this B vitamin.
Vitamin B7 (biotin)	30 mcg d-biotin	The *d-* in front of *biotin* means it is the preferred natural form, *dl-* means it is synthetic.
Vitamin B9 (folate)	400 mcg 5-MTHF (methyltetrahydrofolate), quatrefolic, or ([6S]-5-methyltetrahydrofolic acid glucosamine salt	5-MTHF is the bioactive form of B9. Because of the large population with the genetic enzyme defect (known as the MTHFR mutation) that makes it difficult for them to convert both folate and folic acid into biologically active 5-MTHF, 5-MTHF is a more effective method of folate supplementation.
Vitamin B12 (cobalmin)	2.4 mcg methylcobalamin	The standard source of B12, cyanocobalamin, is not a natural source. In fact, it's not found anywhere in nature and must be converted by the liver into methylcobalamin in order to be usable by humans (and all other animals). Cyanocobalamin is typically found in inexpensive, inferior products. Methylcobalamin is the preferred bioactive form of vitamin B12.

Essential Micronutrient	Beneficial Quantities (DV) and Forms	Why Is This Superior?
Vitamin C	90 mg ascorbyl palmitate	This fat-soluble form of vitamin C is highly absorbable and is more stable than water-soluble forms of vitamin C. It doesn't flush out of the body as quickly as ascorbic acid and can be stored in cell membranes until the body needs it. It has also been shown to be protective of other fat-soluble antioxidants. Cell membranes enriched with ascorbyl palmitate are more resistant to oxidative damage, which means they are better protected against disease and aging.
Vitamin D	2,000 IU vitamin D3	Two forms of vitamin D are available in supplements: vitamin D2 (ergocalciferol) and vitamin D3 (cholecalciferol). D3 is the form that is produced in our skin when we are exposed to sunlight and is biologically superior for supplementation. In fact, research published in the *American Journal of Clinical Nutrition* found that vitamin D2 supplementation caused a reduction in overall serum concentrations of vitamin D over twenty-eight days, with serum levels actually falling below baseline (starting) levels. The researchers concluded that vitamin D2 should no longer be regarded as a nutrient appropriate for supplementation or fortification of foods.

Essential Micronutrient	Beneficial Quantities (DV) and Forms	Why Is This Superior?
Vitamin E	22.35 IU mixed tocopherols and mixed tocotrienols	Vitamin E is split into two families: the tocopherols and the tocotrienols, each containing four unique derivatives (alpha, beta, gamma, and delta). Look on the label for "full spectrum d-tocopherols and d-tocopherolss." Additionally, avoid the synthetic form of this vitamin, which starts with *dl-*. According to a study published in the *American Journal of Clinical Nutrition,* researchers found that levels of natural vitamin E (d-tocopherol) in the blood and in the organs were double that of synthetic vitamin E (dl-tocopherol) when compared, showing that natural vitamin E is better retained and more biologically active than the synthetic form.
Vitamin K	120 mcg vitamin K1 and vitamin K2 (MK-4 and MK-7) (as K2 VITAL Delta)	It is important for a supplement to include both K1 and K2 and even more superior and rare if it also includes both forms of vitamin K2 (MK-4 and MK-7). Vitamin K1 plays a role in blood clotting, whereas K2 is a more important inducer of bone mineralization in human osteoblasts (bone-building cells). The MK-7 form of K2 is optimal for dietary supplementation because it has

Essential Micronutrient	Beneficial Quantities (DV) and Forms	Why Is This Superior?
		a long half-life of two to three days, compared to the one to two hours of MK-4. *Most products contain unprotected vitamin K2 MK-7, which is susceptible to degradation in formulations containing minerals, such as calcium, magnesium, and multivitamin formulations. A specially protected form of MK-7 called K2 VITAL Delta protects the K2 in formulation.*
Boron	2 mg boron citrate	A highly absorbable citrate form of boron.
Calcium	500–600 mg *Pills and capsules:* Calcium potassium phosphate citrate, calcium citrate, or calcium malate *Liquids and powders:* Same as above, or calcium carbonate + citric acid (non-GMO) can convert to calcium citrate. Avoid algae-based calcium products for their poor absorption and high heavy metal reports.	This is the only micronutrient that should be less than 100 percent RDI on your supplement facts. Calcium needs an acidic stomach environment to properly be absorbed, which is why we recommend calcium potassium phosphate citrate, calcium citrate, or calcium malate, as they are more absorbable when taken away from food. Since bone mineral is predominately calcium phosphate, we recommend the calcium potassium phosphate citrate form because it comes with the bone-building micronutrients potassium and phosphate, similar to how it comes in dairy products. Studies have found that calcium that contains phosphate helps maintain strong bones and reduce the risk of osteoporosis.

Essential Micronutrient	Beneficial Quantities (DV) and Forms	Why Is This Superior?
Chromium	35 mg chromium polynicotinate	The most absorbable form of chromium is chromium polynicotinate. Unlike chromium picolonate, which research suggests may be linked to causing DNA damage, chromium polynicotinate is a pure niacin-bound form of chromium, identified by U.S. government researchers as the active component of true GTF (glucose tolerance factor), which regulates the body's use of glucose and helps balance blood sugar levels.
Copper	Should not be included in supplement. If you need to supplement copper because of a copper deficiency, take it separately from your multivitamin.	Taking a multivitamin that contains copper is generally not recommended because too much can hinder your body's ability to destroy the proteins that form the plaques found in the brains of Alzheimer's patients. According Neal D. Barnard, MD, president of the Physicians Committee for Responsible Medicine, many Alzheimer's patients have elevated levels of copper, and in studies, it was determined that many of those affected took multivitamins with copper. Additionally, pregnant women should avoid copper in multivitamins because copper levels can nearly double during pregnancy, making toxicity a concern. Cramps, abdominal pain, vomiting, nausea, and diarrhea are all common when taking supplements that include copper.

Essential Micronutrient	Beneficial Quantities (DV) and Forms	Why Is This Superior?
Iodine	150 mcg potassium iodide	Because of our polluted waters, kelp is no longer considered a safe source of iodine. We recommend potassium iodide.
Iron	Should not be included in supplement. If you need to supplement iron because of an iron deficiency, take it separately from your multivitamin.	Iron is an essential mineral your body needs to function normally. However, the National Institutes of Health's Office of Dietary Supplements has indicated that too much iron can cause serious health complications. Because of this, we recommend an iron-free multivitamin to avoid iron overload, a medical condition that causes excess iron to be stored in vital organs, such as the liver and heart. Too much iron may be toxic— and even fatal. In general, iron supplementation is not recommended for adult males and postmenopausal women. If you are a premenopausal woman, an athlete who works out for more than six hours a week, or a strict vegan/ vegetarian, you may want to consider iron supplementation. *(In the "C Stands for Micronutrient Competitions" section, you will uncover another important reason that iron should be omitted from multivitamin formulations.)*

Essential Micronutrient	Beneficial Quantities (DV) and Forms	Why Is This Superior?
Magnesium	420 mg *Pills and capsules:* magnesium citrate, glycinate, or L-thronate *Liquids and powders:* Same as above, or magnesium carbonate + citric acid (non-GMO) can convert to magnesium citrate.	Most multivitamins supply inadequate amounts of magnesium because of its bulky size. We prefer magnesium citrate for its high bioavailability.
Manganese	2.3 mg manganese gluconate	Manganese gluconate is a highly bioavailable form of manganese.
Molybdenum	45 mcg molybdenum glycinate	Molybdenum glycinate is the best absorbed, most highly bioavailable form of molybdenum.
Potassium	Although the RDI is 4,700 mg, the U.S. government restricts supplementation in pill or capsule form to 99 mg.	Supplements that contain calcium potassium phosphate citrate naturally deliver potassium.
Silicon	4 mg horsetail extract	Horsetail is a natural herbal extract that is rich in silica.
Selenium	70 mcg selenomethionine	Selenomethionine is a superior bioavailable organic form of selenium.
Zinc	11 mg zinc glycinate	Zinc glycinate is a well-absorbed, highly bioavailable form of zinc.

Fixing Flaw 2: Beneficial Quantities and Forms

Can you now see how important it is to take supplements that are formulated with both the beneficial quantities and beneficial forms of each micronutrient? Your money could really be wasted otherwise. This information about beneficial quantities and forms goes a long way toward explaining why many studies on multivitamins have been unsuccessful at providing health benefits. After all, how could a multivitamin with insufficient quantities of calcium or magnesium, the wrong form of vitamin D, and no vitamin K2 promote bone health? It is also important to make sure all the ingredients in your multivitamin are non-GMO. Table 6.4 provides another quick little checklist we want you to use when evaluating a multivitamin; it covers all of the B aspects of our ABCs of Optimal Supplementation Guidelines.

TABLE 6.4 Identifying Whether Your Supplement Follows the Rules for Beneficial Quantities and Forms

Make Sure Your Multivitamin . . .	✓ if Yes
Does contain at least 100% of the Daily Value (DV) for all of the following 20 essential micronutrients? **Note:** Many supplement companies don't list the specific forms for each vitamin and mineral on the supplement facts. You may have to look below in the ingredients to identify the forms that they are using.	

Vitamin A	Vitamin C	Vitamin D
Vitamin E	Vitamin K	B1 (thiamin)
B2 (riboflavin)	B3 (niacin)	B5 (pantothenic acid)
B6	B7 (biotin)	B9 (folate/5-MTHF)
B12	Magnesium	Zinc
Selenium	Manganese	Iodine
Molybedenum	Chromium	

Is delivered twice a day
Is labeled to be non-GMO
Does contain at least 2,500 IU of preformed vitamin A (not beta-carotene)
Does contain thiamine pyrophosphate for B1 (thiamine)
Does contain pantethine for B5 (pantothenic acid)
Does contain ascorbyl palmitate for vitamin C
Does contain chromium polynicotinate (not picolonate)
Does contain selenomethionine for selenium
Does contain 500–600 mg calcium, preferably in the calcium potassium phosphate citrate, citrate, or malate forms
Does contain at least 420 mg magnesium, preferably in the citrate, glycinate, or L-thronate forms

Make Sure Your Multivitamin . . .	✓ if Yes
Does contain 2,000 IU of vitamin D3 (not D2)	
Does not contain more than 100% DV of any micronutrients (vitamin D excluded)	
Does contain methylcobalamin for B12	
Does contain both niacin and niacinamide	
Does contain vitamin K1, vitamin K2 (MK-4), and vitamin K2 (MK-7 as K2 VITAL Delta)	
Does contain 5–MTHF (methyltetrahydrofolate), quatrefolic, or [6S]–5–methyltetrahydrofolic acid glucosamine salt and not folic acid for B9 (folate)	
Does contain pyridoxal-5-phosphate for B6	
Does contain all eight forms of vitamin E (mixed tocopherols and tocotrienols) and does not utilize dl-forms (synthetic)	
Does not contain copper	
Does not contain iron	
Does contain any of the following beneficial but nonessential micronutrients: grapeseed extract, quercetin, CoQ10	
Does contain 6 mg lutein	
Does contain riboflavin-5-phosphate for vitamin B2 (riboflavin)	
Does contain d-biotin (natural)	

C STANDS FOR MICRONUTRIENT COMPETITIONS (AND *S* STANDS FOR SYNERGIES)

Although both the *A* and the *B* in our ABCs can help unlock the amazing benefits of your multivitamin, the *C* and the *s* are truly the game changers! We feel that it is the understanding of the *C* and *s* that unlocked the benefits of supplementation for Mira. Let's use our orchestra analogy again to understand micronutrient competitions and synergies. Imagine that all the musicians in the orchestra arrive at the concert hall to perform a piece of music. All the essential instruments needed for the piece are there. However, for this performance, the musicians are asked to play a brand-new melody without sheet music. Since there is no direction, and they have no idea what the piece is supposed to sound like, they all just end up playing all at once. What do you think that might sound like? Probably just a lot of confusing noises, as the sound of each instrument would compete with the others for your ear. The loud, deep trombone blasts would drown out the delicate strings of the violins, and the booming of the drums would completely negate the heavenly harps. Instead of music, the lack of proper composition would deliver you nothing but chaos.

The same holds true for your micronutrients. Remember, just like instruments, each micronutrient has a unique function (or sound) in the body: some harmonize well and others do not. A typical multivitamin is a lot like the musicians in the orchestra all playing at the same time without any properly composed sheet music (or formulation). Instead of the micronutrients working together as a synergistic unit, they compete with one another for absorption pathways and utilization.

Through our years of research into micronutrient competition, we have uncovered numerous peer-reviewed scientific studies clearly demonstrating that certain micronutrients, when delivered at the same time (like within a multivitamin), greatly reduced or eliminated the ability of other micronutrients to be absorbed or utilized. This is a huge issue if your goal is to improve your bone health by taking a multinutrient product that successfully delivers all the vitamins and minerals your body needs each and every day. In fact, we believe that micronutrient competitions are the main reason researchers have not seen as many health benefits associated with multivitamin use when compared to research using individual or small groupings of micronutrients.

As we dug deeper, we discovered that four types of micronutrient competitions can occur when taking a typical multivitamin: chemical competition, biochemical competition, physiological competition, and clinical competition. Let's take a moment to look closer at each.

Chemical competition occurs during the manufacturing of all nutritional supplements, including multivitamins. When manufacturers combine competing micronutrients in one formulation, a chemical battle can ensue within the formulation itself, leaving the competing micronutrients unable to be absorbed. For example, vitamin B9 (folate) forms an insoluble complex with zinc when both are put together in a nutritional supplement or multivitamin. Additionally, when most forms of vitamin K2 MK-7 are put in a formulation (such as a multivitamin or bone-building complex) with minerals such as calcium and magnesium the K2 is rapidly degraded. When either of these chemical competitions occurs, the absorption of these nutrients is compromised (as are their bone-rebuilding benefits).

Biochemical competition happens after ingestion, but before the micronutrients have been absorbed. An example of this is when copper and zinc are taken at the same time; they duke it out for domination of the receptor site. These receptor sites, or absorption pathways, act as docking locations for specific micronutrients and are found throughout the entire gastrointestinal tract. This also occurs between many other micronutrients, such as lutein and beta-carotene.

Physiological competition happens after micronutrient absorption when one or more micronutrients cause decreased utilization of competing micronutrients. For instance, in some studies, copper has been shown to reduce the activity of vitamin B5 (pantothenic acid). So having copper in your multivitamin may reduce vitamins B5's ability to reduce both stress and cortisol levels.

Clinical competition occurs when the presence of one micronutrient masks the deficiency of another, making it difficult for even trained health professionals to detect a deficiency. The classic example here is vitamin B9 (folate) and vitamin B12. Folate can mask B12 anemia, a condition of inadequate red blood cells that can lead to depression, dementia, high homocysteine levels, and osteoporosis.

You don't have to memorize these micronutrient competitions. They are listed here to illuminate just how frequently competitions can occur from the beginning of a micronutrient's journey at the manufacturing stage all the way through to utilization. In fact, when you illustrate all the competitions that may occur between the thirty-four micronutrients most often included in a multivitamin supplement, it looks like a huge spiderweb. Thus far, our research has identified forty-eight competitions that can occur between those thirty-four micronutrients, with thirty of the thirty-four (88 percent) having at least one competition, fifteen of the thirty-four (44 percent) having at least three competitions, and one micronutrient, iron, having competitions with ten other micronutrients. How do some of our major bone-building nutrients fare where competition is concerned? Let's take a look:

Micronutrients That Have Competitions with Calcium

- **Vitamin B2 (riboflavin):** Calcium can chelate with riboflavin, decreasing riboflavin absorption.
- **Vitamin K2:** Calcium quickly degrades most forms of K2 MK-7 when combined in a formulation.
- **Copper:** Copper shares an absorption carrier with calcium; thus, excess amounts of calcium may antagonize the absorption of copper.
- **Iron:** Calcium can inhibit the absorption of nonheme iron.
- **Magnesium:** Calcium and magnesium compete for absorption.
- **Manganese:** Calcium can slightly decrease the absorption of manganese.
- **Sodium:** High intake of sodium can cause an increase in the urinary excretion of calcium.
- **Zinc:** Large doses of calcium can inhibit the absorption of zinc. It is also possible that zinc can inhibit calcium absorption at the binding site.

Micronutrients That Have Competitions with Vitamin K

- **Fat-soluble vitamins (A, D, and E):** Excessive amounts of the fat-soluble vitamins (A, D, and E) interfere with the absorption and utilization of vitamin K. Vitamin A is the least competitive of the fat-soluble vitamins with K.
- **Calcium:** Calcium quickly degrades most forms of K2 MK-7 when combined in a formulation.
- **Magnesium:** Magnesium quickly degrades most forms of K2 MK-7 when combined in a formulation.

Micronutrients That Have Competitions with Vitamin B12

- **Vitamin B9 (folate):** Large doses of B9 can mask an underlying B12 deficiency, which left unchecked can cause irreversible nerve damage and osteoporosis.
- **Vitamin C, vitamin B1 (thiamine), copper, and iron:** When vitamin C, vitamin B1 (thiamine), copper, and iron are put into a formula with B12, the vitamin B12 is turned to useless analogues.

- **Niacin and thiamine:** Cobalt ions (in B12 molecules) can contribute to the destruction of vitamin B1 when left sitting in liquid formulations. This may be intensified by the presence of nicotinamide, a form of niacin. The combination of vitamins B1 (thiamine) and B12 in a formulation could increase the likelihood of allergic reactions caused by thiamine.
- **Potassium:** Potassium supplements can reduce the absorption of vitamin B12 in some people and may contribute to vitamin B12 deficiency.

Micronutrients That Have Competitions with Iron
- **Vitamin E:** Iron can bind with vitamin E and inactivate it.
- **Calcium:** Calcium can inhibit the absorption of nonheme iron.
- **Chromium:** Chromium may compete with iron for binding to apo-transferrin (during absorption).
- **Copper:** Iron inhibits the absorption of copper. These two compete for protein binding sites. Some sources say that this may occur only when vitamin C is present.
- **Manganese:** High levels of iron or manganese will inhibit the absorption of the other.
- **Molybdenum:** Iron and molybdenum compete for the same intestinal brush-border receptor sites.
- **Phosphorus:** Iron and phosphorus compete for absorption.
- **Selenium:** Iron adversely affects the body's selenium status.
- **Zinc:** Iron and zinc both decrease the absorption of the other.

Micronutrients That Have Competitions with Magnesium
- **Vitamin K2:** Magnesium quickly degrades most forms of K2 MK-7 when combined in a formulation.
- **Calcium:** Calcium and magnesium compete for absorption.
- **Iron:** Magnesium intake inhibits nonheme iron absorption.
- **Manganese:** Magnesium may decrease manganese absorption.
- **Phosphorus:** High intake of phosphorus competes with magnesium.
- **Zinc:** High zinc intake may decrease magnesium absorption.

Shocking, right? We thought so, too. We couldn't believe how many of the vitamins and minerals that Mira needed to increase her bone density were competing within her multivitamin. The more we looked, it seemed that every bone-building supplement on the market was putting many of these competing micronutrients into a single formulation. We were shocked to discover that most of the supplement industry was well aware of micronutrient competitions, but even more shocked to find that no one seemed to care enough to do anything about it.

Many years ago, when we stumbled across the topic of micronutrient competition on the website of a large pharmacy chain, of all places, the problem suddenly became clear. According to their website, "Another area of controversy is whether all of the nutrients in a multiple would be better utilized if they were taken separately. Although certain nutrients compete with each other for absorption, this is also the case when the nutrients are supplied in food. For example, magnesium, zinc, and calcium compete; copper and zinc also compete. However, the body is designed to cope with this competition, which should not be a problem if multiples are spread out over the day."

Did you catch that? To begin, the article's author agreed with us regarding *beneficial quantities* by suggesting that their consumers take a multivitamin multiple times through out the day. Additionally, they acknowledged that micronutrient competitions exist and even gave a few great examples. However, then they simply disregarded the problem, stating that because competitions take place when you eat certain foods, they are not really a problem within your supplementation, as your body is designed to cope with them. This is completely the opposite of what researchers have discovered. Because the goal of taking a multivitamin or any other multinutrient supplement is to achieve micronutrient sufficiency by filling in the vitamin- and mineral-deficiency gaps in one's Rich Food diet, it is self-sabotaging to take a multivitamin that disregards micronutrient competition and instead combines all the micronutrients that are known to compete for absorption and utilization into a single formula. How could the bone-remodeling process that Mira needed to improve her bone health be supported when many of the micronutrients' bone benefits were being reduced or eliminated by micronutrient competitions?

Whereas other formulators simply threw up their hands and said,

"Well, the competitions take place in food, so we'll keep them in our multivitamin," we felt that by carefully separating any known competitors we could create our own multivitamin formulation that would have as few competitions as possible and thus enhanced absorption and utilization potential.

Because the foods we eat vary from day to day, we don't know which micronutrients our diet may leave us deficient in. The job of a well-formulated multivitamin is to cover the bases and do everything possible to ensure you absorb and utilize as many micronutrients as possible. Think of it this way: if you know that a certain micronutrient will reduce or eliminate the absorption or utilization of one or more micronutrients, then by eliminating that competitive micronutrient from the formulation, you have, by definition, enhanced the absorption and utilization potential for the micronutrients that would have been affected.

But it wasn't enough to simply believe. Although we felt the science behind our Anti-Competition Technology theory was sound, we needed proof that it would work in a clinical setting. So we began combing the medical and nutrition journals for any studies that would support our anti-competition theory. After all, we would have to overcome this third flaw in multivitamin formulation if we were going to have any success reversing Mira's osteoporosis. Luckily, our research led us to two studies that worked together to strengthen our belief in our anti-competition theory. The first was published back in 1998 in the *American Journal of Clinical Nutrition*; in it, researchers showed that "lutein negatively affected beta-carotene absorption when the two were given simultaneously." Science had determined that two nutrients, lutein and beta-carotene, compete, but what was still undetermined was if separating these competitive micronutrients could make any real difference. In 2002, the TOZAL study on age-related macular degeneration (AMD), an eye condition that leads to blindness and affects over two million people over age fifty, gave us this answer. For years, it was accepted in scientific circles that both lutein and beta-carotene individually had beneficial effects on patients with AMD. However, for the first time, in the TOZAL study, the competition between lutein and beta-carotene was accounted for. Supplementation that was previously unsuccessful was able to either improve or stabilize vision in 76.7 percent of patients. The study's developer, Edward Paul, OD, PhD, of the

International Academy of Low Vision Specialists, called the discovery "ground shaking," stating that this information "will really turn the way we look at nutrition on its ear." According to Dr. Paul, this new understanding of micronutrient competition represents a "huge paradigm shift when you consider that we had been recommending lutein be combined with other antioxidants, which is a reasonable thing to recommend. But when these two nutrients [lutein and beta-carotene] are competing for the same receptor site, they're only neutralizing one another."

This meant that when the competing micronutrients were separated, the beneficial effects of the individual micronutrients were finally realized—exactly the type of evidence we were looking for. With as many as forty-eight micronutrient competitions in a typical multivitamin, we felt that this was the reason numerous potential benefits were currently being unrealized by most multivitamin takers. We knew that our method of separating competing micronutrients to enhance absorption and utilization was truly innovative, but, amazingly, we discovered still a *fourth* overlooked factor that enhanced micronutrient absorption and utilization even more when paired with our anti-competition theory. It's called *micronutrient synergy*, and it's represented by the *s* in the ABCs of Optimal Supplementation Guidelines.

OPENING THE DOOR FOR SYNERGY

It turns out that micronutrient synergy is like a mirror image of micronutrient competition. Although micronutrient competitions can reduce or eliminate the benefits of certain micronutrients, micronutrient synergies can enhance the beneficial effects of certain micronutrients. But remember (and this is key): micronutrient synergies can offer enhanced absorption and utilization only if all of the micronutrient competitions that could affect their absorption have been eliminated. They cannot reverse or eliminate the effects of micronutrient competitions on their own. The *A*, *B*, and *C* in our ABCs are all capitalized, but we have left the *s* for synergies lower case. It is only when *A*, *B*, and *C* have all been accounted for that micronutrient synergies work to enhance overall results. You can think of micronutrient synergy as the icing on the ABCs of Optimal Supplementation cake. It is an important aspect for enhanced formulation, but one that can be realized only if *A*, *B*, and *C* are in place.

Let's refer to our trusty orchestra analogy once again. If our musicians stopped playing their instruments over one another and began following the sheet music again (i.e., the micronutrient competitions were accounted for), then the concerto could once again benefit from the composer's intentional synergistic pairing of certain instruments. In other words, if the trombones were no longer drowning out the melody of the violins, and the drums were no longer masking the sound of the harps, then when the violin and harps were played together as the composer intended, the synergistic harmony created would enhance the musical piece. Even if the violins and harps were both synergistically playing the musical piece exactly as the composer had intended, if all the other instruments, including the trombones and drums, were all still randomly playing (i.e., the competitions were not accounted for), then the synergy between the violins and harp would not be realized. Directly stated, the benefits of synergistic micronutrients can be realized only when the competitions are eliminated.

Just as there are four types of micronutrient competitions, there are also four types of micronutrient synergies:

Chemical synergy is the opposite of chemical competition. It occurs in the nutritional supplement itself, prior to ingestion, when two micronutrients are put into the same multivitamin to form an advantageous complex that can help increase the absorption of one or both micronutrients. Vitamin B2 (riboflavin) and zinc share such a relationship.

Biochemical synergy is the opposite of biochemical competition. Here, rather than competing for a receptor site or absorption pathway, one micronutrient aids in the absorption of the other. An example is when vitamin D enhances the absorption of calcium.

Physiological synergy is the opposite of physiological competition. Instead of two micronutrients decreasing each other's utilization, one micronutrient aids in the performance of a second micronutrient. This can happen when one micronutrient needs to perform a specific function in order for a second micronutrient to do its job. For example, vitamin K2 is required to direct calcium out of the blood and into the bone, where it is needed to combat osteoporosis.

Clinical synergy is the opposite of clinical competition. Clinical synergy occurs when two or more micronutrients work together to create an observable yet unexpected beneficial change in the body. For example, when vitamins B6, B9 (folate), and B12 are all present in adequate quantities, they have been shown to lower homocysteine levels (a known marker of osteoporosis) by converting homocysteine into cysteine and methionine.

In fact, when you draw out all the synergies that can occur between thirty-four of the micronutrients most often included in a multivitamin supplement, like the micronutrient competitions, the synergies also look like a big spiderweb—but this time, the web represents potential benefits. In all, our research has identified thirty-two synergies that can occur between those thirty-four micronutrients, with twenty-three of the thirty-four (68 percent) having at least three synergies, and seventeen of the thirty-four (50 percent) having at least five synergies. Missing out on these incredible, benefit-boosting synergies can slow down or even impair your bones' ability to remodel. When we go into osteoporosis chat rooms on Facebook, as many of you likely do, we often read posts about individuals supplementing with only a few micronutrients, such as vitamin D or extra calcium, while completely disregarding others. If you remember back in Chapter 2, we showed you that all of the essential micronutrients are required for bone health in some way. By taking a multivitamin that has not eliminated the competitions or by just taking a few bone-building supplements without adequate amounts of all of their synergistic micronutrients, you may be missing out on all the bone-boosting benefits that micronutrient synergies can deliver. Let's take a brief look at how beneficial these synergies can be. (We will look at the same bone-building nutrients as earlier in our discussion on competitions.)

Micronutrients That Are Synergistic with Calcium

- **Vitamin B12:** Calcium is required for the proper absorption of vitamin B12.
- **Vitamin D:** Vitamin D increases the intestinal absorption of calcium and regulates metabolism and the efficiency of its utilization.

- **Vitamin K:** Vitamin K and calcium share a physiological synergy in that vitamin K2 must be present in the body when calcium arrives. This is essential for the formation of bone tissue.
- **Boron:** Boron converts vitamin D to its more active form, which in turn indirectly helps in the absorption of calcium for bone health.
- **Magnesium:** Magnesium helps retain serum blood calcium. This physiological synergy may be why slight magnesium deficiencies have been shown to elicit decreased serum calcium concentrations.
- **Omega-3:** Omega-3 increases both calcium absorption and retention.
- **Potassium:** High consumption of potassium reduces the urinary excretion of calcium.
- **Silicon:** Dietary silicon helps calcium absorption.

Micronutrients That Are Synergistic with Vitamin K

- **Vitamin E:** Vitamin E helps the body utilize vitamin K.
- **Calcium:** Calcium and vitamin K share a physiological synergy, in that vitamin K2 must be present in the body when calcium arrives. This is essential for the formation of bone tissue.
- **Manganese:** Manganese functions with vitamin K in the formation of prothrombin (a blood-clotting protein).

Micronutrients That Are Synergistic with Vitamin B12

- **Vitamin B6:** Vitamin B6 works synergistically with vitamin B12 to lower homocysteine levels. Vitamin B6 is required for vitamin B12 to be absorbed properly. A deficiency of B6 will impair B12 absorption and likely cause a deficiency of B12.
- **Vitamin B9 (folate):** Vitamin B9 works synergistically with vitamin B12 to lower homocysteine levels. Vitamins B9 and B12 and iron work synergistically to improve the hematosis process. Folate works along with vitamin B12 and vitamin C to help the body break down, use, and create new proteins. Additionally, a deficiency in B12 can generate a large pool of methyl-THF

that is unable to undergo reactions and will mimic a folate deficiency.

- **Vitamin C:** Vitamin C works with B12 and folate to help the body break down, use, and create new proteins.
- **Vitamin E:** Vitamin E is required for vitamin B12 to convert from its nonactive form to its biologically active form. Individuals at risk for vitamin E deficiency may show signs of vitamin B12 deficiency as well.
- **Calcium:** Calcium is required for proper absorption of B12.
- **Iron:** Vitamins B9 and B12 and iron work synergistically to improve the hematosis (formation of blood cells) process.

Micronutrients That Are Synergistic with Iron

- **Vitamin A:** Vitamin A increases the absorption of iron. Vitamin A deficiency causes anemia; this shows that although it is not fully understood, vitamin A impacts the metabolism of iron, most likely by affecting the transport of iron and the production of red blood cells. It may be because vitamin A may prevent the depletion of iron caused by phytates.
- **Vitamin B2 (riboflavin):** Riboflavin is necessary for the absorption of iron. Riboflavin deficiency may impair the absorption and utilization of iron.
- **Vitamin B9 (folic acid):** Vitamins B9 and B12 and iron work synergistically to improve the hematosis process.
- **Vitamin B12:** Vitamins B9 and B12 and iron work synergistically to improve the hematosis process.
- **Vitamin C:** Elevated vitamin C levels can cause increased absorption of nonheme iron. Vitamin C may also influence the storage and transport of iron.
- **Copper:** Copper shares a physiological synergy with iron. The transport of iron around the body relies in many ways on the presence of copper. This relationship is extremely important because iron-deficiency anemia may sometimes reflect the more basic underlying problem of copper deficiency.
- **Iodine:** The effects of a deficiency of iodine can be exacerbated by a deficiency of iron.

Micronutrients That Are Synergistic with Magnesium

- **Vitamin B6:** High amounts of vitamin B6 increase magnesium retention, resulting in a high-magnesium/low-calcium ratio. Too much B6 results in a calcium deficiency.
- **Vitamin D:** Vitamin D slightly increases the intestinal absorption of magnesium. Magnesium has been found to influence the body's utilization of vitamin D in the following ways: magnesium activates cellular enzymatic activity. In fact, it appears that all the enzymes that metabolize vitamin D require magnesium. Additionally, low magnesium has been shown to decrease production of vitamin D's active form, 1,25(OH)2D (calcitriol).
- **Boron:** Boron plays an important role in the metabolism of magnesium.
- **Calcium:** Magnesium helps retain serum blood calcium. This physiological synergy may be why slight magnesium deficiencies have been shown to elicit decreased serum calcium concentrations.
- **Potassium:** Potassium and magnesium share a physiological synergy because magnesium regulates the movement of potassium in and out of the cells.
- **Omega-3:** Magnesium is required for delta-6-desaturase to convert ALA to EPA.
- **Omega-6:** Magnesium is required for delta-6-desaturase to convert LA to GLA.

Fixing Flaws 3 and 4: Micronutrient Competitions and Synergies

Like **A**bsorption and **B**eneficial quantities and forms (flaws 1 and 2), you can see how important it is to take a multivitamin formulated to separate the known micronutrient **C**ompetitions and pair the **s**ynergistic micronutrients. Remember, understanding micronutrient competitions and synergies can help us understand why many of the benefits often associated with individual micronutrients are often unrealized when those same micronutrients are paired randomly within a typical multivitamin or bone-building formulation. According to the late Derek H. Shrimpton, PhD, scientific advisor to the European Federation of Health Product Manufacturers, the benefits of a multivitamin "may not be fully realized in those instances where the possibility of micronutrient interaction [competitions and synergies] has been ignored." When evaluating your supplement, use Table 6.5, to see how your multivitamin stacks up regarding the *C* and *s* of our ABCs of Optimal Supplementation Guidelines.

TABLE 6.5 Identifying Whether Your Supplement Follows the Rules for Competitions and Synergies

Make Sure Your Multivitamin . . .	✓ if Yes
Does not contain both vitamin B9 (folate) and zinc in the same dose	
Does not contain both calcium and magnesium in the same dose	
Does not contain vitamin K2 and calcium or magnesium in the same dose, or utilizes vitamin K2 VITAL Delta form to ensure potency	
Does not contain both calcium and zinc in the same dose	
Does not contain both lutein and beta-carotene in the same dose	
Does not contain both vitamin B5 and copper in the same dose	
Does not contain both vitamin A and vitamin D in the same dose	
Does not contain both zinc and copper in the same dose	
Does not contain both vitamin B5 and B7 (biotin) in the same dose	
Does not contain iron at all	
Does not contain copper at all	
Does contain both calcium and silicon in the same dose	
Does contain both vitamin B2 and zinc in the same dose	
Does state that it is formulated using patented Anti-Competition Technology on packaging to account for all competitions and synergies	

Putting the ABCs Together

Identifying the four flaws that reduce a multivitamin's overall effectiveness left us with our ABCs of Optimal Supplementation Guidelines. And although our guidelines were originally developed to evaluate the multivitamin, they can really help increase the absorption and utilization potential of any nutritional supplement—especially a supplement you might take for your osteoporosis. When we put the ABCs of Optimal Supplementation Guidelines together, they revealed that the most effective multivitamin would be a single-serving, powdered formula taken in liquid form free of binders, fillers, excipients (bulking and flow agents), artificial flavors and colors, and sugars. It would contain beneficial quantities (approximately 100 percent of the RDI) of each micronutrient, with two exceptions: calcium would be lower than the RDI (around 500 milligrams) and vitamin D would be higher than the RDI (around 2,000 IU). Additionally, where applicable, the multivitamin would also contain a full spectrum of beneficial forms for each micronutrient and be formulated to separate known competitive micronutrients to enhance absorption and utilization. This would require that it contain at least two completely different formulations to be taken at two different times during the day. And lastly, synergistic micronutrients would be paired in each formula to enhance the potential health benefits of each micronutrient.

SOLVING THE ABCS OF SUPPLEMENTATION

Our ABCs of Optimal Supplementation Guidelines had certainly painted a very different picture of what a properly formulated multivitamin should look like. Because we believed that eliminating these four flaws in the multivitamin would be essential to Mira's healing, we were in pursuit of a highly absorbable multivitamin that contained the beneficial quantities and forms we were looking for, eliminated micronutrient competitions, and paired synergistic nutrients. But sadly, there was not even a single multivitamin on the market that came close. If there had been even one other multivitamin that met our guidelines we would have been thrilled to use it (and would likely be suggesting it to you right now).

So out of necessity, we began purchasing the beneficial quantities and most bioavailable forms of each micronutrient separately, and, in order to avoid competitions, we took them in small, noncompetitive groupings before and after each of our four meals, eight times throughout the day. Two or three pills before breakfast, three or four after, and so on, until the thirty-plus pills we had to take each day were gone. We tried to eliminate absorption issues by opening some of the capsules and pouring the contents into water, but frankly, most were not palatable.

If you decide to embark on this anti-competition method as we once did, you will find that separating competing nutrients can bring about amazing results. However, you may also find it to be quite expensive, with the individual nutrients costing you somewhere in the neighborhood of $150 per person per month. You may also find, as Mira did, that taking the required ten thousand-plus pills a year can become tiresome and daunting. Additionally, the science behind mapping all of the competing and synergistic nutrients is complex, and it may be more than you have time to take on.

But after two years of utilizing our anti-competition method, it had worked! The proof was in witnessing Mira's incredible recovery through her follow-up DEXA scan. Because of the success of our anti-competition method, we started all of our clients on a similar regimen, and we were thrilled to see their health improve as well. However, it wasn't long before our clients also started complaining about our anti-competition, pill-stacking method. From global executives to busy moms, they all wanted something simple and convenient. "Why can't *you* just create something that we can take a couple of times a day?" they would ask. So we decided to do just that.

Since there was nothing on the market that followed the ABCs of Optimal Supplementation Guidelines to the letter, we had no choice but to create one ourselves. Our goal was to formulate a complete multivitamin that would eliminate all four of the flaws we had identified in the typical multivitamin, which we believed were responsible for reducing its overall effectiveness. So we worked closely with the U.S. Patent and Trademark Office to validate our anti-competition method for micronutrient absorption, and after six years and countless formulation attempts, we were granted the U.S. patent on Anti-Competition Technology, and used this technology to create our product, Nutreince, which we believe is the modern reinvention of the multivitamin.

We take Nutreince twice daily and instruct our private clients to do the same in order to support bone health. We highly recommend that you do so as well while following the Rebuild Your Bones twelve-week osteoporosis protocol. For those who opt to search for their own multivitamin among the plethora of products lining store shelves from respected manufacturers like Garden of Life, NOW, and Thorne Research, we strongly suggest you take our Multivitamin Stack-Up Quiz (at CompareYourMulti.com). We cannot stress enough the importance of this extremely thorough and free analysis. After filling in some specific information about the multivitamin you're considering, we will give you a fair and objective score and an in-depth, multipage evaluation of its strengths and weaknesses. Remember, the entire objective of the Rebuild Your Bones twelve-week osteoporosis protocol is to help you achieve micronutrient sufficiency, and supplementing with a properly formulated multivitamin is an essential step to achieving that goal.

Although a properly formulated multivitamin has the potential to help you reach sufficiency in your essential vitamins and minerals, it will not do the same for your amino acids or essential fatty acids. This is why, in Chapter 7, we will share with you the best ways to meet these additional requirements. You will also uncover whether higher quantities of specific bone-building micronutrients are beneficial in certain circumstances, as well as additional supplements you may want to consider that have been proven to aid in bone remodeling. We aren't done with our discussion of micronutrient supplementation quite yet. There is still a lot more important information to uncover before beginning the Rebuild Your Bones twelve-week osteoporosis protocol.

Healing Habits Revealed in Chapter 6

34. Choose only supplements that have the highest **A**bsorption potential.
35. Take supplements that deliver **B**eneficial quantities and forms of each micronutrient.
36. Look for supplements formulated to eliminate micronutrient **C**ompetitions.
37. Make sure your supplements pair **s**ynergistic micronutrients.

Whew! That was a lot of technical information on how competitions and synergies occur. In this chapter's "On the Couch" chat, we will simplify this topic a bit to help you fully grasp the importance of taking a properly formulated supplement. We will discuss the four healing habits we introduced you to in this chapter and break the ABCs down, making them simple and easy to understand. It is a good idea to have your current supplementation handy when watching this next video. Join us now at RebuildYourBones.com.

CHAPTER 7

Supplementation and Testing Methods Beyond the ABCs

Research is to see what everyone else has seen, and to think what nobody else has thought.

—ALBERT SZENT-GYÖRGYI, MD, PHD, WINNER
OF THE NOBEL PRIZE FOR MEDICINE, 1973

We spent the last chapter discussing how the ABCs of Optimal Supplementation can affect the absorption and utilization of your essential vitamins and minerals; in this chapter, we will move beyond the benefits of a properly formulated multivitamin to discuss whether, in some cases, higher levels of specific essential micronutrients may be beneficial for bone health. We will also review the other two members of the essential micronutrient family, your amino acids and essential fatty acids, which will both be part of your daily Rebuild Your Bones osteoporosis protocol for the next twelve weeks, and give you the tools to choose properly formulated supplements. Additionally, we'll identify additional nonessential accessory nutrients you may want to consider as icing on your micronutrient supplementation cake, and finally we will share with you the lab tests we recommend to monitor your progress and keep you moving forward, safely and fully informed on your journey to healthy bones.

Upping the Essentials for Maximum Bone Building

Although supplementing with the RDI for each essential micronutrient in combination with a Rich Food diet *should* be enough to put you on a path to better bone health, these levels may not always be adequate for everyone to reverse osteoporosis. Many times, because of age, environmental factors, chosen diet, lifestyle habits, or just poor digestion, some people may need greater quantities of some micronutrients in order to create their desired bone-remodeling effects. Here are a few key micronutrients that have been shown to be beneficial to the bone-building process that you may want to consider adding on top of your daily multivitamin. If you are taking Nutreince, feel free to download the Accessory Supplement Scheduling Chart, which clearly outlines proper timing to reduce nutrient competitions, at RebuildYourBones.com.

- **Vitamin B12:** Individuals following a vegan diet, seniors, and those with reduced stomach acid should consider supplementation with a sublingual vitamin B12. Sublingual supplements can be taken even by those who have less than optimal digestive health, and they will not compete with any other micronutrients in your gut. *When to take:* You can take your extra sublingual B12 anytime (up to 1,000 mcg daily).
- **Vitamin C:** Daily doses of up to 1,000 mg have been shown to be beneficial for bone mass. Be warned: daily doses of 200 mg or more should be avoided if you are on statins. *When to take:* You can take your extra vitamin C supplementation anytime; just be sure to increase your dosage slowly, as too much vitamin C can cause loose stool.
- **Vitamin D3:** If you are deficient in vitamin D, make sure to take at a minimum 2,000 IU. Our clients find that within a month or two, their vitamin D rises to optimal levels because of the anti-competitive formulation. However, should you decide to supplement further, we prefer a liquid vitamin D3. *Warning:* Make sure not to purchase a combination D3 and K2 supplement. The two nutrients will compete. *When to take:* Take away from any supplements that contain competing nutrients.
- **Vitamin K2:** When trying to increase your bone density (and especially if you are taking extra calcium), we suggest taking a liquid vitamin K2 (MK7) supplement at around 120–240 mcg daily, on top of what is in your multivitamin. If your K2 supplement delivers MK4, rather than MK7, research indicates that

larger quantities (15–45 mg, three times per day) will be necessary, because of its short half-life. This will ensure that your calcium will be directed to your bones and not allowed to remain in the arteries. Although many cardiovascular doctors prefer the use of products that don't contain vitamin K for patients on warfarin (Coumadin), we ask that you work with your doctor to find and regulate your prescription levels rather than omit this essential micronutrient with so many bone-building benefits. *Warning:* Most vitamin K products also contain vitamin D. As these two nutrients compete for absorption, they should be taken separately. *When to take:* Take away from any supplements that contain competing nutrients.

- **Boron:** Therapeutic doses for boron range from 3 to 6 mg. Boron is synergistic with both calcium and magnesium. *When to take:* Take with either your calcium or magnesium supplement.

- **Calcium:** Most physicians recommend taking 1,300 mg of calcium a day. If you take Nutreince, you will be ingesting 500 mg through supplementation. It is your choice then if you want to focus on eating another 800 mg a day through calcium-rich foods, or if you want to take an additional calcium supplement. *Remember:* You don't have to worry about the studies where excess calcium caused arterial calcification, as long as you make sure to take your extra vitamin K2. *When to take:* If you take Nutreince and decide to take an additional 500- or 600-mg supplement (remember that calcium cannot be absorbed at over 600 mg in a single serving), you will need to take the extra calcium at midday away from food and both the a.m. and p.m. Nutreince packets (or other multivitamin).

- **GLA:** Although we strive to keep omega-6 levels low and in balance with omega-3s on the Rebuild Your Bones osteoporosis protocol, gamma-linolenic acid (GLA) is an omega-6 fatty acid that has anti-inflammatory properties similar to those of omega-3s (unlike other omega-6s, which are considered inflammatory). Studies show that supplementing with GLA (200–300 mg) can help support healthy progesterone levels and increase bone density. *When to take:* You can take your GLA supplementation anytime.

- **Silica:** Therapeutic doses for silica range from 6 to 20 mg. *When to take:* Extra silica can be taken anytime, as it is noncompetitive. However, we suggest taking silica in the form of horsetail alongside calcium, because silica can aid in the absorption of calcium.

PICKING THE PERFECT PROTEIN POWDER

As we mentioned in Chapter 4, dietary protein supplies us with our amino acids. Just as the body can rob micronutrients such as calcium from your bones when you do not get enough of it through your diet, potentially leading to osteoporosis, the body will also begin to break down muscle tissue to obtain the essential amino acids it needs when they are not obtained through your diet. And just like water-soluble vitamins, the body does not store excess amino acids for later use, so you must get all your essential amino acids through protein-based food or a supplement each day. But don't worry, because getting enough of your essential amino acids during your twelve-week program is as simple as it is delicious. In Chapter 8, we will show you how to incorporate a quality protein powder into your menu plan so that you can get all the wonderful health benefits associated with a diet that includes enough protein. Let's begin by identifying how to choose quality whey- or plant-based proteins.

CHOOSING A QUALITY WHEY PROTEIN

Finding a good whey protein powder can be difficult. Although there are many to choose from, few meet our high standards. We suggest supplementing your protein intake with a 100 percent organic, non-GMO, grass-fed, whey protein concentrate. First, by choosing only organic, grass-fed products you are saving yourself from the vast majority of low-quality protein powders that have been derived from sick cows that have likely been fed GMO corn and soy and given antibiotics and steroids. Next, although all whey protein will provide you with a full spectrum of your essential amino acids, we suggest that you find a product labeled as a protein *concentrate*, not a protein *isolate*. This is because whey protein concentrates deliver the all the key health components naturally found in whey, whereas protein isolates remove the fat from the whey, and by doing so also remove many of its key health components with immuno-logical properties, such as phospholipids and phosphatidylserine.

Whey protein concentrates also naturally contain lactoferrin, which, as we mentioned in Chapter 4, has been proven to positively affect both the osteoclasts and the osteoblasts in the remodeling activity of bone. You wouldn't want that removed if your goal is bone building, right? Finally, all of the igG immunoglobulins, which are an excellent source of glutamine and cysteine (amino acids), are also bound to the natu-rally occurring fat. Removing them reduces the ability of the essen-tial micronutrients to act as the precursors of a spectacular antioxidant called glutathione.

Although you may have never heard of glutathione before, it is your body's most powerful antioxidant and it works amazingly well as a scav-enger of free radicals. Remember, free radicals cause oxidative dam-age, and this has been directly linked to adulterated bone remodeling. Not only is glutathione a powerful antioxidant that can help us heal our bones, but glutathione levels are also one of the greatest predictors of overall health. When researchers studied the relationship between glutathione levels and overall health, the individuals with the highest levels of glutathione were the healthiest. Those with the lowest levels were the sickest and often hospitalized. In fact, nearly ninety thousand medical articles have been written about this one disease-preventing micronutrient alone because it is so important to your ability to achieve optimal health.

Glutathione protects your cells from oxidative damage and helps:

- Build strong bones
- Build a strong immune system
- Reduce inflammation
- Optimize your central nervous system
- Fight infections
- Prevent cancer
- Help in the treatment of AIDS
- Detoxify your body

- Protect your body from alcohol damage
- Promote heart health
- Increase strength and endurance
- Shift metabolism from fat producing to muscle building
- Flush out heavy metals including mercury
- Promote longevity and protect from chronic illness

However, glutathione is one micronutrient that doesn't appear to be as effective in supplement form as it is in real food. In fact, supplemental glutathione may interfere with your body's ability to naturally produce glutathione over time. So it is crucial to get glutathione from your food, and although foods such as onions, garlic, and cruciferous vegetables like broccoli, cauliflower, and Brussels sprouts can help increase your levels naturally, the best food for truly maximizing your glutathione levels is organic whey protein concentrate.

Because of the power of glutathione, an organic grass-fed whey protein concentrate is a true superfood, and one that we strongly suggest you incorporate into your Rebuild Your Bones twelve-week osteoporosis protocol so that you can take advantage of all the amazing health benefits it has to offer. Although advances in manufacturing have recently created some specialized protein isolates that still contain the key health components commonly found in whey concentrates, don't be fooled: these proteins are still not from organic non-GMO grass-fed cows. Because of this, as well as the multiple processes these proteins must undergo, at this time we still recommend using a natural, minimally processed whey protein concentrate.

CHOOSING A QUALITY PLANT PROTEIN

Now, if you are one of our vegan nutrivores or if you can't tolerate whey, don't think that we forgot about you. Instead of whey, we encourage you to use a high-quality plant protein powder during your twelve-week program. However, it is going to be a little harder to get all of your essential amino acids. That is because soy protein is the only plant-based protein to have a complete amino acid profile like whey protein. But as we mentioned before, soy protein is often derived from

GMO soy (94 percent of all US-grown soy is GMO) and is not rec-ommended by most health professionals for several reasons. First, soy contains a class of compounds called isoflavones, which are phytoestro-gens and have been shown to mimic the effects of the female hormone estrogen. Although some experts recommend soy for this reason, for people with osteoporosis, high estrogen levels have been associated with increased risk of certain cancers in both men and women. Addition-ally, increased estrogen levels in men can lead to sexual dysfunction, reduced body hair, and even the development of gynecomastia (female breasts). And lastly, in addition to the fact that soy is full of antinutrients (including phytic acid, oxalic aid, lectins, and trypsin inhibitors), it also contains goitrogens, substances that suppress the function of the thyroid gland and can interfere with the absorption of iodine. This can result in lower metabolism and weight gain. Because of these reasons, we feel it is best to use a combination of pea, rice, or hemp protein. Remember, only by combining plant proteins can you build a plant protein that has a full spectrum of bone-building and muscle-building essential amino acids. For plant proteins, try to source sprouted proteins to reduce their naturally occurring antinutrients.

BEWARE OF FILLERS AND TOXINS

Regardless of whether you choose a whey or plant protein, you need to look for a high-quality product. Look for certified organic non-GMO products that are third-party tested for heavy metals. Recently, several studies testing protein powders have uncovered potentially dangerous levels of heavy metals in many popular brands—levels exceeding the limits proposed safe by United States Pharmacopeia (USP). Daily use can allow these heavy metals to accumulate in the body over time, making it important to ask the manufacturer for heavy metal test results. Also, make sure the protein you choose is free of fillers, artificial colors, artificial flavors, artificial sweeteners, sugar, soy lecithin, maltodextrin, modified food starch, and carrageenan. Lastly, try to find environmen-tally sustainable products that were grown/raised in the United States and have minimal processing to protect the proteins. To make things easy for you, we developed our organic IN.POWER grass-fed whey and sprouted plant protein powders. If you choose to use another brand, you can use Table 7.1 below to help you choose a safe, high-quality protein.

TABLE 7.1 Identifying Whether Your Protein Powder Follows the Rules

Make Sure Your Protein Powder . . .	✓ if Yes
Does not contain heavy metals (ask for a heavy metal report)	
Is labeled as USDA organic or similar	
Does contain the full spectrum of amino acids (this would require that multiple plants be combined if utilizing plant protein)	
Is grass fed (if whey)	
Is a concentrate (important for both whey and plant)	
Is sprouted (if plant)	
Does not contain artificial colors, artificial flavors, artificial sweeteners, sugar, soy lecithin, maltodextrin, or carrageenan	
Does not contain vitamins and minerals (you don't want them to compete with Nutreince)	

BUY A BONE-TASTIC OMEGA-3 SUPPLEMENT

In Chapter 4, you learned a lot about the bone benefits associated with having an omega-6 to omega-3 ratio of approximately 1:1. You also learned the importance of taking an omega-3 supplement that delivers beneficial quantities of both EPA and DHA. Now we are going to take a more in-depth look at how to purchase the best omega-3 supplements on the market to make sure you get all of the earlier reported benefits. There are four things to consider before purchasing an omega-3 supplement.

1: Is Your Omega-3 Supplement in the Beneficial Triglyceride Form?
Here we go again . . . talking about beneficial forms. Just as with your vitamins and minerals, the form of the omega-3 you purchase will also determine if your product is high-quality or low-quality. First, you should know that many omega-3 products on the market today are using the less expensive, inferior *ethyl ester* form over the superior *triglyceride*

form. Put plainly, although ethyl esters are seemingly safe for human consumption, scientific research consistently confirms three facts:

1. **Ethyl esters are not efficient.** The metabolism of an ethyl ester is less efficient than triglycerides. In, fact, it takes the digestive enzyme lipase as much as fifty times longer to break the ethyl ester bond compared to the triglyceride bond, and longer still in individuals with digestive disorders.
2. **Ethyl esters are poorly absorbed.** The triglyceride form of omega-3 is at least 70 percent better absorbed in the gut than the ethyl ester form. One study showed the EPA and DHA from triglycerides being 340 percent and 271 percent better absorbed, respectively.
3. **Ethyl esters are less stable.** The triglyceride form of omega-3 is far more stable than an ethyl ester. That stability protects against oxidation and makes it safer for a longer period of time.

Wondering if your fish oil is delivered in triglyceride or ethyl ester form?

Visit us at RebuildYourBones.com/FishOilTest to do a quick at-home experiment. You might be shocked by what you discover.

2: Does Your Omega-3 Supplement Deliver the Beneficial Quantities of EPA and DHA?

Most omega-3 supplements also don't deliver beneficial quantities of both EPA and DHA. They have either no EPA and DHA or such small quantities that the consumer would never be able to reach the dosage shown in published research to be beneficial. There are two distinct types of omega-3 supplements, each with its own set of possible drawbacks: plant sources (flaxseed and chia), and fish, krill, and algae sources.

As we stated earlier, although popular plant-derived omega-3s (like flaxseed and chia) do have anti-inflammatory effects and will help you achieve a lower ratio of omega-6 to omega-3 in your diet, they *do not* contain EPA or DHA. Instead, they contain only alpha-linoleic acid (ALA), which the body has to convert into EPA and then into DHA. The problem with plant-based omega-3 supplements is that studies on ALA metabolism in healthy young men indicate that only 5 to 10 percent of dietary ALA is converted to EPA and 2 to 5 percent is then converted to DHA. Women can convert ALA to EPA and then to DHA approximately 2.5 times better than men can. This means that even at the highest conversion rates, a 1,000-mg plant-derived omega-3 capsule would produce only approximately 100 mg (10 percent) of EPA and 50 mg (5 percent) of DHA in men, and 210 mg (21 percent) of EPA and 90 mg (9 percent) of DHA in women. These quantities are nowhere near what is considered beneficial by the medical and nutritional communities.

Omega-3 supplements from fish, krill, or algae (a vegan source) all contain EPA and DHA, but that doesn't mean it's enough to be effective either. Many omega-3 supplements advertise high levels of omega-3 (ALA), but upon closer examination, they supply only minimal levels of EPA and DHA. This makes it important to read the supplement facts carefully. Most research states that between 1.5 and 4 grams (1,500–4,000 mg) of EPA and DHA are required per day to be anti-inflammatory and have a positive effect on bone metabolism—far more than many fish, krill, or algae supplements provide.

3: Does Your Omega-3 Supplement Separate EPA and DHA?

Lastly, let's discuss perhaps the most important issue of all: the fact that even if an omega-3 supplement were delivered in a superior triglyceride form and contained beneficial quantities of both EPA and DHA, if the EPA and DHA were combined in the same dose, your ability to absorb them would be greatly reduced because of inherent micronutrient competitions. Amazingly, the competition between EPA and DHA is widely known throughout the scientific communities but is virtually unknown by the consumer.

Much like the vitamin and mineral competitions you uncovered in the previous chapter, the competition between EPA and DHA can make the process of omega-3 absorption more like an epic battle scene than a harmonious event. Because EPA has a relatively similar structure to DHA, they compete for occupation of active binding sites and reduce their activity. Unfortunately, most supplement companies simply over-look this competition for absorption when formulating their omega-3 supplements. Scientists agree that separating EPA and DHA increases their ability to have desirable biological effects. Because recent research from the journal *Nutrition Research* determined that "both EPA and DHA are probably necessary to optimize osteoblastogenesis and slow bone resorption," it is important to choose an omega-3 supplement that separates EPA from DHA.

4: Is Your Omega-3 Supplement Oxidized or Rancid?

Oxidation occurs when the unsaturated fatty acids found in fats and oils are exposed to oxygen. Upon reaction with oxygen from the air, the chemical bonds in the fatty acid molecules break down to form new molecules. All lipids containing unsaturated fatty acids oxidize over time, regardless of whether they come in the form of cooking oils or fish oil capsules, and this can ultimately lead to the oil becoming rancid.

This oxidation in fish oil products is usually to blame for the fishy taste or odor. But oxidation also affects fish oil in other negative ways. When fish oil is oxidized it has lower levels of EPA and DHA, supplies fewer health benefits, and may actually cause negative health conditions. Oxidized fish oil not only fails to deliver the promised health benefits of omega-3 fatty acids, but it actually produces a negative impact on cholesterol levels for women.

So how rampant is rancidity? Although we don't want to sound alarmist, the published reports out of New Zealand, South Africa, Nor-way, and Canada analyzing oxidation in popular omega-3 products are concerning. New Zealand researchers found that 83 percent of the prod-ucts tested exceeded recommended industry peroxide levels—a measure of primary oxidation. A similar study from South Africa reported the number at 80 percent for their over-the-counter fish oil supplements. In Norway, where fish oil supplementation originated, the results were even worse. A 2012 study demonstrated that over 92 percent of the products analyzed exceeded recommended industry levels. Yet the most upsetting results come from a recent Canadian study, which found that children's omega-3 products had the highest oxidation values of all. The study determined that encapsulated products without flavor ad-ditives had significantly lower oxidation levels than bulk oils and flavored products. *(This is because manufacturers use natural flavors and scents to cover up oxidation.)* Never purchase omega-3 supplements without asking the manufacturer for a TOTOX score, which reports the markers and guidelines for oxidation safety.

OMEGA-3 FOR VEGANS

If you have decided to use a plant-based omega-3, you may want to consider a two-pronged approach—getting some of your omega-3 from flaxseed oil and some from a supplement derived from algae. Like fish and krill oil, algae contains both EPA and DHA (more DHA than EPA), but as you just learned, because of the competition between the two, it is better to separate them. However, there are very few pure EPA algae products on the market, and those that exist not only contain very small amounts of EPA but are also extremely expensive. Because of this, we recommend taking flaxseed oil for your EPA and a separate pure DHA algae product. This approach would give you the potential of converting as much as 21 percent of your flaxseed-oil-derived omega-3 to EPA (if you are a woman) and getting your DHA from your algae supplement. Additionally, research shows that the human body converts DHA to EPA at a rate of approximately 12 percent, so it is possible to get some EPA by simply taking a high-potency DHA supplement.

PUTTING IT ALL TOGETHER

Now that you know the four questions to ask before purchasing an omega-3 supplement, you can choose to search out and find a high-quality, triglyceride-form EPA and a separate DHA product or you can try our product—Origin Omega—which has done the work for you. Using our patented Anti-Competition Technology, we split the more than 1,500 mg of EPA and DHA in Origin Omega into separate morning and evening servings, naturally eliminating their competition. This allows you to rest assured that your omega-3 product is formulated for optimal absorption and extraordinary results. And, because Origin

Omega is made exclusively for Calton Nutrition, we can guarantee its freshness and are happy to share our glowing TOTOX results with you.

Whether you are looking for a fish, krill, or algae supplement, use the following rules from Table 7.2 to identify a high-quality supplement.

TABLE 7.2 Identifying Whether Your Omega-3 Supplement Follows the Rules

Make Sure Your Omega-3 Supplement . . .	✓ if Yes
Is delivered in triglyceride form	
Does contain beneficial quantities of both EPA and DHA	
Does separate the EPA from the DHA in two separate doses	
Is not oxidized (make sure to ask for a TOTOX report)	

HEALTHY FATS TO REDUCE INFLAMMATION

Remember back in Chapter 4, we learned that although increasing omega-3 intake through supplementation is key, it is equally essential to greatly reduce your intake of omega-6. This requires you to ditch oils that are high in omega-6 such as grapeseed, olive, sunflower, and avocado and replace them with oils that have low or no omega-6.

You've probably already heard about the scientifically proven, heart-healthy, cholesterol-normalizing, immune-supportive, thyroid-boosting, antibacterial, and antiviral properties of organic coconut oil. Coconut oil is a great alternative to those omega-6 heavy oils listed earlier for many recipes. Keep in mind, though, that because it's solid at room temperature, it's not the best choice for cold recipes like salad dressings and smoothies. Additionally, some people find the flavor off-putting.

If you haven't heard about MCT oil yet, you're going to love this: MCT simply stands for *medium-chain triglycerides*, specialized fats that have been naturally extracted from coconut or palm oil. Not only is it nearly impossible for your body to store MCT oil as body fat, but peer-reviewed published research also shows that MCT oil increases metabolism, reduces body fat, and improves insulin sensitivity and glucose tolerance. These benefits are fantastic in shakes, dressings, and food cooked at very low temperatures (below 350°F). However, new users of MCT oil sometimes report upset stomach as a side effect. You can avoid this by starting with smaller doses and increasing your intake slowly as your body learns to tolerate it.

Coconut oil and MCT oil are both great ways to help reduce your levels of inflammatory omega-6. An additional option is SKINNY Fat—an incredibly healthy oil that we created by blending these beneficial oils in carefully chosen ratios to deliver the maximum benefits with none of the drawbacks. It's flavorless (although an olive oil option is also available), stays liquid at room temperature, and heats to 350°F safely, making it versatile for use in hot or cold dishes. If you're interested in learning more, visit RebuildYourBones.com.

HEALTHY FATS HELP YOU ABSORB YOUR MICRONUTRIENTS TOO!

Whether on a salad or when taking your multivitamin, fat is required for proper absorption of essential micronutrients. It is key, regardless of which multivitamin you decide on, to take it both on an empty stomach (to reduce micronutrient competitions from food) and with a healthy fat (which is required for nutrient absorption). Long-chain triglycerides (LCTs) are necessary to stimulate the release of the bile acids needed for proper absorption and utilization of the fat-soluble vitamins A, D, E, and K as well as other essential micronutrients, including carotenoids, calcium, and magnesium. MCT oil alone does not contain LCTs. Although most of the fat in SKINNY Fat comes from MCTs, which bypass the normal process of digestion, it was specially formulated to contain just the right amount of LCTs needed for superior nutrient absorption.

PROBIOTICS

Probiotics are bacteria that colonize in your gut and have been shown to benefit your health, including your bone health. Creating a strong probiotic environment (microbiome) inside you can be a challenge in our modern, sterilized world. A healthy microbiome relies on you ingesting the right bacterial blend. Recent studies have demonstrated a close relationship between intestinal bacteria and bone metabolism, providing evidence that the intestinal microbiome may serve as a potential therapeutic target for the treatment of osteoporosis. One recent study determined that age-related bone loss was halved in elderly women who received a regular dose of probiotics, compared to women who received only a placebo.

Here are some of the bone-building benefits a quality probiotic supplement can provide:

- Produce lactic acid. This lactic acid reduces the pH in your gut so that you can absorb your calcium, magnesium, and vitamin B12.
- Produce short-chain fatty acids, such as butyrate, that reduce inflammation.
- Empower your gut cells to do their job to reduce your risk of leaky gut.
- Make milk products more digestible (reducing lactose).
- Reduce the impact of dietary phytates and other antinutrients that limit mineral absorption.
- Produce important vitamins, such as most B vitamins and vitamin K2.
- Reduce stress levels.

Since we want to give you every possible advantage in your fight against osteoporosis, it's important to build a strong microbiome. Fermented foods like kimchi, sauerkraut, and yogurt are great ways to get probiotics from your food, but during your Rebuild Your Bones twelve-week osteoporosis protocol, we also suggest a high-quality probiotic supplement. When choosing a supplement, both the quantity and variety of probiotics are important. Look for a probiotic that supplies a minimum of 5 billion CFUs (colony-forming units—this is how probiotics are measured) and at least five different probiotic strains (spanning both *Lactobacillus* and *Bifidobacterium* families), because each strain produces different benefits. Additionally, there are two types of probiotics, spore-forming (soil-based) and non–spore-forming (from fermented food). We recommend taking a probiotic that contains both, with at least 1 billion spore-forming CFUs. Spore-forming probiotics will be those listed as *Bacillus* on the supplement facts.

DIGESTIVE ENZYMES

We're continually shocked by the number of people with osteoporosis who are taking prescription antacid drugs or OTC antacids for their digestive issues. We reviewed the micronutrient-robbing effects of these drugs with you back in Chapter 5, so you know how damaging they can be. The problem of poor digestion has two main culprits: a lack of digestive enzymes and a lack of stomach acid, or sometimes both!

Let's start with the first one. When the body doesn't make enough digestive enzymes, this can slow the digestion process and lead to poor micronutrient absorption and uncomfortable symptoms. Many people have decreased digestive enzymes due to leaky gut, chronic stress, inflammation, food allergies, low stomach acid, and aging.

The second problem is one of too little stomach acid. Ironically, most people who are taking an antacid for heartburn or digestive issues are taking them to reduce stomach acid—but in reality, their problem is probably too little stomach acid, not too much. In fact, according to some physicians, 90 percent of their patients with osteoporosis have low stomach acid and digestive discomfort.

Here is how it works: your stomach produces hydrochloric acid (HCl), which is used to digest food. However, sometimes the stomach's capacity to secrete hydrochloric acid becomes impaired and this results in lower acid, impaired digestion, and heartburn. You grab an antacid thinking the burning you feel is from too much acid, but in fact you have too little. Adding insult to injury, if your stomach acid is low, then your body won't be able to absorb the calcium, magnesium, and other minerals critical to good bone health. Remember, your bone health is determined not only by what you eat but also by what you absorb. It shouldn't surprise you to see this correlation between poor digestion and bone deterioration. If you think you may have a lack of digestive enzymes, a lack of stomach acid, or both, you may want to try taking a digestive enzyme, perhaps one that contains Betaine HCl.

MELATONIN

Melatonin is a hormone produced by the pineal gland, located in the lower back part of the brain. The best-known function of melatonin is to regulate sleep, but it also helps regulate the immune system, sex hormones, and, according to recent research, bone health. Increasing age, sleep deprivation, changes in sleep patterns, some blood pressure and pain medications, and low levels of zinc, magnesium, and folate can all reduce the amount of melatonin produced by the pineal gland. As we mentioned in our discussion of sleep earlier, there is evidence that lack of sleep increases the risk of osteoporosis. Melatonin, which is used as a sleep aid, has also been shown to be deficient in individuals with osteoporosis. One important clinical trial showed that supplementation with melatonin for one year had significant bone-related benefits—those taking 1 mg of melatonin saw a 0.5 percent increase in femoral neck bone density, but those taking 3 mg saw a significant 2.3 percent increase in bone density. Melatonin promotes osteoblast differentiation and bone formation. This suggests that taking melatonin on a regular basis may not only improve sleep but may also be protective against the bone fractures associated with osteoporosis. Melatonin has been shown to renormalize bone marker turnover in perimenopausal women and increase bone density in postmenopausal women with osteopenia. If you decide to take melatonin, make sure to cycle on and off (perhaps three weeks on and two weeks off, followed by two weeks on and one week off, then repeat). Taking too much of this hormone for too long can limit your body's natural ability to make it.

DHEA

DHEA (dehydroepiandrosterone) is considered a "pro-hormone" tied to longevity, lean muscle mass, and a strong body. Although both men and women create DHEA naturally, levels decline rapidly after age thirty. By the time someone reaches age seventy-five, they produce only about 10 to 20 percent of the original DHEA they created in their youth. This is problematic because DHEA plays a role in more than 150 metabolic functions. It lowers inflammation, protects against depression, decreases body fat, increases lean muscle mass, improves heart health, lowers diabetes risk, increases libido, and has been proven to increase BMD. One study found that taking a DHEA supplement in conjunction with calcium and vitamin D could reduce the risk of spine fractures in older women by 30 to 50 percent. Another study found that both men and women benefited from a mere six months of DHEA supplementation: not only did their total body BMD increase by 1.6 percent, but their lumbar spinal BMD increased by a significant 2.5 percent. Researchers also found that DHEA supplementation increased lean muscle mass (increasing balance and reducing sarcopenia) and caused a natural weight-loss effect (fat loss). Estradiol, IGF-1, and testosterone increased with DHEA supplementation, and bone turnover markers decreased as well.

We recommend DHEA supplementation for those over age 30 who have been found to have low DHEA levels from a blood test. According to the National Institutes of Health, research suggests that taking 20 to 50 milligrams of DHEA daily should be sufficient and safe for most adults over age 30. Scientific studies usually give 50 mg per day for those attempting to build bone.

SAY NO TO STRONTIUM

Don't be duped by the advertised benefits of strontium for bone health. We want you to steer clear of taking this supplement. That's because in the case of strontium, quantity does not equal quality. Bone naturally contains minerals such as calcium, magnesium, and phosphorus. However, the mineral strontium has a similar electric charge to calcium and can take its place in bone. In terms of bone density, the more mineral in bone matrix, the denser the bone. When strontium takes calcium's place in the bone matrix, it increases bone density, especially the thickness of the outer, or cortical, layer of bone. Although this increases bone's compressive strength, *it does not improve and can actually lower bone's tensile strength*—the ability to elongate and flex under pressure. Lacking elasticity, bone infused with strontium rather than calcium becomes brittle, like a dried-up tree branch. And as you may imagine, your fracture risk is higher with more brittle bone. Moreover, strontium is heavier than calcium, so lots of strontium in bone artificially increases your score on a BMD test without improving tensile strength.

Strontium supplementation can also compromise your recovery from osteoporosis by blocking the absorption of other important bone-building minerals. Magnesium and calcium compete for absorption not only with each other but also with many other minerals of similar charge (such as iron . . . and strontium!). Above and beyond causing micronutrient competitions and micronutrient depletions, strontium has also been linked to heart attacks and blood clots. We recommend skipping any supplements that contain strontium—why take something that could hurt you, especially when it hasn't been shown to help you either?

Monitoring and Testing for Micronutrient Sufficiency

We are often asked, "If micronutrient deficiency is so common, and supplementation is so important, then why don't more doctors test micronutrient levels?" Some doctors do test levels of a few micronutrients, and as pertinent research showing the health-producing power of vitamins and minerals is seen more frequently in the news, more and more doctors are starting to test for micronutrient deficiencies. However, the testing typically done through physicians' offices, called serum testing, is often limited to iron, vitamin D, vitamin B12, calcium, and magnesium.

This type of testing has a few innate problems. First, analyzing blood levels of these five micronutrients leaves one in the dark about the more than twenty other essential vitamins and minerals that were not tested. Second, because serum testing measures only the amount of the micronutrient in the sample of blood taken, these tests don't always show the full picture. Here's how.

As you can see, serum testing—the common blood testing done by most physicians—can produce false calcium readings. It can also produce false B12 readings. Studies have proven that even though some patients' serum blood levels of B12 may appear normal, they may still have a B12 deficiency if their bodies do not produce enough of a salivary gland protein called transcobalamin-2. So here again, an individual might have a blood test that shows sufficient levels of B12 and still have a B12 deficiency, which can lead to fatigue, memory problems, and osteoporosis.

A third problem with serum blood testing is that the results can vary depending on how much inflammation the body is experiencing. Scientists have determined that a reliable clinical analysis of plasma (in blood) micronutrients can be made only when the degree of inflammation in the body is known. This is because the levels of several vitamins and minerals decrease by up to 40 percent when inflammation is present. Thus, low values do not necessarily indicate deficiency. So if your body is fighting an infection, for example, this causes an inflammatory response, which will make your blood levels of certain micronutrients appear lower. Although this can be temporary, it may lead you to think you are more deficient than you really are, causing you to perhaps contemplate megadosing the deficient micronutrients (not good) or trying other more serious interventions. The bottom line is that, at least in these circumstances, serum blood testing can fall short.

A Cautionary Tale of Measuring Blood Levels of Calcium

Darcie, a forty-seven-year-old vegan, contacted us and wanted to share a story about how information she had learned from us had made her question her physician's lab results. Darcie, who had followed a vegan diet for twenty-five years and was an avid triathlete, went to her physician for her annual exam. After her blood tests were run, her physician told her that she was very low in vitamin D but her calcium levels were perfect. Having learned from us about foods and lifestyle habits that deplete calcium (information we shared in previous chapters) and realizing that her diet was very high in these EMDs, as well as recognizing that her vegan diet was not supplying a great amount of calcium in the first place, Darcie began questioning how her blood calcium levels could have possibly come back in the sufficient range. Curious now about her bone strength and her doctor's lab results, Darcie decided she wanted a DEXA scan to measure her BMD. The results were devastating. Darcie, a seemingly healthy, athletic woman, was diagnosed with osteoporosis and degenerative scoliosis. She also learned that she was no longer 5 feet, 8 inches tall, but rather 5 feet, 6$^1/_2$ inches. Had Darcie not questioned the perfect calcium levels reported in her blood work, this deficiency would have gone unchecked for a longer period and likely left her in far worse shape.

So is there a better test? We recommend a micronutrient analysis—and a company called SpectraCell Laboratories performs it using patented technology.

SPECTRACELL MICRONUTRIENT TESTING

Similar to serum testing, the process begins with a prick of the needle and blood being drawn. However, traditional serum testing only checks the amount of a specific micronutrient in the sample, whereas Spectra-Cell uses a method called essential metabolic analysis, which doesn't simply test the amount present in the sample but also measures how well your micronutrients are working. Through this, SpectraCell can determine the functionality of a specific micronutrient within a cell. That information is far more important than the measurements given with a serum test, and it more closely estimates the status of a micronutrient, because the reason our cells use that micronutrient is to perform one of the functions necessary for life.

We all know someone (or maybe you are that someone) who likes to analyze data and measures progress by crunching the numbers. We call these clients (who, by the way, are often some of the most successful) our "calculating clients." These individuals feel best when things are precise, so they thrive by turning in meticulous food journals, lab tests, and exercise and supplement information. For this group, a chart that shows quantified health improvements is a great motivator for continued success on the plan. If you can see yourself in this category, then a micronutrient analysis prior to starting the Rebuild Your Bones protocol may be right for you. If you do the blood work before starting and then retest a few months later, you will be able to see the progress you have made toward becoming sufficient in all of your bone-building micronutrients.

OMEGACHECK

The next test that we mandate for clients and recommend to you is called the OmegaCheck. It is also a SpectraCell test, but this one will determine your current levels of omega-6 and omega-3. As you learned in Chapter 4, your omega-6 to omega-3 ratio can determine whether your bone-building osteoblasts function properly or your osteoclasts break down bone and cause osteoporosis. You already know the importance of creating an anti-inflammatory diet with as close to a 1:1 ratio of omega-6 to omega-3 as possible. An OmegaCheck test is essential to see the current ratio in your body. Most clients find this test eye-opening, and it motivates them toward making real changes day by day.

YOUR HORMONES, THYROID, AND ADRENALS

Throughout this book, you have heard us talk about the important hormones that play a role in bone building. But do you know how well they're functioning? Perhaps your DHEA is low; should you be supplementing? Where do your estrogen or testosterone levels fall? The SpectraCell hormone, thyroid, and adrenal test is a specialized blood test that will give you a clear picture of your current hormone functions so that you will be able to identify areas that may be causing bone loss and work to improve them. We suggest taking this comprehensive test prior to beginning the Rebuild Your Bones protocol and then again in three to six months.

All of these SpectraCell tests can be purchased online at Spectra-Cell.com or at RebuildYourBones.com. Additionally, many forward-thinking physicians also offer these tests to their patients, allowing your insurance to cover their costs.

You are finally ready to put all of the incredibly powerful healing habits that you have learned throughout this book to use. In Chapter 8, we will reveal our complete Rebuild Your Bones twelve-week osteoporosis protocol that we created to help you achieve micronutrient sufficiency and, ultimately, improve your bone health. You've read the research . . . there is nothing more to learn. Now it's time to put your new knowledge into practice—get ready for extraordinary results.

38. Amp up your healing with accessory supplements.
39. Test for success and monitor your progress.

Join us On the Couch for an in-depth chat about Chapter 7

Make sure to join us for our next "On the Couch" chat, where we discuss the two healing habits we introduced you to in this chapter (additional supplementation and testing) and help you create a simple plan of action that won't break the bank. Join us now at RebuildYour Bones.com.

CHAPTER 8

The Rebuild Your Bones Twelve-Week Osteoporosis Protocol

Commitment is the foundation of great accomplishments.
—HEIDI REEDER (PROFESSOR, AUTHOR,
AND NATIONAL SPEAKER)

Congratulations! You are now ready to begin your Rebuild Your Bones twelve-week osteoporosis protocol. We have covered a lot of information and discovered some pretty incredible things along the way. On this journey together, we have proven how important reaching a state of micronutrient sufficiency is to building bone health. We've identified how following our three steps—switching to Rich, driving down depletion, and smart supplementation—will guide you down the road to micronutrient sufficiency. And, as promised, you have been introduced to thirty-nine clinically proven healing habits that you should incorporate into your daily regimen in order to prevent further bone loss and start to rebuild your bones. (We will introduce number forty later in this chapter!) Let's start by reviewing a final list of our healing habits, and then we will introduce you to the twelve-week protocol itself so that you can get started on rebuilding your bones.

Your Forty Healing Habits That Have Been Clinically Proven to Prevent and Reverse Bone Loss

1. Avoid the dangers of osteoporosis medications: page 24
2. Make micronutrient sufficiency your chosen path to bone health: page 35
3. Choose Rich Foods and avoid Poor Foods: page 58
4. Say so long to sugar: page 60
5. Halt the high-fructose corn syrup (HFCS): page 63
6. Skip the sinister sugar substitutes: page 64
7. Whack the wheat: page 66
8. Move away from MSG: page 71
9. Fix the phytates (phytic acid): page 74
10. Evade the oxalates (oxalic acid): page 75
11. Lose the lectins through pressure cooking: page 76
12. Take the time to cook out trypsin inhibitors: page 77
13. Flee from phosphoric acid: page 78
14. Escape from excessive alcohol intake: page 79
15. Curb the caffeine: page 79
16. Tame the tannins: page 81
17. Overcome the deficiencies of your chosen dietary doctrine: page 94
18. Pick up the protein: page 104
19. Increase your omega-3 intake: page 110
20. Eliminate omega-6-rich foods: page 111
21. Pitch the plastics: page 119
22. Mind the heavy metals: page 121
23. Toss toxic household products: page 123
24. Stave off stress with de-stressing exercises: page 131
25. Sleep eight to nine hours a day: page 132
26. Stop smoking or exposing yourself to secondhand smoke: page 133
27. Combat the negative effects of smog: page 134
28. Use sunscreen sparingly: page 135
29. Be smart about your smartphone: page 137
30. Minimize micronutrient loss due to excessive cardio and sweating: page 138

31. Perform a weight-bearing, osteogenic-loading exercise routine: page 139
32. Minimize your prescription medications (if possible): page 142
33. Reduce the use of OTC medications: page 142
34. Choose only supplements that have the highest **A**bsorption potential: page 163
35. Take supplements that deliver **B**eneficial quantities and forms of each micronutrient: page 168
36. Look for supplements formulated to eliminate micronutrient **C**ompetitions: page 182
37. Make sure your supplements pair **s**ynergistic micronutrients: page 189
38. Amp up your healing with accessory supplements: page 200
39. Test for success and monitor your progress: page 218
40. Let your Desire, Drive, Discipline, and Determination keep you on a committed path to Rebuild Your Bones (will be introduced on page 237)

The Rebuild Your Bones Osteoporosis Protocol

You've read the studies, and now the real work begins. In Chapter 1, we told you that preventing and reversing bone loss is like running a marathon. Having read this book is much like having attended a great seminar on marathon running: you've been given a lot of information, but up until this point, it has all been educational rather than practical experience. It's now time for you to take the proverbial "first jog around the block." You need to suit up with the right gear and start the hard work and daily dedication it will take to get you to the finish line. Although you may have already started incorporating some of our healing habits into your daily routine, we have found that adding them slowly is the best way to avoid becoming overwhelmed. You wouldn't tell a brand-new runner to run five miles their first day out, would you? You would ease them in slowly so they don't burn out and quit. The same is true for all the changes you will be making in your life to improve your bone health. With the Rebuild Your Bones twelve-week osteoporosis protocol, we recommend adding new habits every few weeks (as we will outline) so that you can adjust to them comfortably and become more surefooted on your journey to prevent and reverse osteoporosis.

The fact that you're here in Chapter 8 indicates that you have already decided to make micronutrient sufficiency your chosen path to bone health (healing habit 2). Great job! Although we made a case in Chapter 2 to avoid the dangers of prescription osteoporosis medications (healing habit 1), if you have decided to take one of the medications, that decision is a personal one. It in no way makes any of the other healing habits less important. In fact, if you have chosen to take osteoporosis medications, becoming sufficient in essential micronutrients is even *more* important for you. Micronutrient sufficiency can help you overcome their prescription-induced depletions. Regardless of your decision, we know that by taking on the Rebuild Your Bones twelve-week osteoporosis protocol you have made a life-changing decision that will have positive effects on your bone health for years to come.

START THESE TASKS *AT LEAST SEVEN DAYS* BEFORE "GO DAY"

If you were actually running a race, there would be a whole slew of products that you'd need to purchase that, when all used together, would make it possible for you to achieve your goal of finishing the marathon. Things like running shoes, running shorts, good socks, and maybe even a watch to monitor your pace and heart rate. The same is true for the Rebuild Your Bones protocol: you will need the correct assortment of gear to set you up to succeed. That's why we want you to pick a "go day" *at least* seven days in the future. This will allow you plenty of time to acquire your collection of bone-building goodies. Here is a quick checklist of things that should be accomplished at least seven days before your "go day":

1. Get Your Pretesting Blood Work Done

Healing habit 39 reminds us that awareness is key when it comes to the current status of our bone health. This is why we suggest having your lab work done before you begin your program. You can find all the SpectraCell tests we talked about in Chapter 7 at SpectraCell.com or RebuildYourBones.com, or you can ask your physician if they offer these tests. If finances allow, we highly suggest having at least a micronutrient analysis and an OmegaCheck before you begin so that you can clearly see your progress when you retest at the end of the twelve weeks. Do this task first, as tests may take up to a week to arrive at your house.

2. Complete Your Reading and Watch the "On the Couch" Coaching Videos

Make sure to read (and reread) Chapters 1–7 for a full understanding of each healing habit you will be integrating into your life for the next twelve weeks, and watch all of the end-of-chapter "On the Couch" videos. These chats offer additional information and bonus materials not covered in the book. (The videos are available at RebuildYourBones .com.)

3. Stock Up on Smart Supplementation

This will require you to review healing habits 18, 19, and 20, as well as healing habits 34 through 39. We've broken them down here to make it easy.

a. **Multivitamin** (pages 163–198): Choose a multivitamin that is formulated using the ABCs. You can test any multivitamin you plan on using during your twelve-week program for free at CompareYourMulti.com to see how well it performs using the ABCs of Optimal Supplementation Guidelines. As we said in Chapter 6, you can purchase high-quality individual micronutrients and separate them throughout the day, or you can check out our multivitamin choice formulated with Anti-Competition Technology, Nutreince, at RebuildYourBones.com.

b. **Omega-3 supplement** (pages 207–212): Find a high-quality omega-3 supplement that supplies high levels of triglyceride form EPA and DHA that have been separated to naturally eliminate competition and increase absorption. We like our Origin Omega.

c. **Omega-6 reduction** (pages 212–213): Make sure to have an oil source on hand that has low or zero omega-6 content, like SKINNYFat Oil.

d. **Protein powder** (pages 203–207): *If choosing whey protein,* choose an organic, non-GMO, grass-fed, single-ingredient whey protein concentrate that has also been tested to prove that it is low in heavy metals. *If choosing plant protein,* find a combination of organic nonsoy plant proteins (to supply a full spectrum of amino acids) that are sprouted to reduce antinutrients; make sure the protein has been tested to prove that it is low in heavy metals. Our IN.POWER protein powders are available in both whey and plant varieties.

e. **Accessory supplements** (pages 201–203, 213–217): Consider purchasing additional essential micronutrients (vitamins B12, C, D, and K2, as well as boron, calcium, and silica) if you feel you need them at levels higher than delivered by your multivitamin. Stock up on accessory supplements that have been shown to benefit bone health such as probiotics, digestive enzymes, melatonin, DHEA, and GLA. Avoid products that contain strontium.

We're chipping in to pay for your supplements!

We know that purchasing supplements can get expensive, and we want to help you make supplementation an affordable addition to your lifestyle. For more, visit RebuildYourBones.com.

START THESE TASKS *ONE TO TWO DAYS* BEFORE "GO DAY"

1. *Review the Supplied Week 1 Menu Plan and Go Shopping!*

Review healing habits 3 to 17 in the preceding list. It is time to shop for Rich Foods that are high in micronutrients and low in antinutrients. If you haven't done so yet, we highly recommend going to Rebuild YourBones.com and grabbing a copy of *Rich Food Poor Food* and the free Rich Food, Poor Food Osteoporosis Grocery Guide that comes with it. This is must-have information that will make shopping during your twelve-week program a snap. Additionally, spend some time reviewing the proper preparation methods for reducing antinutrients so that you will have a clear plan when food preparation begins. Although all of our Rebuild Your Bones recipes in Chapter 9 follow best preparation guidelines, if you choose to create your own dishes you will need to keep these preparation methods in mind. Review the supplied week 1 menu plan (page 242), swap out any foods or recipes you don't love, make a Rich Food shopping list, and go shopping. To make your life even easier, if you are following our recommended menu plan, we provide a week 1 shopping list you can download for free at Rebuild YourBones.com.

2. *Soak and Sprout*

It is time to soak or sprout any nuts, seeds, or grains you plan on using in the first week, unless you purchased them already soaked or sprouted.

3. *Prepare Your Healthy-Fat Oils*

Make any oil infusions, butters, condiments, and salad dressings that you may want to enjoy during the plan (see pages 252–255 for recipes). Here's a tip: you can freeze your butters and pesto in ice cube trays to reduce your meal prep time.

4. *Prepare Triple Threat Puddings and Cheesecakes*

Variety is the spice of life, so try all of the Triple Threat Treats—you will read about these shortly! These delicious recipes (pages 248–251) make great grab-and-go treats, so making them in advance and stocking up is super smart and timesaving.

IT'S "GO DAY"! WEEKS 1 AND 2 (DAYS 1–14)

For the first two weeks on the Rebuild Your Bones protocol, we want you to focus on two things: filling your recipes with Rich Foods and getting comfortable with your supplement schedule. If your dietary philosophy allows, we feel it would be best to follow the menu plan we outline in this book for at least the first week (page 242 in Chapter 9). That can help reduce any stress you might feel about having to create meals on your own from the get-go. The menu plans as outlined are filled with flavorful meals that follow a low-carb, Mediterranean, Primal diet philosophy. This style of diet naturally reduces the antinutrients found in many of the vegetables and legumes, as it is lower in carbohydrates.

If you are following a dietary doctrine that does not allow for the use of our menu plans, then just pay special attention to building micronutrient content into every bite. This means choosing the most micronutrient-rich ingredients, properly preparing them to reduce antinutrients, and avoiding foods high in omega-6. We've even supplied information on how you can alter our favorite recipes for vegan, vegetarian, and ketogenic diets. In Chapter 9, we provide a list of preferred fruits, vegetables, starches, and proteins that you can choose from, as well as our recommendations on how often to enjoy each.

IDENTIFYING YOUR IDEAL DAILY PROTEIN INTAKE FOR BONE GROWTH

When it comes to timing your meals, the Rebuild Your Bones protocol recommends eating every three to five hours, four hours being optimal. The primary reason for this is to make sure you can easily ingest the amount of protein required to build bone. Remember, as you learned in Chapter 4, research suggests that your body requires at least 1.2 times the RDA for protein in order to best build bone. To determine your personal ideal daily protein intake, simply multiply your weight in pounds by 0.545. This number will represent the number of grams of protein you must eat each day. Divide that number by the number of meals you plan to eat each day to calculate the number of grams of protein to strive for in each meal.

For example: a 130-pound woman needs to eat 130 × 0.545 = 71 grams of protein per day. That equals 24 grams in each meal if she chooses to eat three meals, or 18 grams in each meal if she eats four meals a day.

Remember, not all of your meals have to contain the same amount of protein. This is just the total grams of protein required throughout each day. For example, if you require 71 grams of protein per day then you may have a breakfast of 11 grams, a lunch of 24 grams, a snack of 11 grams, and a dinner of 25 grams, which by the end of the day would equal your ideal 71 grams of protein. It is important not to try to ingest all your daily protein in a single meal, as the body can't utilize all that protein at one time.

If you choose to follow a three-meal, high-quality, Rich Food diet, your day might look something like this:

- Breakfast: One 7-ounce container organic Greek yogurt (18 grams protein) with one organic pasture-raised egg (6 grams protein) or one serving of French Onion Egg Tart (page 255)
- Lunch: 4 ounces wild-caught salmon (24 grams protein) with a side dish or one serving of Chicken, Broccoli, and Cheese Soup (page 263)
- Dinner: 2 organic chicken drumsticks or half an organic chicken breast (24 grams protein) with a side dish or one serving of Shepherd's Pie (page 265)

Although this is pretty simple and completely doable, in our experience, cooking and preparing high-quality, protein-rich meals day after day can get overwhelming and tiresome for some people, not to mention expensive. If you find this to be true, having shakes and meal replacements can help simplify the program. If you don't eat a lot of high-quality protein, because you just don't have time or it doesn't fit into your dietary doctrine, adding protein shakes or snacks to reach your ideal daily protein intake can be helpful. Unfortunately, most protein-based bars and puddings on the market contain loads of inflammatory nuts and seeds and other undesirable ingredients. This is why we created something that you can make at home—we call them Triple Threats.

They are in no way mandatory to complete the Rebuild Your Bones protocol, but having them premade in the fridge and using them as one or two of your meals fills your day with yummy, rich, dessertlike treats that save you time and simplify both your life and your supplementation schedule.

Our daily, micronutrient-dense, bone-strengthening, muscle-building Triple Threats cover all the bases. They combine vitamins and minerals from Nutreince with amino acids from IN.POWER protein and micronutrient-absorbing, anti-inflammation power from SKIN-NYFat. Basically, they take three of our foundational products and create a meal replacement that is perfectly formulated for all-day energy and lasting micronutrient coverage.

SHAKES SAVE YOU MONEY

A bonus: using our Triple Threat meal replacements for one or two of your meals rather than eating three or four regular meals actually saves you quite a bit of money when you look at what you are getting. The cost of each Triple Threat meal replacement is less than $3.00 per meal! So enjoying two Triple Threats costs less than a *single* White Chocolate Mocha at Starbucks or a *single* 20-ounce Smartwater at a movie theater. So don't miss out on our delicious Triple Threat Shakes and other Triple Threat treat recipes, including pudding, cheesecake, and ice cream, in Chapter 9.

If you decide to use Triple Threats in your Rebuild Your Bones menus (as Mira did), then your day might look something like this: If you wake up at 6:30 a.m., you might grab a cup of coffee or tea and have a Triple Threat Shake at 7:00 a.m. Then, at 11:30 a.m., you could have lunch, and at 3:00 p.m. you would make and enjoy another Triple Threat Shake or grab a Triple Threat Pudding. Lastly, at around 7:00 p.m., you would enjoy dinner. That would be one example. However, most of us lead ever-changing lives with daily routines that are, well, anything but routine. This means that your schedule might vary from one day to another.

We provide a suggested Rebuild Your Bones daily menu plan in Chapter 9; however, if you want to make alterations and move meals or Triple Threats around on any of the days, feel free. Just remember that in our menu plans, you will have two meals and two Triple Threats a day and eat every three to five hours. And again, because neither Nutreince nor our Triple Threats are mandatory on the Rebuild Your Bones protocol, if you use an alternative multivitamin or meal replacement, you should consume that chosen meal replacement and multivitamin supplement whenever you see "Triple Threat" in the menu plan.

FOLLOWING THE SAME KETOGENIC DIET THAT MIRA FOLLOWED FOR YOUR REBUILD YOUR BONES PROTOCOL

As you have learned, you can follow any type of dietary philosophy you like while on the Rebuild Your Bones protocol. Most dietary philosophies do not require a specific ratio of macronutrients (carbohydrates, fats, and protein), but a ketogenic diet does. Those who are replicating the exact program we used for Mira should shoot to maintain a ratio of at least 70–80 percent fat, 20 percent protein, and up to 5 percent carbohydrates in each meal. To make your life easier, all of the Triple Threats are already set at this optimal ketogenic ratio, and for most of the recipes listed on the weekly menu plan, we have supplied detailed instructions as to how to make them ketogenic. However, should you want to create your own ketogenic meals, you can follow the ratio given here to guarantee keto success. For more information on how to follow the Rebuild Your Bones meal plan on a ketogenic diet, go to Rebuild YourBones.com/keto.

Midweek Homework: By the end of week 1, you should be getting into the groove. As you continue to become more comfortable with your chosen Rebuild Your Bones diet and supplementation schedule, take time during week 2 to plan your exercise routine. Planning is the key to success, and we want you to be successful!

WEEKS 3 AND 4 (DAYS 15–28)

Now that you are on a roll with your chosen diet and supplementation protocols, you are ready to add two more key bone-building healing habits (30 and 31) into your program. It is time to reduce your exercise intensity and focus on osteogenic loading. Quite often, this is where people fail in their quest for better bones. In almost every case, when we get an email or phone call from someone who did not see a positive improvement in their bone density, we ask them if they followed our exercise recommendations and they reply "no" or "not often." Don't make this mistake. As we stated in Chapter 5, osteogenic loading is mandatory if you want to build bone. You may be able to slow down or slightly improve your bone density without exercise, but we feel very strongly that it would be nearly impossible to reverse your osteoporosis without some form of osteogenic loading. The loading acts as a stimulus for bone growth. The idea of rebuilding weak osteoporotic bone without osteogenic loading is like a weak, unfit person asking if they could become a bodybuilder without lifting a weight. Each of the forty healing habits is like an individual link in your chain-mail armor against osteoporosis, but the armor is only as strong as the weakest link; if you skip or disregard several of the habits, your likelihood of success will be greatly compromised. The healing habits work synergistically to produce a result greater than their individual benefits. We hope we have made it clear that these next two weeks are crucial in getting your body accustomed to the osteogenic load that you must practice for the rest of your life in order to prevent and reverse osteoporosis.

The first habit you will add this week is to minimize micronutrient loss due to excessive cardio and sweating. This is the perfect example of the old adage—more is not always better. Although we still want you to be physically active, we also want you to change your routine to include a form of cardio that is load-bearing and that you can perform safely at your level of bone health. You can hold on to the back of a chair and hop in your living room during the commercials of your favorite show; you can take long walks, dance in Zumba class, do a low-intensity step class, or push your lawn mower—it doesn't matter what you choose. Choose a loading routine that you enjoy and can enjoy safely. But don't overdo it! Intense cardio and heavy sweating isn't the goal here . . . in fact, it will work against your ability to achieve micronutrient sufficiency.

Additionally, a weight-bearing exercise routine (preferably one that is performed on an osteogenic-loading machine) should also be added. This healing habit will improve your muscle strength and your balance as well as your bone density! Visit RebuildYourBones.com to learn more about how to incorporate osteogenic loading into your exercise routine. Remember, to reduce calcium loss from your bones during exercise, make sure to take your calcium-containing multivitamin thirty minutes before your workout.

Midweek Homework: As you move into week 4, it is time to go shopping again. This time we want you to focus on purchasing household products to pitch the plastics, mind the heavy metals, and toss household toxins (review our purchasing guidelines on pages 119–127).

WEEKS 5 AND 6 (DAYS 29–42)

By week 5 you are likely hitting your stride. You know how to prepare your favorite micronutrient-rich meals, your supplementation schedule is on track, and your exercise program should be shaping up. That means that you're well on your way to experiencing incredible bone-building benefits from the diet- and exercise-related healing habits you have implemented so far. Now it is time to implement the remaining lifestyle habits (healing habits 21–23, 25–29, 32, and 33). If you did your midweek homework, your shelves should now be stocked with healthy, nontoxic personal care and household cleaning products. Bravo! Using these products will really start reducing your toxic load, giving your antioxidants a chance to attack inflammation head-on. Don't worry if you're not "in love" with each of your initial picks for these healthier goods—there are a lot of great products to discover. With a little time and effort, you will find the perfect ones to suit your personal preferences.

During the next two weeks, we also really want you to start paying attention to reducing EMF exposure, not only from your cell phone but also from tablets, microwave ovens, and other electrical devices. Keeping your cell phone out of the bedroom at night is a great way to not only reduce EMF exposure but also improve the quality of your sleep. Remember, your goal is to get eight to nine hours of uninterrupted sleep each night. Depending on your schedule, this may mean going to bed a bit earlier than normal to clear your head and ready yourself for a good night's sleep. Lastly, if you are a smoker and you haven't quit smoking yet, make sure you are at least looking into options that might assist you in quitting. Our clients have reported great success with behavior modification therapy and hypnosis.

Midweek Homework: As you move into week 6, we want you to decide which de-stressing techniques you will be practicing. (Review our de-stressing techniques on pages 131–132.)

WEEKS 7 AND 8 (DAYS 43–56)

It is now time to put healing habit number 24 into practice and stave off stress. You've been making a lot of changes over the past six weeks, but now it's time to clear your head and de-stress from it all. We would like you to start with at least five minutes of conscious de-stressing every morning when you wake, and the same amount each night before bed. If you can do more, that's great, but these ten minutes are the bare minimum needed to lower your stress-induced cortisol levels and decrease micronutrient depletion. Although we mentioned a few of our favorite options on pages 131–132, don't let us limit you. Perhaps there is an audio meditation series that really helps you relax, or maybe you love those really cool adult coloring books and can get lost for hours at a time in the beautiful patterns and colors. You may also be one of the many people out there who have been caught up in the yarn craze sweeping the country and love to relax by doing needlework or knitting. Regardless of the de-stressing technique you choose, it is important to make stress reduction a healing habit that you do every day. We know that life is stressful enough on its own, but being diagnosed with osteoporosis or osteopenia and having to learn how to reorganize your life to focus on micronutrient sufficiency has undoubtedly added to that stress. Although it may sound corny, you really need this special "you time" twice a day to reduce stress and build stronger bones.

WEEKS 9–12 (DAYS 57–98)

Although you will use most of your time during these last four weeks of your twelve-week program to focus on incorporating all of the thirty-nine healing habits we have covered thus far, we want to introduce one new healing habit (number 40): committing yourself fully to Rebuild

Your Bones. This final healing habit will help you accomplish your goal.

Healing Habit 40: Let your Desire, Drive, Discipline, and Determination keep you on a committed path to Rebuild Your Bones.

Let's face it, it's one thing to dream about being healthy or accomplishing a lifelong goal, and it's a completely different thing to actually do it. Anyone who has accomplished anything in their life knows that it takes desire, drive, discipline, and determination, day in and day out, to make your goal a reality. The bottom line is that achieving and maintaining a state of micronutrient sufficiency is hard work; anyone who tells you differently is lying. Yes, there are tools that can make your journey easier and techniques that can make your efforts more productive, but in the end, without commitment—true commitment, the kind of commitment that most people run away from—most dreams, including that of rebuilding your bones, never come true. We know you have the *desire* to heal your bones, or you wouldn't have picked up this book in the first place. Your *drive* and *discipline* have also been proven by coming this far and incorporating all thirty-nine healing habits into your life during the last eight weeks. Now you are in the home stretch of your Rebuild Your Bones protocol, and finishing strong will prove your *determination*. Although we may not have a scientific study to clinically prove that this fortieth healing habit will increase your bone density, we have included it on our list because we know that commitment is the foundation of great accomplishments.

These last four weeks are the time to ask yourself: have you skipped over any of the healing habits, or do you need to pay more attention to any of them? Have you been preparing your chosen foods properly to reduce antinutrients? Are you doing your osteogenic-loading exercises? Have you remembered to take your supplements every day? These last four weeks are your time to shine, to turn your healing habits into a lifestyle that you can commit to. Keep up the great work; the finish line is right in front of you.

Conclusion: Your Marathon for Life: Rebuild Your Bones and Beat Osteoporosis

As you have seen, Rebuild Your Bones doesn't require you to take pharmaceutical medications. Nor does it ask you to change your chosen dietary philosophy. The Rebuild Your Bones twelve-week osteoporosis protocol is a completely different kind of plan; it requires that you work toward a state of micronutrient sufficiency by making real changes in just about every area of your life—from the food you put into your shopping cart, to your lifestyle habits, to your choice of multivitamin and even the soap you wash your dishes with. All of your new healing habits add up in the end, and every positive step you make along the way will bring you one step closer to the better bone health you deserve. The Rebuild Your Bones protocol requires something else of you too—it requires faith. Faith in the scientific research that shows that your osteoporosis stems from a deficiency in essential micronutrients. Faith that all forty healing habits will work together synergistically to reverse those deficiencies and create an environment within your body where healing can take place. And, finally, faith that when you have done the hard work, your bone health will truly improve.

As with any act of faith, the hardest part is that no one can offer you any real guarantee. However, we can tell you with complete certainty that the healing habits we have outlined within the Rebuild Your Bones protocol, when followed correctly, *will improve your bone health*. We have witnessed it time and time again. The Rebuild Your Bones protocol works because it focuses on reversing the condition that has been shown to be the root cause of osteoporosis—micronutrient deficiency. When the deficiencies causing the body to manifest a health condition or disease are eliminated, the body can heal itself and the health condition or disease improves or is eliminated completely. This is the embodiment of our micronutrient sufficiency hypothesis of health, first mentioned back in Chapter 1. You now have the foundational knowledge you need to heal your body and bring your bone health to a level you may never have dreamed of achieving.

It's time for you to reverse the damage of the past, reclaim your bone health, and start living the extraordinary life you deserve. We are proud of you for making a commitment to improve your bone health and sticking to it! We know it isn't easy at first, and that it requires sacrifice and effort to complete the twelve-week program. And even if you might have erred once or twice when dining out or grocery shopping, or you perhaps missed a training or de-stressing session now and again, we are sure that in the end, you will be surprised by just how easy all of the healing habits actually were to implement and follow.

Keep in mind, the osteoporosis you have now did not magically appear overnight. It took a while to develop. Be patient with yourself; your healing may take just as long. Even halting or slowing down your bone loss is a win, because it means that a positive change has occurred within your body. You are putting yourself on the path to healing—a road that you were meant to discover so that you could attain the extraordinary life that you were born to live. This same path will likely shower you with additional, unexpected health benefits as well. As you move through your twelve-week program, take time to evaluate your overall health. Are you sleeping better? Has your blood pressure, blood sugar level, or digestion improved? Perhaps your skin has a new glow or your energy seems more balanced. These are all great signs that your body is absorbing the micronutrients you're giving it and using them for a multitude of health-enhancing functions. Pay attention as this starts to happen, and use this positive reinforcement to further motivate you. Some of you may decide to keep on cutting out the sugar, wheat, and other micronutrient-depleting and health-robbing foods and lifestyle habits after finishing your twelve-week program. You may think that these permanent changes fit your lifestyle perfectly. Others may feel that adding in some of the eliminated foods once in a while, for special occasions, is the right path. Both are OK—the Rebuild Your Bones protocol gives you the power of choice. As long as you stick to its core philosophies most of the time, it can help you build strong, flexible bones for years to come. However, if you choose to allow Poor Foods and detrimental lifestyle habits back in, just beware: many of these foods and lifestyle habits can be addictive and cause you to backslide rather quickly.

Remember, the further you stray from our Rebuild Your Bones protocol, the more likely you are to experience micronutrient deficiencies and potentially a declining bone density. But don't worry; regardless of the path you take from this point on, we know that the forty healing habits you now have in your possession, and will implement during your twelve-week plan, have the power to improve your health in truly exceptional ways. You are about to embark on a great journey—the journey to becoming the best possible you, to rebuilding your bones and beating osteoporosis and experiencing extraordinary health. Now get out there and do it—we can't wait to hear about your success!

CHAPTER 9

The Rebuild Your Bones Week 1 Menu Plan and More Than 40 Delicious Recipes

Those who have no time for healthy eating will sooner or later have to find time for illness.

—EDWARD STANLEY, FORMER PRIME MINISTER OF THE UNITED KINGDOM

Get ready to enjoy some of the most delicious food you have ever eaten—we mean it! We collected many of these incredible recipes during our travels around the world during the Calton Project. Although we tweaked some a bit here and there to fit into our Rebuild Your Bones protocol, these recipes still include a wide variety of enticing and deeply satisfying flavors for you to enjoy. The first week's menu plan takes your taste buds traveling to India, Greece, England, Italy, and Mexico—so bon appétit and bon voyage!

Remember to put all the information we covered in Chapter 3 into practice when purchasing ingredients for the recipes in this chapter. Do your best over the next twelve weeks to locate and purchase the highest-quality local, organic, pasture-raised, grass-fed, non-GMO food you can—and watch how you prepare them too! As you make your way through the recipes, feel free to change things up a bit to fit your personal taste preferences using the list and guidelines supplied later in this chapter. Although not all recipes can be adapted for all dietary philosophies, if you are vegan, vegetarian, or ketogenic, we have added suggestions for how you might choose to alter our recipes. Whenever we offer more than one option for a meal, if you see an asterisk (*), that recipe can be followed on a ketogenic protocol.

Oh, and one last thing: Each of the recipes clearly states the serving size and how many grams of protein each serving will deliver, but we find that many people following the Rebuild Your Bones protocol enjoy doubling the recipes and either eating that meal several times over the week or freezing a portion for later use. This makes things really easy when you find yourself in a time crunch, so you may want to consider this time-saving tactic as well.

Your Week 1 Menu Plan

Day 1 (Sunday)

9:00 a.m. Protein-Packed Morning Muffins (page 258)

1:00 p.m. Traditional Triple Threat Shake (page 248)

5:00 p.m. Buffalo Chicken Chili (page 259) with optional Ridiculously Simple Wraps (page 268) for dipping [omit wraps for keto]

9:00 p.m. Triple Threat Chocolate Lava Pudding (page 250)

Day 2 (Monday)

7:30 a.m. Cinnamon Spice Triple Threat Shake (page 249)

12:00 p.m. Leftover Buffalo Chicken Chili

3:30 p.m. Traditional Triple Threat Shake (page 248)

7:30 p.m. Grilled Tandoori Skewers (page 260) with Cooling Cucumber Raita (page 271) and optional Indian Garlic-Butter Cheese Non-Naan (page 269) [omit the Non-Naan for keto]

Day 3 (Tuesday)

7:30 a.m. Triple Threat Cheesecake (page 251)

12:00 p.m. Big salad with leftover Grilled Tandoori Skewers and choice of SKINNYFat salad dressing (page 274) or Cooling Cucumber Raita (page 271) [replace the big salad with a plate of lettuce for keto]

3:30 p.m. Traditional Triple Threat Shake (page 248)

7:30 p.m. Greek Chicken (page 262) *or* a baked chicken thigh with optional Buffalo Wing Sauce (aka Jayson's Red Hot) (page 272) and Really Creamy SKINNYFat Blue Cheese Dressing (page 275)★ [use 2–3 tablespoons of the dressing for keto]

Day 4 (Wednesday)

7:30 a.m. Traditional Triple Threat Shake (page 248)

12:00 p.m. Leftover Greek Chicken *or* leftover rotisserie/baked chicken with Buffalo Wing Sauce (aka Jayson's Red Hot) (page 272) and Really Creamy SKINNYFat Blue Cheese Dressing (page 275)★ [use 2–3 tablespoons of the dressing for keto]

3:30 p.m. Triple Threat Chocolate Lava Pudding (page 250)

7:30 p.m. Shepherd's Pie (page 265) *or* Micronutrient-Packed Meat Loaf (page 264)★ and a $^1/_2$ cup side of fibrous vegetables (if not ketogenic) steamed or sautéed in your choice of SKINNYFat butter or oil infusion (pages 252–255)

Day 5 (Thursday)

7:30 a.m. Triple Threat Cheesecake (page 251)

12:00 p.m. Leftover Shepherd's Pie *or* leftover Micronutrient-Packed Meat Loaf★

3:30 p.m. Triple Threat Chocolate Lava Pudding (page 250)

7:30 p.m. 4 ounces salmon steaks and choice of vegetable with choice of a SKINNYFat pesto or butter (pages 252–254) [use at least 2 tablespoons pesto or butter and omit vegetable for keto]

Day 6 (Friday)

7:30 a.m. Traditional Triple Threat Shake (page 248)

12:00 p.m. Chicken, Broccoli, and Cheese Soup (page 263)

3:30 p.m. Traditional Triple Threat Shake (page 248)

7:30 p.m. Rustic Portobello Pizza Caps (page 266)

Day 7 (Saturday)

9:00 a.m. French Onion Egg Tart (page 255)

1:00 p.m. Traditional Triple Threat Shake (page 248)

5:00 p.m. Fabulous Fajitas (page 267) with Holy Moly Guacamole (page 276) and salsa

9:00 p.m. Triple Threat Chocolate Lava Pudding (page 250)

Making Your Own Menus Using Healthy Rich Food Options

Before we get to the Rebuild Your Bones recipes, here are some general tips for how to keep the meals you make yourself in line with the Rebuild Your Bones guidelines:

The Rich Foods listed in this section are high in the essential micronutrients shown to be beneficial for bone building. We have included many of these Rich Food choices in your week 1 menus. Choose these Rich Foods when designing personalized menus or eating out, and don't forget to properly prepare foods that contain EMDs.

Healthy Protein Options

Beef	Oysters
Bone broth	Pork
Chicken	Rainbow trout
Clams	Salmon
Cod	Sardines
Crab	Scallops
Dungeness crab	Shrimp
Flounder	Snapper
Herring	Tuna
Lamb	Turkey
Mussels	Venison
Organ meats	

Healthy Dairy Options

Cheese, especially Gouda★

Cottage cheese

Cream★

Kefir

Milk

Sour cream

Yogurt

★ = approved for ketogenic diets

Healthy Fat Options

Butter

Chocolate (100 percent cocoa)

Cocoa butter

Coconut oil

Eggs (with yolks)

Ghee

Lard

SKINNYFat

Healthy Nonstarchy Vegetable Options (Preferable to Starches)

Enjoy a variety of colorful vegetables. Unlike fruits and starches, we want to see tons of great vegetables on your plate. Here is a list of our go-to vegetables, which tend to be on the low-carbohydrate side. They won't cause that fat storage you are trying to avoid, and they are loaded with a variety of fabulous accessory nutrients that are not readily available in supplements. For the next twelve weeks, try to eat vegetables that deliver all the colors of the rainbow. A vegetable's color can tell you a lot about what micronutrients it will deliver, so choosing vegetables with varied colors delivers the greatest variety of benefits.

Note: Individuals on ketogenic protocols should keep approved vegetables to a minimum. Either choose half servings or eliminate them entirely from one or both meals in order to best achieve ketosis.

Artichokes

Asparagus

Avocado

Bok choy

Broccoli

Brussels sprouts

Cabbage

Cauliflower

Celery

Cucumbers

Dark leafy greens

Garlic

Green beans

Kale

Mushrooms

Mustard greens

Onions	Snow peas
Peppers	Spinach (cooked; use infrequently)
Pumpkin	Sprouts
Romaine lettuce	Swiss chard
Sauerkraut	Tomatoes

Healthy Starchy Vegetables and Fruits

While you are on the Rebuild Your Bones plan, we want you to limit your fruit and starch intake to two servings a week *at most*. You can choose the foods that you like best so you don't feel like you are missing out on your favorites. For example, you may choose fruit with your breakfast on Monday and a potato with your dinner on Thursday, or you might opt for wheat-free pasta twice in one week. But keep in mind that you can't just load up with restricted foods on those two chosen days: remember, you're permitted *two servings total each week*. Regardless of your sweet or salty preferences, this allows you to really savor your favorite treats. You will also find that you will lose your cravings and reliance on your favorite forbidden foods in only a short time.

Note: Individuals on ketogenic protocols should omit all starch and fruit options.

STARCH OPTIONS

Brown rice (fermented or soaked)	Lima beans
Buckwheat (sprouted)	Potatoes (with skin)
Corn (non-GMO)	Quinoa
Garbanzo beans	Specialty wheat-free pasta
Green peas	Squash (acorn, butternut, or winter)
Jicama	Sweet potatoes
Lentils	Yams

FRUIT OPTIONS

Apples	Coconut water (counts as a fruit, not as a beverage; check carefully for sugar)
Bananas	
Berries	
Cherries	Dates

Dried apricots
Grapefruit
Lemons
Mangoes
Melons
Nectarines
Oranges

Papaya
Peaches
Pears
Pineapple
Plums
Prunes
Raisins

NUTS AND SEEDS

We highly suggest removing all nuts and seeds (and all nut- and seed-based products) from your diet to reduce omega-6 overload except for the following:

Chia seeds
Flaxseeds

Macadamias (if you simply cannot give up nuts, then these are the best once in a great while)

Daily Beverages

Feel free to enjoy as much water, sparkling water (unsweetened or with approved sugar substitiutes), and decaffeinated coffee and tea as you would like.

ALCOHOL

Enjoy up to two servings of alcohol per day. Those following a ketogenic protocol must limit alcohol to no more than three servings per week and should omit beer, hard cider, mead, and sweet wine.

Gluten-free beer
Hard alcohol
Hard cider

Mead
Wine

CAFFEINE

Make sure to add cream or milk to caffeinated coffee or tea to reduce the calcium-leaching effect.

TRIPLE THREAT RECIPES

If you are new to SKINNYFat, begin by adding only 1 teaspoon to shakes or coffees and slowly increase to the required amount. It may take about a week for your stomach to become accustomed to this oil.

Traditional Triple Threat Shake

SERVES 1   11 GRAMS OF PROTEIN PER SERVING

8 ounces cold water

1 packet Nutreince AM or PM

1 tablespoon SKINNYFat Original

1 scoop IN.POWER protein

1. Place the water in a blender (or a Calton Nutrition Triple Threat Tornado cup). On low speed, add the Nutreince while blending.

2. Add the SKINNYFat while continuing to blend. Finally, add the IN.POWER while blending.

Optional: Substitute chilled coffee for the water. If you have only hot coffee, use $1/2$ cup hot coffee and 1 cup ice in lieu of the 8 ounces water. This option is delicious with AM Vanilla Chai or PM Chocolate Lava.

Double Chocolate Mocha Triple Threat Shake

SERVES 1   11 GRAMS OF PROTEIN PER SERVING

8 ounces chilled organic fair-trade coffee

1 scoop IN.POWER protein

1 packet Nutreince PM Chocolate Lava

1 teaspoon Stevita Delight chocolate drink mix

1 tablespoon SKINNYFat Original

Combine all of the ingredients in a blender (or a Calton Nutrition Triple Threat Tornado cup).

Optional: Want a Double Chocolate Mocha Triple Threat Shake in the morning? No problem. Simply make this recipe with a Nutreince AM Vanilla Chai or AM Unflavored packet and add more chocolate Stevita Delight to taste.

Cinnamon Spice Triple Threat Shake

SERVES 1   11 GRAMS OF PROTEIN PER SERVING

8 ounces cold water

1 packet Nutreince AM Vanilla Chai

1 scoop IN.POWER protein

$^1/_2$ teaspoon organic cinnamon

1 tablespoon SKINNYFat Original

Combine all of the ingredients in a blender (or a Calton Nutrition Triple Threat Tornado cup).

Gingerbread Triple Threat Coffee

SERVES 1   11 GRAMS OF PROTEIN PER SERVING

8 ounces warm organic fair-trade coffee

1 scoop IN.POWER protein

1 packet Nutreince AM Vanilla Chai

5 to 10 drops toffee-flavored Stevita

1 tablespoon SKINNYFat Original

$^1/_2$ teaspoon organic vanilla extract

$^1/_2$ teaspoon organic cinnamon

$^1/_8$ teaspoon organic ground ginger

Combine all of the ingredients in a blender (or a Calton Nutrition Triple Threat Tornado cup). If you are an iced coffee fan, you can use chilled coffee for the same delicious treat.

Triple Threat Chocolate Lava Pudding

MAKES 4 PUDDINGS (TO BE USED AS MEAL REPLACEMENTS)

14 GRAMS OF PROTEIN PER PUDDING

3/4 tablespoon grass-fed gelatin (we like the Great Lakes brand in the red-orange can)

1 cup full-fat coconut milk (BPA-free can) or organic grass-fed heavy cream

1/2 tablespoon organic vanilla extract

1/2 tablespoon organic cinnamon (optional)

1 tablespoon Stevita Delight chocolate drink mix (optional)

1 tablespoon organic grass-fed salted butter (the salt helps bring out sweetness in desserts)

1 tablespoon SKINNYFat Original

4 packets Nutreince PM Chocolate Lava (that's right, the multivitamin is in the pudding!)

4 scoops IN.POWER protein

1. In a small saucepan over low heat, dissolve the gelatin in 1 cup water.

2. Pour the milk into a blender, then add the vanilla, cinnamon, Stevita Delight (if using), butter, and SKINNYFat and blend.

3. Add the gelatin mixture to the blender while blending on low speed.

4. Add the Nutreince and IN.POWER to the blender while blending on low speed. Blend thoroughly.

5. Pour the mixture into four ramekins, cover, and chill.

Tip: You can easily create vanilla chai breakfast puddings by using Nutreince AM Vanilla Chai and omitting the Stevita Delight chocolate.

Note: If you are not following a ketogenic program, and trying to up your protein, you may want to add an additional 4 scoops IN.POWER so that you will have a total of 2 scoops in each of the four puddings.

Ketogenic Option: Make with heavy cream instead of coconut milk.

Triple Threat Cheesecake

MAKES 4 CHEESECAKES (TO BE USED AS MEAL REPLACEMENTS)

17 GRAMS OF PROTEIN PER CHEESECAKE

$^3/_4$ tablespoon grass-fed gelatin (Great Lakes or similar)

1 block (16 tablespoons) organic cream cheese

$^1/_2$ tablespoon organic cinnamon

$1^1/_2$ teaspoons organic vanilla extract

$1^1/_2$ teaspoons Stevita Delight chocolate drink mix (if using Nutreince PM Chocolate Lava)

4 packets Nutreince AM or PM

4 scoops IN.POWER protein

1 tablespoon SKINNYFat Original

1. In a small saucepan over low heat, dissolve the gelatin in 1 cup water.

2. Place all of the remaining ingredients in a blender, add the gelatin mixture, and blend thoroughly.

3. Pour the mixture into 4 four ramekins, cover, and chill.

Triple Threat Ice Cream

MAKES 4 SERVINGS (TO BE USED AS MEAL REPLACEMENTS)

17 GRAMS OF PROTEIN PER SERVING

1. Start with the recipe for the Triple Threat Pudding or Triple Threat Cheesecake.

2. Make the pudding or cheesecake (using any Nutreince flavor you love), but do not place the mixture in ramekins.

3. Place the mixture in an ice cream maker and follow the machine's instructions.

Tip: Make these fabulous fats ahead of time—freeze them in ice cube trays or silicone molds, and then pop them out when you need them. They add a punch of flavor to any recipe.

Basil SKINNYFat Pesto (Dairy-Free, Nut-Free)

4 cups packed fresh organic basil leaves

Juice of $^1/_2$ organic lemon

2 large garlic cloves, quartered

Unrefined sea salt to taste

$^1/_4$ cup SKINNYFat Olive

1. Combine all of the ingredients in a blender or food processor and blend or process until smooth.

2. Refrigerate or freeze in ice cube trays to use later in recipes.

Sun-Dried Tomato SKINNYFat Pesto (Dairy-Free)

1 cup organic dry-packed sun-dried tomatoes

Handful of organic macadamia nuts

2 garlic cloves

Unrefined sea salt and organic pepper to taste

$^1/_4$ cup SKINNYFat Olive

1. Reconstitute the dried tomatoes by soaking them in warm water for 30 minutes.

2. Combine all of the ingredients in a blender or food processor and blend or process until smooth. Add extra SKINNYFat if necessary.

3. Refrigerate or freeze in ice cube trays to use later in recipes.

Herb SKINNYFat Butter

Choose fresh organic herbs if available. If not, then use dried organic herbs.

$^1/_2$ tablespoon organic thyme

$^1/_2$ tablespoon organic sage

$^1/_2$ tablespoon organic rosemary

$^1/_2$ tablespoon organic parsley

2 tablespoons SKINNYFat Olive

8 tablespoons (1 stick) organic grass-fed salted butter, room temperature

1. Combine the herbs with the SKINNYFat in a blender or food processor and blend or process until smooth.

2. Add the butter and blend or process until smooth.

3. Refrigerate or freeze in ice cube trays to use later in recipes.

Can't Get Enough Curry SKINNYFat Butter

2 teaspoons organic curry powder

2 teaspoons organic turmeric

2 teaspoons freshly grated ginger

2 tablespoons SKINNYFat Original

8 tablespoons (1 stick) organic grass-fed salted butter, room temperature

1. In a skillet over low heat, toast the curry and turmeric for about 2 minutes.

2. Combine all of the ingredients in a blender or food processor and blend or process until smooth.

3. Refrigerate or freeze in ice cube trays to use later in recipes.

Garlic-Parmesan SKINNYFat Butter

$^1/_2$ cup freshly grated organic Parmesan cheese

1 teaspoon organic garlic powder

$^1/_2$ teaspoon organic onion salt

$^1/_4$ teaspoon organic pepper

2 tablespoons SKINNYFat Olive

8 tablespoons (1 stick) organic grass-fed salted butter, room temperature

1. Combine all of the ingredients in a blender or food processor and blend or process until smooth.

2. Refrigerate or freeze in ice cube trays to use later in recipes.

Avocado Potassium-Packed SKINNYFat Butter

2 small avocados, halved, pitted, and peeled

Juice of 1 lemon

1 garlic clove, minced

2 teaspoons organic ground cumin

Unrefined sea salt and organic pepper to taste

2 tablespoons SKINNYFat Olive

4 tablespoons ($^1/_2$ stick) organic grass-fed salted butter, room temperature

1. Combine all of the ingredients in a blender or food processor and blend or process until smooth.

2. Refrigerate or freeze in ice cube trays to use later in recipes.

Spicy SKINNYFat Butter

$^1/_2$ teaspoon organic chili powder

$^1/_2$ teaspoon organic paprika

$^1/_2$ tablespoons organic garlic powder

$^1/_4$ teaspoon organic onion powder

$^1/_4$ teaspoon organic cayenne pepper

2 tablespoons SKINNYFat Olive

8 tablespoons (1 stick) organic grass-fed salted butter, room temperature

1. Combine the seasonings with the SKINNYFat in a blender or food processor and blend or process until smooth.

2. Add the butter and blend or process until smooth.

3. Refrigerate or freeze in ice cube trays to use later in recipes.

SKINNYFat Pizza-in-a-Bottle Italian Infused Oil

1 ounce fresh organic basil leaves

1 ounce fresh organic oregano leaves

1 (25-fluid-ounce) bottle SKINNYFat Olive

3 garlic cloves, chopped

1 to 2 hot peppers, halved (optional)

1. Preheat the oven to 300°F.

2. Clean the basil and oregano and place all of the ingredients in an oven-safe bowl or baking dish. Cover with the SKINNYFat.

3. Bake for 40 minutes.

4. Let cool, then strain the oil before pouring it back into the glass SKINNYFat bottle.

Tip: Make sure to label the bottle. You don't want to accidentally use this for your Triple Threat Shake!

BREAKFAST IDEAS

French Onion Egg Tart

SERVES 4   17 GRAMS OF PROTEIN PER SERVING

1 tablespoon organic grass-fed salted butter, plus more to cook the eggs

2 medium organic yellow onions, cut into 1- to 2-inch pieces

1 large garlic clove (or 2 small cloves), minced

3 sprigs fresh organic thyme

$1/2$ teaspoon organic crushed red pepper flakes, or to taste (we use 1 teaspoon because we like it spicy)

$1/4$ teaspoon unrefined sea salt

$1/4$ teaspoon organic pepper

4 large organic pasture-raised eggs

2 tablespoons freshly grated organic Parmesan cheese (or a similar cheese)

1 cooked, leftover, organic boneless chicken thigh, diced (if you don't have one in the fridge, you can substitute another leftover meat or quickly dice and brown a thigh in an additional skillet)

3 ounces freshly grated organic Gouda cheese

1. Melt 1 tablespoon butter in a $10^1/_2$-inch ceramic skillet or similar pan over medium to high heat.

2. Add the onions, garlic, thyme, red pepper flakes, salt, and pepper.

3. Cook until the onions are caramelized. Remove the thyme stems.

4. Remove the onions from the heat and set them aside in a small bowl.

5. Crack the eggs into a bowl and beat them with a fork. Add the Parmesan.

6. Place the skillet over medium heat and add a little butter.

7. Pour the egg mixture into the skillet so that it covers the bottom.

8. Cover and cook until the egg solidifies like a pancake, 2 to 3 minutes.

9. Distribute the cooked chicken evenly over the egg and cover with the caramelized onions.

10. Sprinkle the shredded Gouda over the whole tart.

11. Cover and cook for approximately 5 minutes, or until the cheese is melted.

Ketogenic Option: Use 2 tablespoons butter. When scrambling the eggs in step 5, use 4 whole eggs, 1 egg yolk, and $^1/_4$ cup heavy cream. Use only one onion and substitute 2 links cooked sausage for the chicken thigh. *22 grams of protein per serving.*

Salmon (or Sausage) Cake Egg Sandwich

MAKES 4 OPEN-FACED SANDWICHES
30 GRAMS OF PROTEIN PER SANDWICH

Salmon Cake

2 (6-ounce) cans wild-caught salmon (we love the wild red sockeye salmon from Vital Choice)

2 large organic pasture-raised eggs

1 scoop IN.POWER protein

$^1/_2$ organic onion

2 teaspoons seafood seasoning

2 teaspoons organic Cajun spice

Unrefined sea salt and organic pepper to taste

1 tablespoon organic grass-fed salted butter

Topping

2 ounces organic cream cheese

4 large organic pasture-raised eggs

1. Preheat the broiler.

2. Combine all the salmon cake ingredients except the butter in a bowl. Form the mixture into 4 large salmon cakes.

3. In a large skillet, melt the butter. Brown the salmon cakes over medium heat on one side, then flip to cook on the other side.

4. Remove from the heat.

5. Place the cooked salmon cakes on a baking sheet and top each cake with $^1/_2$ ounce cream cheese. Broil until the cheese is melted.

6. In the skillet, fry 1 egg per salmon cake over medium heat. Place the fried eggs on top of the cakes to serve.

Ketogenic Option: Use 4 sausage links rather than the salmon cake ingredients to create the cakes. Remove each sausage from its casing and flatten them to form 4 patties. In a large skillet, melt 1 tablespoon butter. Brown the sausage patties on one side, then flip to cook on the other side. Remove from the heat. Place the cooked sausage patties on a baking sheet and top each patty with 1 ounce cream cheese. Broil until the cheese is melted. In the skillet, fry 1 egg per sausage patty. Place the fried eggs on top of the patties to serve. *26 grams of protein per sandwich.*

Protein-Packed Morning Muffins

MAKES 6 MUFFINS   9 GRAMS OF PROTEIN PER MUFFIN

EAT AS MANY AS FIT FOR YOUR PROTEIN INTAKE.

6 slices organic pasture-raised bacon

$^1/_3$ organic onion, finely diced

1 garlic clove, chopped

5 large organic pasture-raised eggs

$^1/_4$ cup organic sour cream (you choose the fat content—full fat for keto)

$^2/_3$ cup freshly chopped or grated organic cheese

Unrefined sea salt and organic pepper to taste

Organic cayenne pepper to taste

Organic seasonings, as desired

$^1/_3$ organic tomato, chopped

$^1/_3$ cup cooked organic spinach or asparagus

1. Preheat the oven to 325°F.

2. Grease a muffin tin with ghee, coconut oil, SKINNYFat, butter, or retained and collected fat, or use a nonstick tin. You will use only six of the muffin cups (perhaps seven, depending on the bulk of the vegetables and bacon).

3. In a small nonstick skillet, brown the bacon over medium heat. Remove from the heat and chop the bacon. Use the remaining bacon fat to cook the onion and garlic until the onion is translucent, 2 to 3 minutes.

4. In a small bowl, beat the eggs and combine them with the sour cream, cheese, and seasonings.

5. Divide the egg mixture among the muffin cups, filling each one two-thirds full, keeping enough room on top for the bacon and vegetables.

6. In the bowl that was used for the egg mixture, combine the cooked onion and garlic, tomato, spinach, and bacon. Distribute evenly among the filled muffin cups.

7. Bake for approximately 25 minutes, or until cooked through. Allow the muffins to cool completely before removing them from the muffin tin.

Tip: You can use up any of your leftovers in these muffins to create delicious and freezable portable morning treats.

Ketogenic Option: Use 4 whole eggs and 1 yolk instead of 5 whole eggs. Omit the onions and tomato. Use half the amount of vegetables and top with cream cheese to serve. *9 grams of protein per muffin.*

Vegetarian/Vegan Option: Omit the bacon and add your choice of beans or a meat alternative.

ENTRÉES

Buffalo Chicken Chili

SERVES 6   33 GRAMS OF PROTEIN PER SERVING

4 tablespoons SKINNYFat Original

$1^1/2$ pounds organic pasture-raised ground chicken

1 large organic onion, chopped

2 organic celery stalks, chopped

2 large organic carrots, chopped

4 garlic cloves, chopped

1 (28-ounce) can organic fire-roasted diced tomatoes (BPA-free can)

2 tablespoons organic chili powder

1 teaspoon organic ground cumin

1 teaspoon organic dried oregano

$1/2$ teaspoon organic cayenne pepper

Unrefined sea salt and organic pepper to taste

$1/2$ cup organic crumbled blue cheese (gluten-free!)

3 tablespoons organic white vinegar

1. In a large ceramic pot over medium–high heat, heat the SKINNYFat.

2. Add the chicken and cook until brown, about 10 to 15 minutes.

3. Stir in the onion, celery, carrots, garlic, tomatoes, and seasonings.

4. Cover and simmer over low heat for approximately 4 hours. (Or, after browning the chicken in the pot, place all of the ingredients in a slow cooker and cook on low for 4 hours.)

5. Mix in the cheese and vinegar just before serving.

Note: To reduce/eliminate the lectin content of the tomatoes, cook them in a pressure cooker before adding them to the recipe.

Ketogenic Option: Substitute ground chuck for the ground chicken and omit the vegetables and tomato when cooking on the stove. Then add in $1/2$ cup Buffalo Wing Sauce (aka Jayson's Red Hot) (page 272), with butter added, and 8 ounces cream cheese. Top each serving with $1/4$ cup sour cream. *26 grams of protein per serving.*

Vegetarian/Vegan Option: Substitute organic sprouted black beans for the organic chicken.

Grilled Tandoori Skewers

SERVES 6   35 GRAMS OF PROTEIN PER SERVING

$1^1/4$ cups organic plain Greek yogurt

2 tablespoons fresh lemon juice

2 tablespoons SKINNYFat Olive

3 tablespoons freshly grated ginger

1 teaspoon unrefined sea salt

1 teaspoon organic turmeric

1 teaspoon organic garam masala (Indian spice; we use Frontier brand)

1 teaspoon organic cayenne pepper, or more for extra spiciness

1 teaspoon organic paprika

2 garlic cloves, minced

$1/2$ head organic broccoli, cut into large florets

$1/2$ head organic cauliflower, cut into large florets

1 large organic yellow onion, cut into about 8 pieces

| 1 organic zucchini or summer squash, cut into $^3/_4$-inch slices | 2 pounds high-quality protein, cut into 1- to 2-inch squares (choose one or a combination: chicken, shrimp, fish, or beef) |

1. In a large mixing bowl, combine the yogurt, lemon juice, SKINNYFat, ginger, salt, turmeric, garam masala, cayenne, paprika, and garlic.

2. Place the broccoli, cauliflower, and onion in a steamer on the stove or in a microwave oven and lightly steam. Do not cook all the way through—simply soften.

3. Add the softened vegetables, zucchini, and protein to the yogurt mixture and combine well.

4. Cover and refrigerate for at least 30 minutes.

5. Heat a grill or broiler to medium-high heat.

6. Thread the yogurt-coated proteins and vegetables onto eight skewers.

7. Grill the skewers until lightly charred.

Tip: These skewers can be accompanied by Cooling Cucumber Raita (page 271) and Indian Garlic-Butter Cheese Non-Naan (page 269).

Ketogenic Option: Omit the broccoli, cauliflower, and tomatoes and use 6 portobello mushrooms instead. Closely follow the ketogenic adaptation for Cooling Cucumber Raita (page 271). *31 grams of protein per serving.*

Vegetarian/Vegan Option: You can substitute plain coconut yogurt for the Greek yogurt. Vegans can make these with no protein and serve with a bowl of organic sprouted cooked beans.

Greek Chicken

SERVES 6   37 GRAMS OF PROTEIN PER SERVING

Spinach Layer

1 tablespoon SKINNYFat Olive

10 ounces organic spinach

4 ounces organic feta cheese

2 large organic pasture-raised eggs

1 medium organic onion, diced

Chicken Mixture

2 tablespoons SKINNYFat Olive

1 1/2 pounds organic pasture-raised chicken thighs, cut into 1-inch pieces

2 teaspoons organic garlic powder

2 teaspoons organic dried oregano

Topping

3 ounces organic feta cheese

1/2 to 1 cup organic sugar-free tomato sauce

1. Preheat the oven to 325°F.

2. Coat a 9 × 13 baking dish with a thin layer of SKINNYFat.

3. Create the spinach layer by first boiling the spinach for 15 minutes to remove oxalates. In a mixing bowl, combine the spinach with the feta, eggs, and onion. Spread the mixture on the bottom of the prepared dish.

4. For the chicken mixture, in a skillet over medium heat, heat the SKINNYFat. Add the chicken, garlic, and oregano and cook until the chicken is no longer pink.

5. Spoon the chicken layer over the spinach layer in the baking dish.

6. To make the topping, layer the feta and tomato sauce over the chicken.

7. Bake for 30 minutes. Let stand for 5 minutes before serving.

Ketogenic Option: This recipe is not suitable for a ketogenic diet.

Vegetarian/Vegan Option: The flavors in this dish match perfectly with large, raw sprouted butter beans, lima beans, tofu, or eggplant.

You can replace the feta with a soy-free, nut-free option. We like the Paleo-friendly versions by Urban Cheesecraft.

Chicken, Broccoli, and Cheese Soup

SERVES 6   26 GRAMS OF PROTEIN PER SERVING

1 (9-ounce) chicken thigh

1 tablespoon SKINNYFat Original or organic grass-fed salted butter

1 head organic broccoli, chopped into pieces (you can use the stems too)

3 cups chicken broth (homemade or an organic sugar-free store-bought version)

8 ounces organic cream cheese

2 tablespoons organic grass-fed salted butter

1 cup organic grass-fed heavy cream

2 cups shredded organic Cheddar cheese (buy a block and shred it yourself to avoid added cellulose powder)

Unrefined sea salt and organic pepper to taste

1. Cut the chicken thigh into $^1/_2$-inch pieces. In a small nonstick sauté pan, sauté the chicken pieces in the SKINNYFat. When the chicken is cooked through, remove it from the heat, drain, and set aside.

2. In a large pot, cook the broccoli in the broth. By doing this, you will preserve the nutrients that broccoli loses during boiling.

3. When the broccoli is cooked through (fork-soft), transfer about half of the florets to a small bowl and set aside.

4. Place the broth and the remaining broccoli in a blender or food processor and blend or process until smooth.

5. In the large pot, combine the cream cheese, 2 tablespoons butter, cream, and Cheddar and cook slowly over low heat, stirring frequently to avoid burning.

6. When the cheese mixture is completely melted, add the puréed broccoli and broth and chicken and heat through over low heat.

7. Add the reserved broccoli florets for texture.

8. Add the salt and pepper.

Ketogenic Option: Use half of the broccoli for this recipe. *26 grams of protein per sandwich.*

Vegetarian/Vegan Option: Omit the chicken thigh. Replace the chicken broth with vegetable broth and add 2 cups organic lima or cannellini beans.

Micronutrient-Packed Meat Loaf

SERVES 6   21 GRAMS OF PROTEIN PER SERVING

$1/4$ pound organic liver (or an additional $1/2$ cup ground beef, if you prefer)

1 pound organic grass-fed ground beef

1 cup mushrooms (we like reconstituted dried wild porcini mushrooms), chopped

$1/2$ cup organic crumbled blue cheese (gluten-free!)

1 tablespoon organic garlic powder

1 tablespoon organic onion powder

2 teaspoons organic crushed red pepper flakes

1 tablespoon unrefined sea salt

1 tablespoon organic pepper

1 tablespoon organic chipotle powder

$3/4$ cup organic tomato sauce

$1/4$ cup freshly grated or finely sliced organic cheese (optional, but we love Port du Salut for this!)

1. Preheat the oven to 350°F.

2. Liquefy the liver in a blender or food processor.

3. Place the ground beef and mushrooms in a baking pan or glass baking dish and pour in the liver. Add the blue cheese, garlic powder, onion powder, red pepper flakes, salt, pepper, and chipotle.

4. Use your hands to combine the ingredients and shape the mixture into a loaf. Bake for 30 minutes.

5. Remove from the oven and cover with the tomato sauce and grated cheese. Return to the oven for an additional 10 minutes to allow the cheese to melt.

Ketogenic Option: This recipe is already ketogenic.

Vegetarian/Vegan Option: This recipe is not suitable for a vegetarian diet. Consider making a chickpea meat loaf or similar.

Shepherd's Pie

SERVES 6   23 GRAMS OF PROTEIN PER SERVING

Top Layer
1 recipe Cauliflower Mash
   (page 270)

Bottom Layer

2 tablespoons SKINNYFat Olive

2 organic onions, chopped

2 garlic cloves, minced

1^1/$_2$ pounds organic grass-fed ground beef

2 tablespoons organic curry powder

2 tablespoons organic turmeric

1 tablespoon organic ground cumin

^{1}/$_2$ teaspoon organic ground ginger

^{1}/$_2$ tablespoon organic cinnamon

^{1}/$_2$ to 1 teaspoon organic cayenne pepper

1 (3-ounce) bag organic frozen peas

1 organic carrot, cut into small cubes

1. Prepare the Cauliflower Mash and set it aside. Preheat the oven to 350°F.

2. In a large skillet over medium heat, heat the SKINNYFat. Add the onions and garlic and cook until the onions just begin to become translucent, 2 to 3 minutes.

3. Add the ground beef and cook until browned, about 5 minutes.

4. Add the spices, peas, and carrots. Reduce the heat to medium-low and cook for 15 minutes.

5. Spread the meat mixture across the bottom of a 9 × 13-inch baking dish. Create a second layer on top with the Cauliflower Mash. You can refrigerate until needed or pop it in the oven until piping hot.

Ketogenic Option: This recipe is not suitable for a ketogenic diet.

Vegetarian/Vegan Option: Replace the ground beef with 1^1/$_2$ cup raw lentils or 3^3/$_4$ cups cooked lentils or cooked sprouted organic lentils. They give the recipe a hearty, earthy flavor. Add one extra carrot and a larger (12-ounce) bag of peas. *15 grams of protein per serving.*

Rustic Portobello Pizza Caps

SERVES 8   14 GRAMS OF PROTEIN PER SERVING

8 large portobello mushroom caps, stems and gills removed

6 tablespoons SKINNYFat Pizza-in-a-Bottle Italian Infused Oil (page 255)

Unrefined sea salt and organic pepper

^{1}/$_2$ cup organic pizza sauce of your choice (sugar-free)

8 to 16 organic black olives, sliced

2 anchovy fillets, chopped (optional, but preferred for flavor and omega-3 content)

30 slices organic pepperoni

^{1}/$_2$ pound cooked organic Italian sausage (optional)

8 garlic cloves, roasted and smashed

2 cups shredded organic mozzarella cheese (buy a block and shred it yourself to avoid added cellulose powder)

Organic crushed red pepper flakes (optional)

1. Preheat the oven to 425°F.

2. Brush each mushroom cap with ^{3}/$_4$ tablespoon of the SKINNYFat and sprinkle with a pinch of salt and a grind of pepper.

3. Roast the caps for 15 to 20 minutes (depending on the size of the mushrooms), or until they are nicely roasted but still holding their general shape.

4. Let the caps cool until they can be handled.

5. Drain or pat dry the caps to remove any excess moisture.

6. Spoon 1 to 2 tablespoons pizza sauce into each cap.

7. Top with the olives, anchovies (if using), pepperoni, sausage (if using), garlic, mozzarella, red pepper flakes (if using), and a small grind of pepper.

8. Place the mushrooms back in the oven until the cheese is melted and beginning to brown, like on pizza, about 5 minutes.

9. Serve immediately. *Buon appetito!*

Ketogenic Option: Limit the pizza sauce to $1/4$ cup. *21 grams of protein per serving.*

Vegetarian/Vegan Option: Leave out the meats and cheese or find protein-filled, soy-free, sugar-free vegan substitutes such as BeyondMeat products.

Fabulous Fajitas

SERVES 6   35 GRAMS OF PROTEIN PER SERVING

4 tablespoons SKINNYFat Olive

1 teaspoon organic chili powder

$1^1/2$ teaspoons organic dried oregano

1 teaspoon unrefined sea salt

1 teaspoon organic paprika

1 teaspoon organic onion powder

1 teaspoon organic garlic powder

$1/2$ to 1 teaspoon organic cayenne pepper (optional)

$1^1/2$ teaspoons organic ground cumin

$1^1/2$ pounds organic pasture-raised chicken thighs, cut into strips (you can also use shrimp, beef, or fish)

2 organic red bell peppers, sliced into strips

2 organic yellow bell peppers, sliced into strips

2 organic onions, thinly sliced into strips

1. Make a marinade by combining 2 tablespoons of the SKINNYFat with the chili powder, oregano, salt, paprika,

onion powder, garlic powder, cayenne (if using), and cumin in a large mixing bowl.

2. Add the chicken and toss to coat well.

3. Cover and chill for 1 to 5 hours.

4. In a large skillet over medium heat, heat the remaining 2 tablespoons SKINNYFat.

5. Add the bell peppers and onions and cook, covered, stirring frequently, until they begin to soften, about 5 minutes.

6. Add the chicken. Stir so the seasonings coat the vegetables as well.

7. Cook until the chicken is thoroughly cooked, about 10 minutes. Remove from the heat.

8. Serve with Holy Moly Guacamole (page 276), organic salsa, shredded organic cheese (Manchego), organic sour cream, and Ridiculously Simple Wraps (optional, page 268).

Ketogenic Option: Omit the bell peppers and wraps and load up on all the toppings. Add 1 tablespoon SKINNYFat to the sour cream to make super keto sour cream. *35 grams of protein per serving.*

Vegetarian/Vegan Option: Omit the protein and serve with a bowl of organic cooked sprouted beans.

SENSATIONAL SIDE DISHES AND RAD WRAPS

Ridiculously Simple Wraps

MAKES 1 LARGE WRAP OR 2 SMALL WRAPS

1 large organic pasture-raised egg

1 tablespoon SKINNYFat Original

1 tablespoon freshly grated organic Parmesan cheese

1 tablespoon IN.POWER protein

$1/2$ tablespoon buckwheat flour

$1/2$ tablespoon coconut flour

1 tablespoon water

1. In a small bowl, mix all of the ingredients together to form the batter.

2. Heat a small ceramic skillet lightly coated with SKINNYFat or another fat over medium heat.

3. Pour in the batter so it forms a thin layer across the bottom of the skillet.

4. Cover and cook until bubbles form; don't hurry this.

5. Flip and cook for 1 minute, or until golden brown.

Tip: These can be made fresh, or make a larger batch and keep them in the refrigerator for grab-and-go meals.

Indian Garlic-Butter Cheese Non-Naan

MAKES 1 WRAP

1 organic pasture-raised egg

1 tablespoon SKINNYFat Original

1 tablespoon freshly grated organic Parmesan cheese

1 tablespoon water

1 tablespoon IN.POWER protein

$^1/_2$ tablespoon buckwheat flour

$^1/_2$ tablespoon coconut flour

$^1/_2$ teaspoon organic garlic powder

1 teaspoon minced garlic

1 ounce organic mozzarella cheese, finely chopped

Organic grass-fed salted butter

1. In a small bowl, mix all of the ingredients together to form the batter.

2. Heat a small ceramic skillet lightly coated with butter over medium heat.

3. Pour in the batter so it forms a thin layer across the bottom of the skillet.

4. Cover and cook until bubbles form.

5. Flip and cook for 30 to 60 seconds more.

Tip: These are amazing with any Indian-spiced meal, such as Grilled Tandoori Skewers (page 260). If making a large batch—say for a family dinner—keep them warm in the oven as you make them. Place shavings of butter in between each piece of naan. Then watch them disappear at the dinner table.

Vegetarian/Vegan Option: Vegans can omit the cheeses.

Cauliflower Mash

SERVES 4

1 head organic cauliflower, chopped

3 tablespoons organic grass-fed salted butter

2 tablespoons organic cream cheese

$^1/_2$ teaspoon organic garlic powder

$^1/_4$ teaspoon organic onion powder

Unrefined sea salt and organic pepper to taste

1. Steam the cauliflower until soft.

2. Place the cauliflower and the remaining ingredients in a blender or food processor and blend or process until smooth. We like to keep it a bit chunky, as the texture more resembles potato.

Ketogenic Option: This recipe is not suitable for a ketogenic diet.

Vegetarian/Vegan Option: Replace the butter and cream cheese with full-fat coconut milk.

Rich and Creamy Alfredo Sauce

SERVES 2 TO 4

4 tablespoons ($^1/_2$ stick) organic grass-fed unsalted butter

1 large organic pasture-raised egg, beaten

$^1/_2$ cup organic grass-fed heavy cream

1 garlic clove, minced

$^2/_3$ cup freshly grated organic Parmesan cheese

Organic pepper to taste

1. In a skillet over low heat, melt the butter.

2. Add the egg and cream and combine. Raise the heat to medium.

3. Add the garlic, then slowly add the cheese, stirring to avoid forming clumps.

4. When the mixture is fully combined, season with pepper.

5. Refrigerate or freeze in ice cube trays to use later in recipes.

Optional: Add sliced portobello mushrooms for an earthy, meatlike quality.

Cooling Cucumber Raita

SERVES 4

2 cups organic plain Greek yogurt (try to find one that has some fat in it)

2 tablespoons SKINNYFat Olive

2 large organic seedless cucumbers, 1 chopped, 1 shredded with a vegetable peeler and drained to remove excess water (leave the skin on for color)

| 1/4 teaspoon organic ground coriander | 1/4 cup fresh organic cilantro, chopped |
| 1/4 teaspoon organic ground cumin | Unrefined sea salt to taste |

Combine all of the ingredients in a large bowl and let sit for at least 30 minutes before serving.

Tip: This cooling, traditionally Indian salad is perfect as an accompaniment to Grilled Tandoori Skewers (page 260) or Indian Garlic-Butter Cheese Non-Naan (page 269).

Ketogenic Option: Use sour cream in place of the Greek yogurt and omit the cucumber.

Buffalo Wing Sauce (aka Jayson's Red Hot)

MAKES 1/2 CUP

2/3 cup organic white vinegar (apple cider, rice, and white wine vinegar work also)

2 teaspoons SKINNYFat Original

2 teaspoons organic chili powder

1/4 teaspoon organic smoked paprika

1/2 teaspoon organic sweet paprika

1 tablespoon organic garlic powder

1/2 teaspoon organic onion powder

1/2 teaspoon organic cayenne pepper

1/4 teaspoon unrefined sea salt

Stevia to taste (Jayson uses 1/2 to 1 scoop stevia using the tiny scooper in the bottle; start with just a little and add to taste)

1 teaspoon grass-fed gelatin (Great Lakes or similar)

2 tablespoons organic grass-fed salted butter, melted

1. In a small pot, stir together all of the ingredients except the gelatin and the butter.

2. Place the pot over medium-high heat. Once the sauce is warm, stir in the gelatin slowly, to avoid clumping. Heat until the sauce starts to bubble and thicken.

3. Remove the sauce from the heat and allow it to cool.

4. Store the sauce in an airtight glass bottle and keep it refrigerated.

5. When you are ready to serve, warm the finished sauce and combine with the butter. Do not add the butter until you are ready to serve; the sauce will not keep well after you add the butter.

5-Minute SKINNYFat Mayonnaise

2 large organic pasture-raised egg yolks

1 large organic pasture-raised whole egg

1 tablespoon organic mustard

$^1/_4$ teaspoon unrefined sea salt

$^1/_4$ teaspoon organic pepper

1 tablespoon fresh lemon juice or organic white vinegar (or apple cider vinegar)

1 cup SKINNYFat Original

1. Combine the eggs, mustard, salt, pepper, lemon juice, and 1 tablespoon cold water in a blender or food processor and blend or process on low to medium speed until smooth.

2. Slowly pour the SKINNYFat into the blender while running at low speed.

3. Once all of the SKINNYFat has been mixed in, you will have a creamy, smooth, homemade mayonnaise.

4. Keep refrigerated.

Note: Never attempt to make mayonnaise using chilled eggs; bring them to room temperature first.

Optional:
- *Curry mayo:* Add organic curry powder and organic cayenne pepper to taste. Great in chicken salad.
- *Cajun mayo:* Add organic Cajun spice and organic cayenne pepper to taste. Tasty on salmon cakes.

Simple SKINNYFat Italian Dressing

²/₃ cup SKINNYFat Olive

1 tablespoon minced garlic

4 tablespoons organic red wine vinegar

Unrefined sea salt and organic pepper to taste

Combine all of the ingredients in a glass jar with a lid that seals tightly. Shake before using.

SKINNYFat Parmesan-Peppercorn Dressing

¹/₂ cup Simple SKINNYFat Italian Dressing (above)

4 heaping teaspoons shredded organic Parmesan cheese (buy a block and shred it yourself to avoid added cellulose powder)

¹/₄ cup organic full-fat sour cream or organic plain Greek yogurt

Freshly cracked organic peppercorns to taste

Use an immersion blender to combine the dressing, Parmesan, and sour cream in a mixing bowl. Add the peppercorns and serve.

SKINNYFat Tartar Sauce

¹/₂ cup 5-Minute SKINNYFat Mayonnaise (page 273)

2 tablespoons diced pickles (we love Bubbies brand)

1 tablespoon organic white vinegar or white wine vinegar

1 teaspoon favorite organic mustard

Juice of ¹/₄ lemon

Pinch of unrefined sea salt

Pinch of organic pepper

Combine all of the ingredients in a small bowl and let sit for at least 30 minutes before serving.

Citrus-Garlic Dipping Sauce for Fish

1 large organic pasture-raised egg, beaten

2 tablespoons organic yogurt or SKINNYFat mayonnaise

1 tablespoon organic Dijon mustard

1/4 teaspoon organic garlic powder

1/8 teaspoon organic cayenne pepper

1/2 teaspoon organic thyme

4 drops in.essence orange essential oil

2 drops in.essence lemon essential oil

Combine all ingredients in a blender and blend until smooth.

Really Creamy SKINNYFat Blue Cheese Dressing (or Dip)

1/2 recipe 5-Minute SKINNYFat Mayonnaise (page 273)

4 ounces organic blue cheese (gluten-free!)

1/3 cup organic sour cream

4 ounces organic cream cheese

Combine all of the ingredients in a blender and blend until smooth. If you prefer chunky blue cheese, mix the mayonnaise with the sour cream and cream cheese and then hand-crumble the blue cheese into the recipe.

Orange Balsamic Vinaigrette

12 ounces SKINNYFat Olive

4 ounces balsamic vinegar

1/2 teaspoon salt (we like Redmond Real Salt)

1/2 teaspoon organic pepper

1 tablespoon organic mustard powder

2 garlic cloves, minced

4 drops in.essence orange essential oil

Combine all ingredients in blender and blend until smooth.

Cuban Avocado Mojo Dressing

1 large avocado, halved, pitted, peeled, and cut into large chunks

Zest and juice from 1 organic orange

Zest and juice from 2 organic limes

3 garlic cloves

1 organic jalapeño pepper, seeded and finely chopped

1 organic green onion (scallion), white and green parts, chopped

1/2 bunch fresh organic cilantro (leaves only), chopped

Organic unrefined sea salt to taste

SKINNYFat Olive, as desired

Combine all the ingredients except the SKINNYFat in a blender and blend until smooth. Serve within 2 hours so that the avocado does not turn brown. Stir in SKINNYFat olive last until the guacamole reaches the desired thickness.

Tip: This can also be used as a delicious dip.

Holy Moly Guacamole

2 avocados

1 small organic onion, minced

1 garlic clove, minced

1 ripe organic tomato, chopped

1 organic jalapeño pepper, chopped

Juice of 1 organic lime

Unrefined sea salt and organic pepper to taste

1. Halve the avocados, remove the pits, and scoop out the flesh into a bowl.

2. Mash the avocado in the bowl and stir in the onion, garlic, tomato, and jalapeño to taste.

3. Season with the lime juice, salt, and pepper and combine.

4. Chill for 30 minutes before serving.

Optional: In a hurry? Mash the avocado and simply add 2 tablespoons organic salsa. It might not be homemade, but it will be a home run!

Killer Ketchup That Won't Kill You!

1 can (12 ounces) organic tomato paste (BPA-free can)

$^1/_2$ cup water

2 tablespoons organic white vinegar

1 teaspoon organic onion powder

1 teaspoon organic allspice

$^1/_2$ teaspoon organic garlic powder

Organic cayenne pepper to taste

Unrefined sea salt and organic pepper to taste

Stevia extract to taste

1. If possible, pressure-cook the tomato paste first to eliminate lectins.

2. In a saucepan over medium heat, combine all of the ingredients and stir until smooth.

3. Cool and store in a canning jar, preferably opaque, in the refrigerator.

Tip: This sugar-free, organic ketchup stores well in the refrigerator—you can keep it for over a week.

Notes

Chapter 1: Micronutrient Deficiency

7   **adequate intake of vitamin D:** Fulgoni VL et al., "Foods, fortificants, and supplements: where do Americans get their nutrients?" *Journal of Nutrition* 141, no. 10 (October 2011):1847–54. doi: 10.3945/jn.111.142257.

7   **increase the risk of osteoporosis:** Bischoff-Ferrari HA et al., "Fracture prevention with vitamin D supplementation: a meta-analysis of randomized controlled trials." *JAMA* 293, no. 18 (2005):2257–2264. See also Kim MH et al., "Osteoporosis, vitamin C intake, and physical activity in Korean adults aged 50 years and over." *Journal of Physical Therapy Science* 28, no. 3 (2016):725–30; Lim LS et al., "Vitamin A intake and the risk of hip fracture in postmenopausal women: the Iowa Women's Health Study." *Osteoporosis International* 15, no. 7 (July 2004):552–9; Tucker KL et al., "Potassium, magnesium, and fruit and vegetable intakes are associated with greater bone mineral density in elderly men and women." *American Journal of Clinical Nutrition* 69, no. 4 (April 1999):727–36; Vicky T et al., "Calcium intake and bone mineral density: systematic review and meta-analysis." *BMJ* 351 (2015):h4183; *Clinical Education.* clinicaleducation.org/news/building-bone-the-novel-role-of-tocotrienols.

8   **according to Mehmet Oz:** Oz M, "Dr. Oz's ultimate supplement checklist." doctoroz.com/videos/dr-ozs-ultimate-supplement-checklist.

8   **number of Americans affected:** *National Osteoporosis Foundation.* cdn.nof.org /wp-content/uploads/2015/12/Osteoporosis-Fast-Facts.pdf. See also Mozaffarian D et al., "Heart disease and stroke statistics—2015 update: a report from the American Heart Association." *Circulation* 131, no. 4 (January 2015):e29–322; American Cancer Society. *Cancer Facts and Figures 2017.* Atlanta, GA: American Cancer Society, 2017; *National Diabetes Statistics Report, 2014.* Atlanta, GA: US Department of Health and Human Services, 2014; *The Heart Foundation.* https://theheartfoundation.org /heart-disease-facts-2.

8   **more than two billion people:** World Health Organization. *World Health Report, 2000.* Geneva: World Health Organization, 2000.

8   **a 2010 study:** Tulchinsky TH, "micronutrient deficiency conditions: global health issues." *Public Health Reviews* 2010, no. 32:243–55.

8   **researchers determined:** Ruston D et al. *The National Diet and Nutrition Survey: Adults Aged 19 to 64 Years.* London: Stationary Office, 2004. See also Derbyshire E, "Micronutrient intakes of British adults across mid-life: a secondary analysis of the UK National Diet and Nutrition Survey." *Frontiers in Nutrition* 5, no. 55 (July 2018):fig. 4. doi: 10.3389/fnut.2018.00055.

9   **is on the rise:** *Daily Mail.* dailymail.co.uk/news/article-2543724/Rickets-soar -children-stay-indoors-Number-diagnosed-disease-quadruples-ten-years.html #ixzz3AYczNJLL.

9   **In the United Arab Emirates:** *Gulf News.* gulfnews.com/going-out/society /90-of-uae-population-vitamin-d-deficient-says-dha-official-1.2113556.

9   **in China:** *World Health Organization.* www.wpro.who.int/nutrition/documents /docs/chn.pdf.

9   **Researchers caution:** Lu HK et al., "High prevalence of vitamin D insufficiency in China: relationship with the levels of parathyroid hormone and markers of bone turnover." *PLoS One* 7, no. 11 (2012):e47264.

9   **In India:** *Times of India.* www.timesofindia.indiatimes.com/life-style/health -fitness/health-news/7-out-of-every-10-Indians-are-vitamin-deficient/article show/49380097.cms.

9   **according to the World Health Organization:** *World Health Organization.* who. int/vmnis/database/vitamina/x/en/.

10   **only 5 to 10 percent:** Anand P et al., "Cancer is a preventable disease that requires major lifestyle changes." *Pharmaceutical Research* 25, no. 9 (September 2008):2097–116.

10   **a statement from the *Journal of the American Medical Association*:** Fairfield KM et al., "Vitamins for chronic disease prevention in adults: scientific review." *JAMA* 287, no. 23 (June 2002):3116–26.

10   **Dr. Mark Hyman:** Hyman M, "How dietary supplements reduce health care costs." drhyman.com/how-dietary-supplements-reduce-health-care-costs-3250/.

11   **a study published in the *Proceedings of the National Academy of Sciences*:** Langsjoen PH et al., "Response of patients in classes III and IV of cardiomyopathy to therapy in a blind and crossover trial with coenzyme Q10." *Proceedings of the National Academy of Sciences* 82, no. 12 (1985):4240–4.

11   **Michael Holick, MD:** Holick MF, "Vitamin D and sunlight: strategies for cancer prevention and other health benefits." *Clinical Journal of the American Society of Nephrology* 3, no. 5 (2008):1548–54.

11   **In a study published in the *European Journal of Neurology*:** Kivipelto M et al., "Homocysteine and holo-trans-cobalamin and the risk of dementia and Alzheimer's disease: a prospective study." *European Journal of Neurology* 16, no. 7 (July 2009):808–13.

11   **Researchers at Erasmus University:** Geleijnse JM et al., "Dietary intake of menaquinone is associated with a reduced risk of coronary heart disease: the Rotterdam Study." *Journal of Nutrition* 134, no. 11 (November 2004):3100–5.

11   **a 2012 study out of Harokopio University of Athens:** Kanellakis S et al., "Changes in parameters of bone metabolism in postmenopausal women following a 12-month intervention period using dairy products enriched with calcium, vitamin D, and phylloquinone (vitamin K1) or menaquinone-7 (vitamin K2): the Postmenopausal Health Study II." *Calcified Tissue International* 90, no. 4 (April 2012):251–62.

13   **more than 50 percent of the people over age fifty:** National Osteoporosis Foundation. cdn.nof.org/wp-content/uploads/2015/12/Osteoporosis-Fast-Facts.pdf.

13   **According to the International Osteoporosis Foundation:** International Osteoporosis Foundation. iofbonehealth.org/facts-statistics.

13   **children are getting osteoporosis too:** Rovner AJ et al., "Vitamin D deficiency and insufficiency in children with osteopenia or osteoporosis." *Pediatrics* 122, no. 4 (October 2008):907–8. See also Khoshhal KI, "Childhood osteoporosis." *Journal of Taibah University Medical Sciences* 6, no. 2 (2011):61–76.

13   **the worldwide incidence:** International Osteoporosis Foundation. iofbonehealth.org/facts-statistics.

13   **And in China:** Chen P et al., "Prevalence of osteoporosis in China: a meta-analysis and systematic review." *BMC Public Health* 16, no. 1(2011):1039. See also Si L et al., "Projection of osteoporosis-related fractures and costs in China: 2010–2050." *Osteoporosis International* 26, no. 7 (July 2015):1929–37.

15   **a bone disorder that occurs with aging:** Cleveland Clinic. https://my.cleveland clinic.org/health/articles/10091-menopause—osteoporosis. See also Taxel P et al., "Differential diagnosis and secondary causes of osteoporosis." *Clinical Cornerstone* 2, no. 6 (2000):11-21.

15   **potential causes of secondary osteoporosis:** Uziel Y et al., "Osteoporosis in children: pediatric and pediatric rheumatology perspective: a review." *Pediatric Rheumatology Online Journal* 7, no. 16 (2009).

16   **including children:** Gebel E, "More kids than ever have type 2 diabetes." *Diabetes Forecast.* November 2012. diabetesforecast.org/2012/nov/more-kids-than-ever -have-type-2-diabetes.html.

16   **more than 132,000 children:** Centers for Disease Control and Prevention. "National Diabetes Statistics Report, 2017." cdc.gov/diabetes/pdfs/data/statistics/national -diabetes-statistics-report.pdf.

16   **According to Laura Bachrach, MD:** Williams S, "Pediatrician's outreach and research are cutting straight to the bones." *Stanford Report*, November 10, 2004. news.stanford.edu/news/2004/november10/med-bones-1110.html.

16   **the medical community is now experimenting:** NIH Osteoporosis and Related Bone Diseases National Resource Center. www.bones.nih.gov/health-info/bone /bone-health/juvenile/juvenile-osteoporosis.

18   **stress itself actually causes deficiencies:** Stough C et al., "Reducing occupational stress with a B-vitamin focussed intervention: a randomized clinical trial: study protocol." *Nutrition Journal* 13, no. 1 (2014):122.

20   **this drug increases the risk of osteoporosis:** Fraser LA et al., "Glucocorticoid-induced osteoporosis: treatment update and review." *Therapeutic Advances in Musculoskeletal Disease* 1, no. 2 (2009):71–85.

20   **These include beta-carotene:** Pelton R et al. *Drug-Induced Nutrient Depletion Handbook*, 2nd ed. Hudson, OH: Lexi-Comp, 2001. See also Pelton R et al. *The*

Nutritional Cost of Prescription Drugs, 2nd ed. Englewood, CO: Morton, 2004; Vaglini F, Fox B. *The Side Effects Bible: The Dietary Solution to Unwanted Side Effects of Common Medications*. New York: Broadway Books, 2005. *InVite Health*. invitehealth.com /Drug-Induced-Nutrient-Depletion.html.

Chapter 2: Osteoporosis Treatment

25   **the most widely prescribed of the osteoporosis drugs:** Wighton K, "Drug used to treat weak bones associated with micro-cracks." *Imperial College London*. March 1, 2017. www.imperial.ac.uk/news/177851/drug-used-treat-weak-bones-associated/.

25   **a meta-analysis of more than thirty studies:** Järvinen TL et al., "Overdiagnosis of bone fragility in the quest to prevent hip fracture." *BMJ* 26, no. 350 (May 2015):h2088.

25   **scientists at Imperial College London:** Shah FA et al., "Micrometer-sized magnesium whitlockite crystals in micropetrosis of bisphosphonate-exposed human alveolar bone." *Nano Letters* 17, no. 10 (October 2017):6210–16.

26   **Side effects of the oral tablets:** *National Osteoporosis Foundation*. nof.org/patients /treatment/medicationadherence/side-effects-of-bisphosphonates-alendronate -ibandronate-risedronate-and-zoledronic-acid.

26   **bisphosphonate use increases the risk of serious atrial fibrillation:** Sharma A et al., "Risk of serious atrial fibrillation and stroke with use of bisphosphonates: evidence from a meta-analysis." *Chest* 144, no. 4 (October 2013):1311–22.

26   **twice as likely to develop esophageal cancer:** Edwards BJ et al., "Bisphosphonates and esophageal cancer: A RADAR report." *Journal of Clinical Oncology* 30, no. 15s (May 2012):4063–4063.

27   **According to findings presented**: Curtis J et al., "The impact of the duration of bisphosphonate drug holidays on hip fracture rates." *Arthritis & Rheumatology*. Supplement 10 (2017); 69. https://acrabstracts.org/abstract/the-impact-of-the-duration -of-bisphosphonate-drug-holidays-on-hip-fracture-rates/.

28   **"When low levels of calcium":** *National Osteoporosis Foundation*. nof.org/patients /treatment/medicationadherence/side-effects-of-bisphosphonates-alendronate -ibandronate-risedronate-and-zoledronic-acid/.

28   *have been shown to have inadequate calcium intakes:* Bailey RL et al., "Estimation of total usual calcium and vitamin D intakes in the United States." *Journal of Nutrition* 140, no. 4 (April 2010):817–22. See also Committee to Review Dietary Reference Intakes for Vitamin D and Calcium, Food and Nutrition Board, Institute of Medicine. *Dietary Reference Intakes for Calcium and Vitamin D*. Washington, DC: National Academies Press, 2010.

28   **when bisphosphonates come into contact:** Koçer G et al., "Basic fibroblast growth factor attenuates bisphosphonate-induced oxidative injury but decreases zinc and copper levels in oral epithelium of rat." *Biological Trace Element Research* 153(2013):251. See also Itoh A et al., "Interaction between bisphosphonates and mineral water: study of oral risedronate absorption in rats." *Biological and Pharmaceutical Bulletin* 39, no. 3 (2016):323–8.

28   **preventing your body from absorbing:** *WebMD*. webmd.com/drugs/2 /drug-63444/ascorbic-acid-vitamin-e-zinc-oral/details/list-interaction-details

/dmid-1660/dmtitle-oral-multivalent-cations-oral-bisphosphonates/intrtype
-drug.

28   **cautions you not to:** *Linus Pauling Institute.* lpi.oregonstate.edu/mic/minerals
/calcium.

28   **a study published in the *Journal of Clinical Endocrinology and Metabolism*:** Kalyan S
et al., "Nitrogen-bisphosphonate therapy is linked to compromised coenzyme Q10
and vitamin E status in postmenopausal women." *Journal of Clinical Endocrinology and
Metabolism* 99, no. 4 (April 2014):1307–13.

30   **this new injectable osteoporosis drug:** Reid IR et al., "Epidemiology and
pathogenesis of osteonecrosis of the jaw." *Nature Reviews, Rheumatolology* 8, no. 2
(November 2011):90–6.

31   **researchers have concluded that chronic elevation of PTH:** Braverman ER
et al., "Age-related increases in parathyroid hormone may be antecedent to both
osteoporosis and dementia." *BMC Endocrine Disorders* 9 (October 2009):21. See also
Lourida I et al., "Parathyroid hormone, cognitive function and dementia: a systematic review." *PLoS One* 10, no. 5 (May 2015):e0127574.

32   **On their website, under side effects:** forteo.com.

32   **"Too much calcium in your blood":** *Mayo Clinic.* mayoclinic.org/diseases
-conditions/hypercalcemia/symptoms-causes/syc-20355523.

32   **in nearly 36 percent of the subjects:** Bégin MJ et al., "Hypomagnesemia during
teriparatide treatment in osteoporosis: incidence and determinants." *Journal of Bone
and Mineral Research* 33, no. 8 (August 2018):1444–9.

32   **over six hundred important metabolic reactions:** de Baaij JH et al., "Magnesium in man: implications for health and disease." *Physiological Reviews* 95, no. 1
(January 2015):1–46.

33   **Low magnesium levels cause:** Tastekin N et al., "Probable osteosarcoma risk
after prolonged teriparatide treatment: comment on the article by Saag et al." *Arthritis and Rheumatism* 62, no. 6 (June 2010):1837.

33   **teriparatide causes a spike in PTH:** Lasco A et al., "Adrenal effects of teriparatide in the treatment of severe postmenopausal osteoporosis." *Osteoporosis International* 22, no. 1 (January 2011):299–303.

33   **Researchers found that cortisol indirectly acts on bone:** Heshmati HM et
al., "Effects of the circadian variation in serum cortisol on markers of bone turnover and calcium homeostasis in normal postmenopausal women." *Journal of Clinical
Endocrinology and Metabolism* 83, no. 3 (March 1998):751–6.

33   **This disruption to serum calcium:** Hardy R et al., "Adrenal gland and bone."
Archives of Biochemistry and Biophysics 503, no. 1 (November 2010):137–45. See also
Raff H et al., "Elevated salivary cortisol in the evening in healthy elderly men and
women: correlation with bone mineral density." *Journals of Gerontology* 54, no. 9
(September 1999):M479–83.

33   **Even a short bout:** Chiodini I et al., "[Role of cortisol hypersecretion in the pathogenesis of osteoporosis]." *Recenti Progressi in Medicina* 99, no. 6 (June 2008):309–13.
[Article in Italian.]

34   **Research shows that teriparatide's dramatic stimulation:** Yu EW et al.,
"Time-dependent changes in skeletal response to teriparatide: escalating vs.

constant dose teriparatide (PTH 1-34) in osteoporotic women." *Bone* 48, no. 4 (April 2011):713–9.

34 **the FDA did mandate a "black box" warning:** Marcus R, "Present at the beginning: a personal reminiscence on the history of teriparatide." *Osteoporosis International* 22, no. 8 (August 2011):2241–8.

34 **This drug received FDA approval:** Subbiah V et al., "Of mice and men: divergent risks of teriparatide-induced osteosarcoma." *Osteoporosis International* 21, no. 6 (June 2010):1041–5. See also Tastekin N et al., "Probable osteosarcoma risk after prolonged teriparatide treatment: comment on the article by Saag et al." *Arthritis and Rheumatism* 62, no. 6 (June 2010):1837.

34 **your odds of getting hypercalcemia are less:** Bach FC et al., "The paracrine feedback loop between vitamin D3 (1,25(OH)$_2$D$_3$) and PTHrP in prehypertrophic chondrocytes." *Journal of Cellular Physiology* 229, no. 12 (December 2014):1999–2014.

35 **the medicine be refused marketing authorization:** *European Medicine Agencies.* www.ema.europa.eu/en/news/meeting-highlights-committee-medicinal-products -human-use-chmp-23-26-july-2018.

40 **Table 2.1: Plays an essential role:** "Vitamin A and your bones." *Harvard Health Publishing.* March 2014. www.health.harvard.edu/newsletter_article/vitamin-a -and-your-bones.

40 **Table 2.1: Both low and excessively high:** Opotowsky AR et al., "Serum vitamin A concentration and the risk of hip fracture among women 50 to 74 years old in the United States: a prospective analysis of the NHANES I follow-up study." *American Journal of Medicine* 117, no. 3 (August 2004):169–74. See also Lim LS et al., "Vitamin A intake and the risk of hip fracture in postmenopausal women: the Iowa Women's Health Study." *Osteoporosis International* 15, no. 7 (July 2004):552–9.

40 **Table 2.1: studies suggest that lutein:** Sahni S et al., "Inverse association of carotenoid intakes with 4-y change in bone mineral density in elderly men and women: the Framingham osteoporosis study." *American Journal of Clinical Nutrition* 89, no. 1 (January 2009):416–24. See also Wattanapenpaiboon N et al., "Dietary carotenoid intake as a predictor of bone mineral density." *Asia Pacific Journal of Clinical Nutrition* 12, no. 4 (2003):467–73.

41 **Table 2.1: Thiamine deficiency reduces stomach acid:** Sipponen P et al., "Hypochlorhydric stomach: a risk condition for calcium malabsorption and osteoporosis?" *Scandinavian Journal of Gastroenterology* 45, no. 2 (2010):133–8.

41 **Table 2.1: increased dietary riboflavin has been associated:** Yazdanpanah N et al., "Effect of dietary B vitamins on BMD and risk of fracture in elderly men and women: the Rotterdam Study." *Bone* 41 (2007):987–94.

41 **Table 2.1: There is a positive significant correlation:** Sasaki S et al., "Association between current nutrient intakes and bone mineral density at calcaneus in pre- and postmenopausal Japanese women." *Journal of Nutritional Science and Vitaminology (Tokyo)* 47 (2001):289–94.

41 **Table 2.1: chronic stress is a risk factor for osteoporosis:** Azuma K et al., "Chronic psychological stress as a risk factor of osteoporosis." *Journal of UOEH* 37, no. 4 (December 2015):245–53.

41 **Table 2.1: by maintaining proper function:** Stachowicz M et al., "The effect of diet components on the level of cortisol." *European Food Research and Technology* 242, no. 12 (2016):2001–9.

41   **Table 2.1: B6 deficiency causes an imbalance:** Sasaki S et al., "Association between current nutrient intakes and bone mineral density at calcaneus in pre- and postmenopausal Japanese women." *Journal of Nutritional Science and Vitaminology (Tokyo)* 47 (2001):289–94.

41   **Table 2.1: Increased dietary B6 intake:** Yazdanpanah N et al., "Effect of dietary B vitamins on BMD and risk of fracture in elderly men and women: the Rotterdam Study." *Bone* 41 (2007):987–94.

42   **Table 2.1: Vitamin B7 (biotin) deficiency affects IGF-1 status:** Báez-Saldaña A et al., "Biotin deficiency in mice is associated with decreased serum availability of insulin-like growth factor-I." *European Journal of Nutrition* 48 (2009):137–44.

42   **Table 2.1: resorption activity was found:** Sasaki S et al., "Association between current nutrient intakes and bone mineral density at calcaneus in pre- and postmenopausal Japanese women." *Journal of Nutritional Science and Vitaminology (Tokyo)* 47 (2001):289–94.

42   **Table 2.1: Dietary folate is a significant predictor:** Rejnmark L et al., "Dietary intake of folate, but not vitamin B2 or B12, is associated with increased bone mineral density 5 years after the menopause: Results from a 10-year follow-up study in early postmenopausal women." *Calcified Tissue International* 82 (2008):1–11.

42   **Table 2.1: proven to have a protective role:** Carmel R et al., "Cobalamin and osteoblast-specific proteins." *NEJM* 319, no. 2 (1988):70–5. See also Dai Z et al., "B-vitamins and bone health—a review of the current evidence." *Nutrients* 7, no. 5 (2015):3322–46.

42   **Table 2.1: Higher vitamin C intake levels:** Kim MH et al., "Osteoporosis, vitamin C intake, and physical activity in Korean adults aged 50 years and over." *Journal of Physical Therapy Science* 28, no. 3 (2016):725–30.

42   **Table 2.1: People with low levels of vitamin D:** Bischoff-Ferrari HA et al., "Fracture prevention with vitamin D supplementation: a meta-analysis of randomized controlled trials." *JAMA* 293, no. 18 (2005):2257–64.

42   **Table 2.1: Vitamin D supplements:** Bischoff-Ferrari HA et al., "Fracture prevention with vitamin D supplementation: a meta-analysis of randomized controlled trials." *JAMA* 293, no. 18 (2005):2257–64.

43   **Table 2.1: can completely prevent the erosion:** Chin KY et al., "The biological effects of tocotrienol on bone: a review on evidence from rodent models." *Drug Design, Development and Therapy* 9 (2015):2049–61. See also *Clinical Education.* clinicaleducation.org/news/building-bone-the-novel-role-of-tocotrienols.

43   **Table 2.1: Deficiency in another form of vitamin E:** Michaelsson K et al., "Intake and serum concentrations of α-tocopherol in relation to fractures in elderly women and men: 2 cohort studies." *American Journal of Clinical Nutrition* 99, no. 1 (January 2014):107–14.

43   **Table 2.1: Vitamin K2 has been proven in studies:** Geleijnse JM et al., "Dietary intake of menaquinone is associated with a reduced risk of coronary heart disease: the Rotterdam Study." *Journal of Nutrition* 134, no. 11 (November 2004):3100–5.

43   **Table 2.1: Vitamin K2 has also been proven to induce:** Kanellakis S et al., "Changes in parameters of bone metabolism in postmenopausal women following a 12-month intervention period using dairy products enriched with calcium, vitamin D, and phylloquinone (vitamin K1) or menaquinone-7 (vitamin K2):

the Postmenopausal Health Study II." *Calcified Tissue International* 90, no. 4 (April 2012):251–62.

43 **Table 2.1: Subjects with the lowest dietary total choline:** Øyen J et al., "Dietary choline intake is directly associated with bone mineral density in the Hordaland Health Study." *Journal of Nutrition* 147, no. 4 (April 2017):572–8.

43 **Table 2.1: One study found that boron:** Xu P et al., "[Therapeutic effect of dietary boron supplement on retinoic acid–induced osteoporosis in rats]." *Nan Fang Yi Ke Da Xue Xue Bao* 26, no. 12 (December 2006):1785–8. [Article in Chinese.]

43 **Table 2.1: Studies determined that increases in BMD:** Tai V et al., "Calcium intake and bone mineral density: systematic review and meta-analysis." *BMJ* 351 (September 2015):h4183.

43 **Table 2.1: reducing the rate of bone resorption:** McCarty MF, "Anabolic effects of insulin on bone suggest a role for chromium picolinate in preservation of bone density." *Medical Hypotheses* 45, no. 3 (September 1995):241–6.

44 **Table 2.1: Reduced copper levels have been shown:** Mir E et al., "Adequate serum copper concentration could improve bone density, postpone bone loss and protect osteoporosis in women." *Iranian Journal of Public Health (A supplementary issue on Osteoporosis)* 36, no. suppl. 1 (2007):24–9.

44 **Table 2.1: iodine deficiency is frequently observed:** Arslanca T et al., "Body iodine status in women with postmenopausal osteoporosis." *Menopause* 25, no. 3 (March 2018):320–3.

44 **Table 2.1: Chronic iron deficiency induces:** Toxqui L et al., "Chronic iron deficiency as an emerging risk factor for osteoporosis: a hypothesis." *Nutrients* 7, no. 4 (April 2015):2324–44.

44 **Table 2.1: Lower magnesium intake is associated:** Tucker KL et al., "Potassium, magnesium, and fruit and vegetable intakes are associated with greater bone mineral density in elderly men and women." *American Journal of Clinical Nutrition* 69, no. 4 (April 1999):727–36. See also Orchard TS et al., "Magnesium intake, bone mineral density, and fractures: results from the Women's Health Initiative Observational Study." *American Journal of Clinical Nutrition* 99, no. 4 (2014):926–33.

44 **Table 2.1: Deficiencies in manganese have been correlated:** Lyn P et al., "Comparative absorption of calcium sources and calcium citrate malate for the prevention of osteoporosis." *Alternative Medicine Review* 4, no. 2 (April 1999):74–85.

45 **Table 2.1: High intake of phosphorus has no adverse effect:** Lee AW et al., "Association between phosphorus intake and bone health in the NHANES population." *Nutrition Journal* 14 (2015):28.

45 **Table 2.1: Studies show that potassium can decrease:** Lambert H et al., "The effect of supplementation with alkaline potassium salts on bone metabolism: a meta-analysis." *Osteoporosis International* 26, no. 4 (April 2015):1311–8.

45 **Table 2.1: researchers noted that at least 40 mg:** Jugdaohsingh R et al., "Dietary silicon intake is positively associated with bone mineral density in men and premenopausal women of the Framingham Offspring cohort." *Journal of Bone and Mineral Research* 19, no. 2 (February 2004):297–307.

45 **Table 2.1: Another study found that individuals:** Schiano A et al., "[Silicon, bone tissue and immunity]." *Revue du rhumatisme et des maladies ostéo-articulaires* 46, no. 7–9 (July–September 1979):483–6. [Article in French.]

45 **Table 2.1: Studies have shown that selenium deficiency:** Moreno-Reyes R et al., "Selenium deficiency-induced growth retardation is associated with an impaired bone metabolism and osteopenia." *Journal of Bone and Mineral Research* 16 (2001):1556–63. See also Cao JJ et al., "Selenium deficiency decreases antioxidative capacity and is detrimental to bone microarchitecture in mice." *Journal of Nutrition* 142 (2012):1526–31.

45 **Table 2.1: Low serum zinc is associated with low BMD:** Bekheirnia MR et al., "Serum zinc and its relation to bone mineral density in beta-thalassemic adolescents." *Biological Trace Element Research* 97, no. 3 (March 2004):215–24.

Chapter 3: Let Thy Food Be Thy Medicine

58 **Research published in the journal** *Environmental Research*: Oates L et al., "Reduction in urinary organophosphate pesticide metabolites in adults after a week-long organic diet." *Environmental Research* 132 (July 2014):105–11.

60 **stevia is currently being researched:** Minoru S et al., United States Patent #6,500,471. December 31, 2002.

60 **xylitol is being researched:** Mattila PT et al., "Effects of a long-term dietary xylitol supplementation on collagen content and fluorescence of the skin in aged rats." *Gerontology* 51, no. 3 (May–June 2005):166–9. See also Sato H et al., "The effects of oral xylitol administration on bone density in rat femur." *Odontology* 99, no. 1 (January 2011):28–33.

60 **sugar makes up 17 percent of the global diet:** *Credit Suisse Research Institute.* "Sugar: consumption at a crossroads." September 2013.

60 **And vitamin C is also affected by sugar:** Chen L et al., "Hyperglycemia inhibits the uptake of dehydroascorbate in tubular epithelial cell." *American Journal of Nephrology* 25, no. 5 (September–October 2005):459–65.

61 **Researchers at the Monell Chemical Senses Center:** Tordoff MG, "Adrenalectomy decreases NaCl intake of rats fed low-calcium diets." *American Journal of Physiology* 270, no. 1 (January 1996):R11–21.

63 **Its popularity has skyrocketed:** Jensen HH et al., "U.S. sweetener consumption trends and dietary guidelines." *Iowa Ag Review Online* 11, no. 1 (Winter 2005).

63 **Recent animal studies:** Yarrow JF et al., "Fructose consumption does not worsen bone deficits resulting from high-fat feeding in young male rats." *Bone* 85 (2016):99–106. See also Krafsig LA, "The relationship between fructose and bone fragility." *LiveScience.* September 7, 2012. livescience.com/23039-fructose-effects -calcium-absorption-nsf-bts.html.

65 **when diet-induced changes:** Weaver CM, "Diet, gut microbiome, and bone health." *Current Osteoporosis Reports* 13, no. 2 (2015):125–30.

65 **Additionally, scientists have discovered:** Mahnam K et al., "A theoretical and experimental study of calcium, iron, zinc, cadmium, and sodium ions absorption by aspartame." *Journal of Biological Physics* 43 (2017):87–103. See also Nguyen UN, "Aspartame ingestion increases urinary calcium, but not oxalate excretion, in healthy subjects." *Journal of Clinical Endocrinology and Metabolism* 83, no. 1 (January 1998):165–8.

66 **According to a study in the** *American Journal of Clinical Nutrition*: Hallberg L et al., "Prediction of dietary iron absorption: an algorithm for calculating absorption

and bioavailability of dietary iron." *American Journal of Clinical Nutrition* 71, no. 5 (May 2000):1147–60.

66   **A study on Pakistani immigrants:** M. R. Wills et al., "Phytic Acid and Nutritional Rickets in Immigrants." *Lancet* 1, no. 7754 (April 1972):771–3.

67   **celiac disease induces micronutrient malabsorption:** Pacheco GG et al., "Deficiencia de micronutrientes y enfermedad celíaca en pediatría." *Archivos Argentinos de Pediatria* 112, no. 5 (2014):457–63. [Spanish.] See also Kupper C, "Dietary guidelines and implementation for celiac disease." *Gastroenterology* 128, no. 4, suppl. 1 (April 2005):S121–7.

67   **zonulin then damages the seals:** S. Drago et al., "Gliadin, zonulin, and gut permeability: Effects on celiac and non-celiac intestinal mucosa and intestinal cell lines." *Scandinavian Journal of Gastroenterology* 41, no. 4 (April 2006):408–19.

68   **New scientific research:** *New York Presbyterian.* nyp.org/pdf/newsletters/2016 -Advances-Winter-Endocrinology.pdf. See also Ducy P et al., "Leptin inhibits bone formation through a hypothalamic relay: a central control of bone mass." *Cell* 100, no. 2 (January 2000):197–207.

70   **eating a slice of whole-wheat bread:** Atkinson FS et al., "International tables of glycemic index and glycemic load values: 2008." *Diabetes Care* 31, no. 12 (December 2008):2281–3.

70   **in the consumption of more than four hundred additional calories:** William Davis. *Wheat Belly Total Health.* Emmaus, PA: Rodale, 2014, 78.

71   **Research shows that laboratory rats given MSG:** *Euroresidentes UK.* "Scientists in Spain link additive to obesity." euroresidentes.com/euroresiuk/news-spain /scientists-in-spain-link-additive-to.

73   **This means it can cross:** Konkel L, "What is glutamate?" *Everyday Health.* October 16, 2015. everydayhealth.com/glutamate/guide.

73   **magnesium, chromium, and zinc are all important protectors:** Blaylock R. *Excitotoxins: The Taste That Kills.* Albuquerque, NM: Health Press, 1997.

75   **According to a 2010 article:** Nagel, R, "Living with phytic acid." *Weston A. Price Foundation.* March 26, 2010. westonaprice.org/food-features/living-with -phytic-acid.

75   **Eighty percent of all kidney stones:** Coe FL et al., "Kidney stone disease." *Journal of Clinical Investigation* 115, no. 10 (2005):2598–608.

76   **a study in the *Journal of Agricultural and Food Chemistry*:** Chai W, "Effect of different cooking methods on vegetable oxalate content." *Journal of Agricultural and Food Chemistry* 53, no. 8 (2005):3027–30.

76   **It causes both an increase:** Goldstein IJ, ed. *The Lectins.* Orlando, FL: Academic Press, 1986, 529–52. See also Shechter Y, "Bound lectins that mimic insulin produce persistent insulin-like activities." *Endocrinology* 113, no. 6 (December 1983):1921–6.

76   **Lectins are present:** Nachbar MS et al., "Lectins in the United States diet: a survey of lectins in commonly consumed foods and a review of the literature." *American Journal of Clinical Nutrition* 33, no. 11 (November 1980):2338–45. See also Ellgen P, *The Lectin Avoidance Cookbook.* Berkeley, CA: Ulysses Press, 2018, chap. 1.

77   **In studies, a deficiency of B6, B9, and B12:** Dai Z et al., "B-vitamins and bone health—a review of the current evidence." *Nutrients* 7, no. 5 (2015):3322–46. See also Herrmann M et al., "Stimulation of osteoclast activity by low B-vitamin concentrations." *Bone* 41 (2007):584–91.

77   **Most of the USDA studies:** Daniel K, "Plants bite back." *Weston A. Price Founda-tion.* March 29, 2010. westonaprice.org/health-topics/plants-bite-back.

77   **when researchers heated sweet potatoes:** Kiran KS et al., "Inactivation of tryp-sin inhibitors in sweet potato and taro tubers during processing." *Plant Foods for Human Nutrition* 58, no. 2 (Spring 2003):153–63.

79   **Alcohol interferes with the pancreas:** Subramanian VS et al., "Uptake of ascor-bic acid by pancreatic acinar cells is negatively impacted by chronic alcohol expo-sure." *American Journal of Physiology, Cell Physiology* 311, no. 1 (July 2016):C129–35. See also Davis JL, "Drink less for strong bones." *WebMD.* webmd.com/osteoporosis /features/alcohol#1.

79   **A recent study out of the University of Oregon:** Marrone JA, "Moderate alcohol intake lowers biochemical markers of bone turnover in postmenopausal women." *Menopause* 19, no. 9 (September 2012):974–79.

79   **Finnish researchers concur:** Sommer I et al., "Alcohol consumption and bone min-eral density in elderly women." *Public Health Nursing* 16, no. 4 (April 2013):704–12.

79   **two Harvard studies:** Camargo CA et al., "Prospective study of moderate alcohol consumption and mortality in US male physicians." *Archives of Internal Medicine* 159, no. 79 (1997):79–85. See also Fuchs CS et al., "Alcohol consumption and mortality among women." *NEJM* 332, no. 19 (1995):1245–50.

80   **A recent study determined:** Barger-Lux MJ et al., "Caffeine and the calcium economy revisited." *Osteoporosis International* 5 no. 2 (March 1995):97–102.

80   **can inhibit the absorption of nonheme iron:** Morck TA, "Inhibition of food iron absorption by coffee." *American Journal of Clinical Nutrition* 37, no. 3 (1983):416–20. See also Hallberg L, "Effect of different drinks on the absorption of non-heme iron from composite meals." *Human Nutrition, Applied Nutrition* 36, no. 2 (1982):116–23.

80   **a Korean study:** Choi EJ et al., "Coffee consumption and bone mineral den-sity in korean premenopausal women." *Korean Journal of Family Medicine* 35, no. 1 (2014):11–8.

80   **Potentially negative effects:** Heaney RP, "Effects of caffeine on bone and the calcium economy." *Food and Cosmetics Toxicology* 40 (2002):1263–70.

80   **high CRP levels are an indicator:** Kotani K et al., "The relationship between usual coffee consumption and serum C-reactive protein level in a Japanese female population." *Clinical Chemistry and Laboratory Medicine* 46, no. 10 (2008):1434–7.

81   **a 2013 study:** Tallis J et al., "Assessment of the ergogenic effect of caffeine supple-mentation on mood, anticipation timing, and muscular strength in older adults." *Physiological Reports* 1, no. 3 (2013):e00072.

81   **UK researchers recommend:** Nelson M et al., "Impact of tea drinking on iron status in the UK: a review." *Journal of Human Nutrition and Dietetics* 17, no. 1 (February 2004):43–54.

Chapter 4: Dietary Doctrine, Alkalinity, and Omega-6 Overload . . . Oh My!

90   **their team of trained nutrition professionals:** *National Agricultural Library, USDA.* nutrition.gov/subject/dietary-supplements/faqs.

90   **The late Shari Lieberman, PhD:** Lieberman S, Burning N. *The Real Vitamin and Mineral Book.* New York: Avery, 2003, 19.

90   **Walter Willett, MD:** *Harvard Health Publishing.* "Multivitamins: should you buy this insurance?" September 2006. www.health.harvard.edu/newsletter_article /multivitamins-should-you-buy-this-insurance.

90   **Dr. Mark Hyman:** Hyman M, "Do you need supplements?" drhyman.com/blog /2015/04/02/do-you-need-supplements/.

91   **the American Dietetic Association had wondered:** Dollahite J et al., "Problems encountered in meeting the recommended dietary allowances for menus designed according to the Dietary Guidelines for Americans." *Journal of the American Dietetic Association* 95, no. 3 (March 1995):341–4.

91   **Jayson's 2010 study:** Calton JB, "Prevalence of micronutrient deficiency in popular diet plans." *Journal of the International Society of Sports Nutrition* 10 (June 2010): 7–24.

94   **Research published by the National Institute of Hygiene in Poland:** Pachocka L, "Changes in vitamins intake in overweight and obese adults after low-energy diets." *Roczniki Państwowego Zakładu Higieny* 53, no. 3 (2002):243–52. [Article in Polish.]

95   **A study published in *Nutrition Journal*:** Truby H et al., "Commercial weight loss diets meet nutrient requirements in free living adults over 8 weeks: a randomized controlled weight loss trial." *Nutrition Journal* 7, no. 25 (2008).

95   **Deficiencies in vitamins B1, B9, B12, and D:** O'Donnell K, "Small but mighty: selected micronutrient issues in gastric bypass patients." *Semantic Scholar.* 2008.

95   **One recent study by investigators:** Yu EW et al., "Two-year changes in bone density after Roux-en-Y gastric bypass surgery." *Journal of Clinical Endocrinology and Metabolism* 100, no. 4 (2015):1452–9.

96   **have been shown to fall short:** Winston JC, "Health effects of vegan diets." *American Journal of Clinical Nutrition* 89, no. 5 (2009):1627S–3S.

96   **Studies show that the vegan diet:** Davey GK et al., "EPIC-Oxford: Lifestyle characteristics and nutrient intakes in a cohort of 33,883 meat-eaters and 31,546 non-meat-eaters in the UK." *Public Health Nutrition* 6, no. 3 (2003):259.

96   **94 percent of all soy:** *United States Department of Agriculture Economic Research Service.* www.ers.usda.gov/data-products/adoption-of-genetically-engineered-crops -in-the-us/recent-trends-in-ge-adoption.aspx.

96   **In one study published in the *Journal of Nutrition*:** Geleijnse JM, "Dietary intake of menaquinone is associated with a reduced risk of coronary heart disease: the Rotterdam Study." *Journal of Nutrition* 134, no. 11 (November 2004):3100–5.

97   **Another study from the Netherlands:** Schurgers LJ, "Vitamin K-containing dietary supplements: comparison of synthetic vitamin K1 and natto-derived menaquinone-7." *Blood* 109, no. 8 (April 2007):3279–83.

97   **in a study published in the *American Journal of Clinical Nutrition*:** Ho-Pham LT, "Effect of vegetarian diets on bone mineral density: a Bayesian meta-analysis." *American Journal of Clinical Nutrition* 90, no. 4 (October 2009):943–50.

97   **BMD was approximately 4 percent lower:** Ho-Pham LT, "Effect of vegetarian diets on bone mineral density: a Bayesian meta-analysis." *American Journal of Clinical Nutrition* 90, no. 4: (October 2009):943-50.

98   **Two recent Australian studies:** Manousou S et al., "A Paleolithic-type diet results in iodine deficiency: a 2-year randomized trial in postmenopausal obese women." *European Journal of Clinical Nutrition* 72, no. 1 (January 2018):124–29. See also Genoni A, "Cardiovascular: metabolic effects and dietary composition of ad-libitum Paleolithic vs. Australian guide to healthy eating diets: a 4-week randomised trial." *Nutrients* 8 (2016):314–27.

99   **more than half of the individuals:** Mariani P et al., "The gluten-free diet: a nutritional risk factor for adolescents with celiac disease?" *Journal of Pediatric Gastroenterology and Nutrition* 27, no. 5 (November 1998):519–23.

100   **According to calcium researcher Randi Wolf:** Wolf RL et al., "Factors associated with calcium absorption efficiency in pre- and perimenopausal women." *American Journal of Clinical Nutrition* 72 (2000):466–71. See also Heaney RP, "The paradox of osteoporosis irreversibility." blogs.creighton.edu/heaney/2014/07/25/the-paradox-of-osteoporosis-irreversibility-2/.

100   **When the Atkins diet:** Truby H et al., "Commercial weight loss diets meet nutrient requirements in free living adults over 8 weeks: a randomised controlled weight loss trial." *Nutrition Journal* 7 (September 2008):25.

101   **when researchers looked at high-fat diets:** Wang T et al., "Effects of a standard high-fat diet with or without multiple deficiencies on bone parameters in ovariectomized mature rat." *PLoS One* 12, no. 9 (September 2017):e0184983. doi: 10.1371/journal.pone.0184983.

101   **studies indicate that high fiber intakes:** Wolf RL et al., "Factors associated with calcium absorption efficiency in pre- and perimenopausal women." *American Journal of Clinical Nutrition* 72(2000):466–71.

103   **Your blood pH is kept in a tight range:** Hamm LL et al., "Acid-base homeostasis." *Clinical Journal of the American Society of Nephrology* 10, no. 12 (2015):2232–42.

103   **there are cultures all over the world:** Ströhle A et al., "Estimation of the diet-dependent net acid load in 229 worldwide historically studied hunter-gatherer societies." *American Journal of Clinical Nutrition* 91, no. 2 (February 2010):406–12. See also Ströhle A et al., "Latitude, local ecology, and hunter-gatherer dietary acid load: implications from evolutionary ecology." *American Journal of Clinical Nutrition* 92, no. 4 (October 2010):940–5; Carrera-Bastos P et al., "The western diet and lifestyle and diseases of civilization." *Research Reports in Clinical Cardiology* 2 (2011):15–35.

104   **According to research published in the** *European Journal of Clinical Nutrition*: Calvez J et al., "Protein intake, calcium balance and health consequences." *European Journal of Clinical Nutrition* 66, no. 3 (March 2012):281–95.

104   **long-term inadequate calcium intake causes osteoporosis:** Institute of Medicine. *Dietary Reference Intakes for Calcium and Vitamin D.* Washington, DC: National Academies Press, 2010.

104   **Scientists have determined that low-protein:** Kerstetter JE, "The impact of dietary protein on calcium absorption and kinetic measures of bone turnover in women." *Journal of Clinical Endocrinology and Metabolism* 90, no. 1 (January 2005):26–31.

104   **but a 2018 study:** Rizzoli R et al., "Benefits and safety of dietary protein for bone health-an expert consensus paper endorsed by the European Society for Clinical and Economical Aspects of Osteopororosis, Osteoarthritis, and Musculoskeletal Diseases and by the International Osteoporosis Foundation." *Osteoporosis International* 29 no. 9 (September 2018): 1933–48.

105   **According to Dr. Heaney:** Heaney R, "The paradox of osteoporosis irreversibility." blogs.creighton.edu/heaney/2014/07/25/the-paradox-of-osteoporosis-irreversibility-2.

105   **A few years ago, a study:** Dawson-Hughes B, "Interaction of dietary calcium and protein in bone health in humans." *Journal of Nutrition* 133, no. 3 (March 2003):852S–4S.

108   **have been shown to promote osteoblast growth and differentiation:** Liu Z et al., "Dose- and glucose-dependent effects of amino acids on insulin secretion from isolated mouse islets and clonal INS-1E beta-cells." *Review of Diabetic Studies* 5, no. 4 (2008):232–44. See also Yang J et al., "Insulin stimulates osteoblast proliferation and differentiation through ERK and PI3K in MG-63 cells." *Cell Biochemistry and Function* 28, no. 4 (2010):334–41.

108   **Arginine has also been shown:** Chevalley T et al., "Arginine increases insulin-like growth factor-I production and collagen synthesis in osteoblast-like cells." *Bone* 23, no. 2 (1998):103–9.

108   **Arginine, lysine, and glycine have been associated:** Fini M et al., "Effect of L-lysine and L-arginine on primary osteoblast cultures from normal and osteopenic rats." *Biomedicine and Pharmacotherapy* 55, no. 4 (2001):213–20. See also Melendez-Hevia E et al., "A weak link in metabolism: the metabolic capacity for glycine biosynthesis does not satisfy the need for collagen synthesis." *Journal of Biosciences* 34, no. 6 (2009):853–72.

108   **Leucine has a direct effect:** Fujita S et al., "Amino acids and muscle loss with aging." *Journal of Nutrition* 136, no. 1 suppl. (2006):277S–80S.

109   **Supplementation with L-arginine:** Goel S et al., "Role of L-arginine in the treatment of osteoporosis." *International Journal of Orthopaedics* 1, no. 4: (2014):177–180.

109   **that science has determined is excellent for bone health:** Blais A et al., "Oral bovine lactoferrin improves bone status of ovariectomized mice." *American Journal of Physiology-Endocrinology and Metabolism* 296, no. 6 (2009):E1281–8. See also Bharadwaj S et al., "Milk ribonuclease-enriched lactoferrin induces positive effects on bone turnover markers in postmenopausal women." *Osteoporosis International* 20, no. 9 (September 2009):1603–11; Cornish J et al., "Lactoferrin is a potent regulator of bone cell activity and increases bone formation in vivo." *Endocrinology* 145, no. 9 (2004):4366–74; Grey A et al., "The low-density lipoprotein receptor-related protein1 is a mitogenic receptor for lactoferrin inosteoblastic cells." *Molecular Endocrinology* 18, no. 9 (2004):2268–78; Grey A et al. "Lactoferrin potently inhibits osteoblast apoptosis, viaan LRP1-independent pathway." *Molecular and Cellular Endocrinology* 251, no. 1–2 (2006):96–102; Guo HY et al., "Orally administered lactoferrin preserves bone mass and microarchitecture in ovariectomized rats." *Journal of Nutrition* 139, no. 5 (2009):958–66; Hou JM et al., "Lactoferrin inhibits apoptosis through insulin-like growth factor 1 in primary rat osteoblasts." *Acta Pharmacologica Sinica* 35, no. 4 (2014):523–30; Lorget F et al., "Lactoferrin reduces invitro osteoclast differentiation and resorbing activity." *Biochemical and Biophysical Research Communications* 296, no. 2 (2002):261–6; Montesi M et al., "Coupling hydroxyapatite nanocrystals with lactoferrin as a promising strategy to fine regulate bone homeostasis." *PloS One* 10, no. 7 (2015):e0132633.; Naot D et al., "Molecular mechanisms involved in hemitogenic effect of lactoferrin in osteoblasts." *Bone* 49, 2 (2011):217–24; Onubushi T et al., "Molecular mechanisms of the inhibitory effects of bovine lactoferrin on lipopolysaccharide-mediated osteoclastogenesis." *Journal of Biological*

Chemistry 287, no. 28 (2012):23527–36; Takayama Y et al., "Effect of bovine lactoferrin on extracellular matrix calcification by human osteoblast-like cells." *Bioscience, Biotechnology, and Biochemistry* 72, no. 1 (2008):226–30; Takayama Y et al., "Effect of lactoferrin-embedded collagen membrane on osteogenic differentiation of human osteoblast-like cells." *Journal of Bioscience and Bioengineering* 107, no. 2 (2009):191-5; Yagi M et al., "Effects of lactoferrin on the differentiation of pluripotent mesenchymal cells." *Cell Biology International* 33, no. 3 (2009):283–9; Ying X et al., "Effect of lactoferrin on osteogenic differentiation of human adipose stem cells." *International Orthopaedics* 36, no. 3 (2012):647–53.

109 **new studies suggest that lactoferrin:** Amini AA et al., "Lactoferrin: a biologically active molecule for bone regeneration." *Current Medicinal Chemistry* 18, no. 8 (2011):1220–9. See also Li W et al., "Bone regeneration is promoted by orally administered bovine lactoferrin in a rabbit tibial distraction osteogenesis model." *Clinical Orthopaedics and Related Research* 473, no. 7 (2015):2383–93; Zhang W et al., "Lactoferrin stimulates osteoblast differentiation through PKA and p38 pathways independent of lactoferrin's receptor LRP1." *Journal of Bone and Mineral Research* 29, no. 5 (2014):1232–43.

109 **scientifically proven health benefits:** Markus R et al., "The bovine protein alpha-lactalbumin increases the plasma ratio of tryptophan to the other large neutral amino acids, and in vulnerable subjects raises brain serotonin activity, reduces cortisol concentration, and improves mood under stress." *American Journal of Clinical Nutrition* 71, no. 6 (June 2000):1536–44. See also Camfield A et al., "Dairy constituents and neurocognitive health in ageing." *British Journal of Nutrition* 106, no. 2 (July 2011):159–74; Gerdes SK et al., "Bioactive components of whey and cardiovascular health." Applications monograph. *U.S. Dairy Export Council.* 2001; LanPidhainy X et al., "The hypoglycemic effect of fat and protein is not attenuated by insulin resistance." *American Journal of Clinical Nutrition* 91, no. 1 (January 2010):98–105; Markus R et al., "Whey protein rich in alpha-lactalbumin increases the ratio of plasma tryptophan to the sum of the other large neutral amino acids and improves cognitive performance in stress-vulnerable subjects." *American Journal of Clinical Nutrition* 75, no. 6 (June 2002):1051–6; Matsumoto H et al. "New biological function of bovine alpha-lactalbumin: protective effect against ethanol- and stress-induced gastric mucosal injury in rats." *Bioscience, Biotechnology, and Biochemistry* 65, no. 5 (May 2001):1104–11; Mierlo A et al., "Weight management using a meal replacement strategy: meta and pooling analysis from six studies." *International Journal of Obesity and Related Metabolic Disorders* 27, no. 5 (May 2003):537–49; Parodi W, "A Role for milk proteins and their peptides in cancer prevention." *Current Pharmaceutical Design* 13, no. 8 (2007):813–28; Shertzer G et al., "Dietary whey protein lowers the risk for metabolic disease in mice fed a high-fat diet." *Journal of Nutrition* 141, no. 4 (April 2011):582–7; Zhang X et al., "Lowering effect of dietary milk-whey protein v. casein on plasma and liver cholesterol concentrations in rats." *British Journal of Nutrition* 70, no. 1 (July 1993):139–46.

110 **Our Paleolithic ancestors:** Simopoulos AP, "An Increase in the omega-6/omega-3 fatty acid ratio increases the risk for obesity." *Nutrients* 8 no. 3 (2016):128.

110 **Today, our diets have skewed:** Simopoulos AP, "The importance of the ratio of omega-6/omega-3 essential fatty acids." *Biomedicine and Pharmacotherapy* 56, no. 8 (October 2002):365–79.

110 **a study published in the *American Journal of Clinical Nutrition*:** Weiss LA et al., "Ratio of n-6 to n-3 fatty acids and bone mineral density in older adults: the

Rancho Bernardo Study." *American Journal of Clinical Nutrition* 81 (2005):934–8. https://www.ncbi.nlm.nih.gov/pubmed/19571226/.

112 **Scientists have determined that omega-6 and omega-3:** Simopoulos AP, "An Increase in the omega-6/omega-3 fatty acid ratio increases the risk for obesity." *Nutrients* 8 no. 3 (2016):128.

114 **research published in the prestigious medical journal *The Lancet*:** de Lorgeril M et al., "Mediterranean alpha-linolenic acid-rich diet in secondary prevention of coronary heart disease." *Lancet* 343 (1994):1454–9.

Chapter 5: It's Time to Play the Game of Life.

119 **the 93 percent of Americans:** Calafat AM et al., "Exposure of the U.S. population to bisphenol A and 4-tertiary-octylphenol: 2003–2004." *Environmental Health Perspectives* 116, no. 1 (2007):39–44.

119 **the 75-plus percent of Americans:** Duty SM et al., "Personal care product use predicts urinary concentrations of some phthalate monoesters." *Environmental Health Perspectives* 113, no. 11 (November 2005):1530–5.

119 **In a 2012 study:** Soriano S et al., "Rapid insulinotropic action of low doses of bisphenol-A on mouse and human islets of langerhans: role of estrogen receptor." *PLoS One* 7, no. 2 (2012):e31109.

119 **Recent studies have also determined:** Stahlhut RW et al., "Concentrations of Urinary phthalate metabolites are associated with increased waist circumference and insulin resistance in adult U.S. males." *Environmental Health Perspectives* 115, no. 6 (June 2007):876–82.

120 **Insulin resistance has been proven:** Srikanthan P et al., "Insulin resistance and bone strength: findings from the study of midlife in the United States." *Journal of Bone and Mineral Research* 29, no. 4 (2014):796–803.

120 **Research published in the *Journal of Clinical Endocrinology and Metabolism*:** Meeker JD et al., "Urinary Phthalate Metabolites Are Associated With Decreased Serum Testosterone in Men, Women, and Children From NHANES 2011–2012." *The Journal of Clinical Endocrinology & Metabolism*, 2014. doi: 10.1210/jc.2014-2555.

120 **testosterone may increase the bone's ability to retain calcium:** *Women's International Pharmacy.* womensinternational.com/portfolio-items/testosterone-for -women/.

120 **up to 30 percent of men:** *National Institutes of Health, Osteoporosis and Related Bone Diseases National Resource Center.* my.clevelandclinic.org/health/diseases/17303 -osteoporosis-in-men.

120 **Both affect calcium absorption:** Deutschmann A et al., "Bisphenol A inhibits voltage-activated Ca(2+) channels in vitro: mechanisms and structural requirements," *Molecular Pharmacology* 83, no. 2 (February 2013):501–11. See also Liu PS et al., "Comparative Suppression of phthalate monoesters and phthalate diesters on calcium signalling coupled to nicotinic acetylcholine receptors." *Journal of Toxicological Sciences* 34, no. 3 (June 2009):255–63.

120 **Each year about six billion pounds:** Perrine S, Hurlock H. *The New American Diet.* Emmaus, PA: Rodale, 2009.

121   **Table 5.1:** Sources for this table include Ballatori N et al., "N-acetylcysteine as an antidote in methylmercury poisoning." *Environmental Health Perspectives* 106, no. 5 (1998):267–71; Ettinger AS et al., "Effect of calcium supplementation on blood lead levels in pregnancy: a randomized placebo-controlled trial." *Environmental Health Perspectives* 117, no. 1 (January 2009):26–31; Flora G et al., "Toxicity of lead: A review with recent updates." *Interdisciplinary Toxicology* 5, no. 2 (2012):47–58; Li YF et al., "Organic selenium supplementation increases mercury excretion and decreases oxidative damage in long-term mercury-exposed residents from Wanshan, China." *Environmental Science and Technology* 46, no. 20 (October 2012):11313–8; Van Barneveld AA et al., "Influence of Ca and Mg on the uptake and deposition of Pb and Cd in mice." *Toxicology and Applied Pharmacology* 7, no. 1 (June 1985):1–10.

121   **Table 5.1: Lead:** Kuzma C, "Lead in rice: what you need to know." *Prevention.* April 10, 2013. prevention.com/food-nutrition/healthy-eating/a20445159/lead-in -rice-what-you-need-to-know/.

121   **Table 5.1: lead uptake is enhanced in iron deficiency:** Smith H. *Diagnosis in Paediatric Haematology.* New York: Churchill Livingstone, 1996, 6–40.

122   **Table 5.1: Mercury:** Dufault R et al., "Mercury from chlor-alkali plants: measured concentrations in food product sugar." *Environmental Health* 8 (2009):2.

122   **Table 5.1: Arsenic:** Singh AP et al., "Mechanisms pertaining to arsenic toxicity." *Toxicology International* 18, no. 2 (2011):87–93. See also Argos M et al., "Arsenic exposure from drinking water, and all-cause and chronic-disease mortalities in Bangladesh (HEALS): a prospective cohort study." *Lancet* 376, no. 9737 (July 2010):252–8.

122   **Table 5.1: High aluminum levels in the bloodstream:** Cannata Andia JB et al., "Aluminum toxicity: its relationship with bone and iron metabolism." *Nephrology Dialysis Transplantation* 2, no. 3 suppl. (1996):69–73.

123   **but teen girls:** *Environmental Working Group Skin Deep.* ewg.org/skindeep/top-tips -for-safer-products/.

123   **However, the bad news is:** Shaofang Cai, Jiahao Zhu, Lingling Sun, Chunhong Fan, Yaohong Zhong, Qing Shen, Yingjun Li, Association between urinary triclosan with bone mass density and osteoporosis in the US adult women, 2005-2010, *The Journal of Clinical Endocrinology & Metabolism,* https://doi.org/10.1210/jc .2019-00576.

125   **Fluoride accumulates in your bones:** *Fluoride Action Network.* fluoridealert.org /studies/bone04.

126   **High levels of PFCs:** Knox SS et al., "Implications of early menopause in women exposed to perfluorocarbons." *Journal of Clinical Endocrinology and Metabolism* 96, no. 6 (June 2011):1747–53.

127   **PFCs have also been shown:** *National Collaborating Centre for Environmental Health.* ncceh.ca/sites/default/files/Health_effects_PFCs_Oct_2010.pdf.

127   **Stress and anxiety:** Gallup poll, December 4–11, 2017. news.gallup.com/poll /224336/eight-americans-afflicted-stress.aspx. See also 2008 Stress in America survey. American Psychological Association.

127   **According to WHO:** Hamer M et al., "The Role of functional foods in the psychobiology of health and disease." *Nutrition Research Reviews* 18, no. 1 (June 2005):77-88.

127   **Although studies have shown:** Matthews KA et al., "Chronic work stress and marital dissolution increase risk of post–trial mortality in men from the multiple risk

factor intervention trial." *Archives of Internal Medicine* 162, no. 3 (February 2002):309–15. See also Heraclides A et al., "Psychosocial stress at work doubles the risk of type 2 diabetes in middle-aged women: evidence from the Whitehall II Study." *Diabetes Care* 32, no. 12 (December 2009):2230–5; Kruk J, "Self-reported psychological stress and the risk of breast cancer: a case-control study." *Stress* 15, no. 2 (March 2012):162–71; Thayer et al., "The relationship of autonomic imbalance, heart rate variability and cardiovascular disease risk factors." *International Journal of Cardiology* 141, no. 2 (May 2010):122–31; Veen G et al., "Salivary Cortisol, serum lipids, and adiposity in patients with depressive and anxiety disorders." *Metabolism* 58, no. 6 (June 2009):821–7.

127   **In a 2018 study:** Catalano A et al., "Anxiety levels predict fracture risk in postmenopausal women assessed for osteoporosis." *Menopause* 25, no. 10 (October 2018):1110–15.

128   **a study conducted by the Mayo Clinic:** Ballentine R. *Diet and Nutrition.* Honesdale, PA: Himalayan Institute Press, 1978.

129   **a 2013 study published in *Psychosomatic Medicine*:** Long SJ et al., "Effects of vitamin and mineral supplementation on stress, mild psychiatric symptoms, and mood in nonclinical samples: a meta-analysis." *Psychosomatic Medicine* 75, no. 2 (2013): 144–53.

129   **the Michigan Bone Health Study:** Sowers M et al., "Bone mineral density and its change in pre- and perimenopausal white women: the Michigan Bone Health Study." *Journal of Bone and Mineral Research* 13, no. 7 (July 1998):1134–40.

129   **Cortisol indirectly acts on your bones:** Chiodini I et al., "Role of cortisol hypersecretion in the pathogenesis of osteoporosis." *Recenti Progressi in Medicina* 99, no. 6 (June 2008):309–13.

129   **The disruption increases bone resorption:** Heshmati HM et al., "Effects of the circadian variation in serum cortisol on markers of bone turnover and calcium homeostasis in normal postmenopausal women." *Journal of Clinical Endocrinology and Metabolism* 83, no. 3 (March 1998):751–6. See also Hardy R et al., "Adrenal gland and bone." *Archives of Biochemistry and Biophysics* 503, no. 1 (November 2010):137–45.

129   **Even a short bout:** Bilanin JE et al., "Lower vetebral bone density in male long distance runners." *Medicine and Science in Sports and Exercise* 21, no. 1 (February 1989):66–70.

130   **According to *Psychology Today*:** "Vitamin C: Stress Buster." *Psychology Today.* April 25, 2003.

130   **according to researchers at the University of Maryland:** Oz M, "Dr. Oz's Cure for Stubborn Belly Fat." *First for Women*, March 14, 2011, 32–37.

130   **Researchers proved that DHA:** Hamazaki T, "The effect of docosahexaenoic acid on aggression in young adults. A placebo-controlled double-blind study." *Journal of Clinical Investigation* 97, no. 4 (1996):1129–33.

130   **Scientists believe that omega-3 supplementation:** Delarue J et al., "Fish Oil prevents the adrenal activation elicited by mental stress in healthy men." *Diabetes and Metabolism* 29, no. 3 (June 2003):289–95.

130   **Studies have also shown that omega-3:** Noreen E et al., "Effects of supplemental fish oil on resting metabolic rate, body composition, and salivary cortisol in healthy adults." *Journal of the International Society of Sports Nutrition* 7 (October 2010):31.

133 **In 2017:** Swanson CM et al., "Bone Turnover markers after sleep restriction and circadian disruption: a mechanism for sleep-related bone loss in humans." *Journal of Clinical Endocrinology and Metabolism* 102, no. 10 (October 2017):3722–30.

133 **Remember that cortisol:** Chiodini I et al., "[Role of cortisol hypersecretion in the pathogenesis of osteoporosis]." *Recenti Progressi in Medicina* 99, no. 6 (June 2008):309–13. [Article in Italian.] See also Heshmati HM et al., "Effects of the circadian variation in serum cortisol on markers of bone turnover and calcium homeostasis in normal postmenopausal women." *Journal of Clinical Endocrinology and Metabolism* 83, no. 3 (March 1998):751–6; Hardy R et al., "Adrenal gland and bone." *Archives of Biochemistry and Biophysics* 503, no. 1 (November 2010):137–45.

133 **The study concluded:** Fu X et al., "Association between sleep duration and bone mineral density in Chinese women." *Bone* 49, no. 5 (November 2011):1062–6.

133 **Other recent studies:** Chen YL et al., "Obstructive sleep apnea and risk of osteoporosis: a population-based cohort study in Taiwan." *Journal of Clinical Endocrinology and Metabolism* 99, no. 7 (July 2014):2441–7. See also Sivertsen B et al., "Insomnia as a risk factor for ill health: results from the large population-based prospective HUNT study in Norway." *Journal of Sleep Research* 23, no. 2 (April 2014):124–32.

134 **Research out of Johns Hopkins:** Alberg AJ et al., "Household Exposure to Passive Cigarette Smoking and Serum Micronutrient Concentrations." *American Journal of Clinical Nutrition* 72, no. 6 (December 2000):1576–82.

134 **According to WHO:** *World Health Organization.* www.who.int/mediacentre/news /releases/2014/air-pollution/en.

134 **Studies show that supplementation of antioxidants:** Zhong J et al., "B-vitamin Supplementation mitigates effects of fine particles on cardiac autonomic dysfunction and inflammation: a pilot human intervention trial." *Scientific Reports* 7 (April 2017):45322.

135 **A recent study in *The Lancet Planetary Health*:** Prada D et al., "Association of air particulate pollution with bone loss over time and bone fracture risk: analysis of data from two independent studies." *Lancet Planetary Health* 8 (November 2017):e337–47.

135 **An estimated 9,320 people:** American Cancer Society. *Cancer Facts and Figures 2018.* Atlanta, GA: American Cancer Society, 2018.

136 **scientifically linked to:** Vimaleswaran KS et al., "Causal relationship between obesity and vitamin D status: Bi-directional Mendelian randomization analysis of multiple cohorts." *PLoS Medicine* 10, no. 2 (2013):e1001383.

136 **The people who are most at risk:** *Harvard School of Public Health.* www.hsph .harvard.edu/nutritionsource/vitamin-d-deficiency-risk.

136 **Dr. Elizabeth Plourde:** Plourde E, "Sunscreens cause cancer instead of protect you from it!" Video. ihealthtube.com/video/sunscreens-cause-cancer-instead -protect-you-it.

137 **According to WHO:** *World Health Organization.* www.who.int/peh-emf/about /WhatisEMF/en.

137 **Martin Pall, PhD:** Pall ML, "Scientific evidence contradicts findings and assumptions of Canadian Safety Panel 6: microwaves act through voltage-gated calcium channel activation to induce biological impacts at non-thermal levels, supporting a paradigm shift for microwave/lower frequency electromagnetic field action." *Reviews on Environmental Health* 30, no. 2 (2015):99–116. See also Pall ML, "How to

Approach the challenge of minimizing non-thermal health effects of microwave radiation from electrical devices." *International Journal of Innovative Research in Engineering and Management* 2, no. 5 (September 2015). Pall ML, "Electromagnetic fields act via activation of voltage-gated calcium channels to produce beneficial or adverse effects." *Journal of Cellular and Molecular Medicine* 17, no. 8 (August 2013):958–65; Pall, ML, "Electromagnetic fields act similarly in plants as in animals: probable activation of calcium channels via their voltage sensor." *Current Chemical Biology* 10, no. 1 (July 2016):74–82; Pall ML, "Microwave frequency electromagnetic fields (EMFs) produce widespread neuropsychiatric effects including depression." *Journal of Chemical Neuroanatomy* 75, pt. B (September 2016):43–51.

138 **keeping your smartphone in your pocket:** Saraví FD, "Asymmetries in hip mineralization in mobile cellular phone users." *Journal of Craniofacial Surgery* 22, no. 2 (March 2011):706–10.

138 **may be increased by up to 20 to 100 times:** Maughan RJ et al., "Role of micronutrients in sport and physical activity." *British Medical Bulletin* 55, no. 3 (1999):683–90.

138 **Individuals who work out less than four hours a week:** Mierlo CA et al., "Weight Management using a meal replacement strategy: meta and pooling analysis from six studies." *International Journal of Obesity and Related Metabolic Disorders* 27, no. 5 (May 2003):537–49.

139 **findings presented at the 2013 meeting:** Klempel et al., "Intermittent fasting combined with calorie restriction is effective for weight loss and cardio-protection in obese women." *Nutrition Journal* 11 (November 2012):98. •

139 **zinc and magnesium can also be depleted:** D. Jakubowicz et al., "Incretin, Insulinotropic and glucose-lowering effects of whey protein pre-load in type 2 diabetes: a randomised clinical trial." *Diabetologia* 57, no. 9 (September 2014):1807–11.

139 **USDA research shows:** Nielsen FH et al., "Update on the relationship between magnesium and exercise." *Magnesium Research* 19, no. 3 (September 2006):180–9.

140 **This is why astronauts:** *NASA.* nasa.gov/mission_pages/station/research /experiments/118.html.

140 **A 2015 study:** Hunte B et al., "Axial bone osteogenic loading-type resistance therapy showing BMD and functional bone performance musculoskeletal adaptation over 24 weeks with postmenopausal female subjects." *Journal of Osteoporosis and Physical Activity* 3 (2015):146.

140 **Scientists in the UK:** Deer K et al., "Habitual Levels of high, but not moderate or low impact activity are positively related to hip BMD and geometry: results from a population-based study of adolescents." *Journal of Bone and Mineral Research* 27, no. 9 (September 2012):1887–95.

140 **You can nearly double this load:** Hunte B et al., "Axial bone osteogenic loading-type resistance therapy showing BMD and functional bone performance musculoskeletal adaptation over 24 weeks with postmenopausal female subjects." *Journal of Osteoporosis and Physical Activity* 3 (2015):146.

141 **Although yoga and Pilates:** Smith EN et al., "Yoga, vertebral fractures, and osteoporosis: research and recommendations." *International Journal of Yoga Therapy* 23, no. 1 (2013):17–23.

142 **The Centers for Disease Control and Prevention (CDC) reports:** Gu Q, et al., "Prescription drug use continues to increase: US prescription drug data for 2007–2008." NCHS Data Brief 42. September 2010.

142   **overdoses involving prescription drugs:** Centers for Disease Control and Prevention (CDC). "Vital signs: overdoses of prescription opioid pain relievers—United States, 1999–2008." *Morbidity and Mortality Weekly Report* 60, no. 43 (November 2011):1487–92.

142   **the average person in the UK:** "Prescriptions dispensed in the community—statistics for England, 2002–2012." *National Health Service.* July 2013.

142   **two-thirds of Australians over age 60:** Elliott RA, "Problems with medication use in the elderly: an Australian perspective." *Journal of Pharmacy Practice and Research* 36, no. 1 (2006).

143   **They interfere with bone formation:** Davidge Pitts CJ et al., "Update on medications with adverse skeletal effects." *Mayo Clinic Proceedings* 86, no. 4 (2011):338–43.

143   **studies have shown that within the first year:** Davidge Pitts CJ et al., "Update on medications with adverse skeletal effects." *Mayo Clinic Proceedings* 86, no. 4 (April 2011):338–43; Mazziotti G et al., "Drug-induced osteoporosis: mechanisms and clinical implications." *American Journal of Medicine* 123, no. 10 (October 2010):877–84.

143   **they inhibit dopamine production:** Damsa C et al., "Dopamine-dependent side effects of selective serotonin reuptake inhibitors: a clinical review." *Journal of Clinical Psychiatry* 65, no. 8 (August 2004):1064–8.

143   **they cause chronic elevation:** Bushe C et al., "Prevalence of hyperprolactinaemia in a naturalistic cohort of schizophrenia and bipolar outpatients during treatment with typical and atypical antipsychotics." *Journal of Psychopharmacology* 21, no. 7 (September 2007):768–73.

144   **increased risk for osteoporosis:** Bolton JM et al., "Risk of low bone mineral density associated with psychotropic medications and mental disorders in postmenopausal women." *Journal of Clinical Psychopharmacology* 31, no. 1 (February 2011):56–60.

144   **osteoporotic fractures:** Bolton JM et al., "Fracture risk from psychotropic medications: a population-based analysis." *Journal of Clinical Psychopharmacology* 28, no. 4 (August 2008):384–91.

144   **Two other antidepressants:** Rauma PH et al., "Effects of antidepressants on postmenopausal bone loss—A 5-year longitudinal study from the OSTPRE cohort." *Bone* 89 (August 2016):25–31.

144   **Research indicates that these medications can deplete:** *Penn State Hershey.* pennstatehershey.adam.com/content.aspx?productId=107&pid=33&gid=000176. See also "Preventing Pharmaceutical-Induced Nutritional Deficiencies." *Life Extension Magazine.* March 2006. lifeextension.com/magazine/2006/3/report_drugs /page-01.

145   **Many studies evaluating PPI use:** Lau Y et al., "Fracture risk and bone mineral density reduction associated with proton pump inhibitors." *Pharmacotherapy* 32(2012):67–79.

145   **Short-term PPI use:** Yang Y et al., "Long-term proton pump inhibitor therapy and risk of hip fracture." *JAMA* 296(2006):2947–53. See also Corley D et al., "Proton pump inhibitors and histamine-2 receptor antagonists are associated with hip fractures among at-risk patients." *Gastroenterology* 139 (2010): 93–101; Roux C et al., "Increase in vertebral fracture risk in postmenopausal women using omeprazole." *Calcified Tissue International* 84(2009):13–19.

145 **Heartburn is almost always a case:** English J, "Gastric balance: heartburn not always caused by excess acid." *Nutrition Review.* November 25, 2018. nutrition review.org/2018/11/gastric-balance-heartburn-caused-excess-acid.

148 **Table 5.2: Micronutrients Depleted:** Pelton R, ed. *Drug-Induced Nutrient Depletion Handbook,* 2nd ed. Hudson, OH: Lexi-Comp, 2001. See also Pelton R, ed. *The Nutritional Cost of Prescription Drugs,* 2nd ed. Englewood, CO: Morton, 2004; Vaglini F, ed. *The Side Effects Bible: The Dietary Solution to Unwanted Side Effects of Common Medications.* New York: Broadway Books, 2005.

Chapter 6: Smart Supplementation

164 **Dr. Löbenberg conducted a research study:** Löbenberg R et al., "Investigation of vitamin and mineral tablets and capsules on the Canadian market." *Journal of Pharmacy and Pharmaceutical Sciences* 9, no. 1 (2006):40–9.

165 **According to a nationwide survey:** Harris Interactive Inc. "Pill-Swallowing Problems in America: A National Survey of Adults." New York, NY: Harris Interactive Inc. for Schwarz Pharma; (2003); 1–39.

166 **Unscrupulous manufacturers:** Kobylewsk S, Jacobson M. *Food Dyes: A Rainbow of Risks.* Washington, DC: Center for Science in the Public Interest, 2010.

169 **"excessive amounts of vitamin A":** *The NIH Osteoporosis and Related Bone Diseases National Resource Center.* https://www.bones.nih.gov/health-info/bone/bone -health/nutrition/vitamin-and-bone-health.

171 **"You want to give your body":** "Dr. Oz's ultimate anti-aging checklist." doctoroz.com/article/dr-ozs-ultimate-anti-aging-checklist.

171 **Research published in the** *American Journal of Epidemiology***:** Botto LD et al., "5,10-Methylenetetrahydrofolate Reductase Gene Variants and Congenital Anomalies: A Huge Review." *American Journal of Epidemiology* 151, no. 9: (May 2000): 862–77.

172 **Table 6.3:** Tang G, "Bioconversion of dietary provitamin A carotenoids to vitamin A in humans." *American Journal of Clinical Nutrition* 91, no. 5 (May 2010):1468S–73S. See also Botto LD et al., "5,10-Methylenetetrahydrofolate Reductase gene variants and congenital anomalies: a huge review." *American Journal of Epidemiology* 151, no. 9 (May 2000):862–77; Heaney RP, "Phosphate and carbonate salts of calcium support robust bone building in osteoporosis." *American Journal of Clinical Nutrition* 92, no. 1(2010):101–5; Iwamoto T et al., "Combined treatment with vitamin K2 and bisphosphonate in postmenopausal women with osteoporosis." *Yonsei Medical Journal* 44, no. 5 (2003): 751–56; Serbinova E et al., "Free Radical recycling and intramembrane mobility in the antioxidant properties of alpha-tocopherol and alpha-tocotrienol." *Free Radical Biology and Medicine* 10, no. 5 (1991):263–75; Willner P et al., "Depression Increases "craving" for sweet rewards in animal and human models of depression and craving." *Psychopharmacology* 136, no. 3 (April 1998):272–83; *Linus Pauling Institute.* lpi.oregonstate.edu/infocenter/vitamins/vitamin; *MedlinePlus.* nlm.nih.gov/medlineplus/druginfo/natural/924.html; *National Institutes of Health.* ods.od.nih.gov/factsheets/Magnesium-HealthProfessional; "Most multivitamin extras don't add up." *Tufts University Health and Nutrition Letter,* February 1, 2010; Institute of Medicine. *Dietary Reference Intakes for Calcium, Phosphorus, Magnesium, Vitamin D, and Fluoride,* vol. 35. Washington, DC: National Academy of Sciences, 2001, 1678–82.

178   **Table 6.3: Copper:** *Physicians Committee for Responsible Medicine.* pcrm.org/health
-topics/alzheimers. See also Main E, "Is there too much copper in your multivitamin?" *Rodalenews.com.* August 25, 2013. prevention.com/health/memory
/a20457994/too-much-copper-in-your-multivitamin/.

183   **numerous peer-reviewed scientific studies:** Tyssandier V et al., "Vegetable-
borne lutein, lycopene, and beta-carotene compete for incorporation into chylomi-
crons, with no adverse effect on the medium-term (3-wk) plasma status of carotenoids
in humans." *American Journal of Clinical Nutrition* 75, no. 3 (March 2002):526–34. See
also Leena M et al., "Selenium iron interaction in young women with low selenium status." *Journal of Human Nutrition and Dietetics* 2, no. 1 (February 1989):39–
42; Micozzi MS et al., "Plasma carotenoid response to chronic intake of selected
foods and beta-carotene supplements in men." *American Journal of Clinical Nutrition*
55, no. 6 (June 1992):1120–5; Watts DL, "Nutrient interrelationships: minerals—
vitamins—endocrines." *Journal of Orthomolecular Medicine* 5, no. 1 (1990):11–19.

185   **Micronutrients That Have Competitions with Calcium:** Watts DL, "Nutrient interrelationships: minerals—vitamins—endocrines." *Journal of Orthomolecular
Medicine* 5, no. 1 (1990):11–19.

185   **Calcium can chelate with riboflavin:** Gaby A. *Nutritional Medicine.* Concord,
NH: Perlberg, 2011.

185   **Copper shares an absorption carrier:** Bland JS, ed. *Clinical Nutrition: A Functional Approach.* Federal Way, WA: Institute For Functional Medicine, 2004, 173.

185   **Calcium can inhibit the absorption:** Bendich A, "Calcium supplementation
and iron status of females." *Nutrition* 17, no. 1 (January 2001):46–51. See also Sand-
ström B et al., "Micronutrient interactions: effects on absorption and bioavailability." *British Journal of Nutrition* 85, no. 2 suppl. (May 2001):S181–5.

185   **Calcium and magnesium compete for absorption:** Hendrix ZJ et al., "Competition between calcium, strontium, and magnesium for absorption in the isolated
rat intestine." *Clinical Chemistry* 12 (December 1963):734–44. See also Alcock N
et al., "Inter-relation of calcium and magnesium absorption." *Clinical Science* 22
(April 1962):185–93; De Swart PM et al., "The interrelationship of calcium and
magnesium absorption in idiopathic hypercalciuria and renal calcium stone disease."
Journal of Urology 159, no. 56 (May 1998):1650; Giles MM et al., "Magnesium metabolism in preterm infants: effects of calcium, magnesium, and phosphorus, and of
postnatal and gestational age." *Journal of Pediatrics* 117, no. 1, part 1 (July 1990):147–
54; Gaby A. *Nutritional Medicine.* Concord, NH: Perlberg, 2011; *PDR for Nutritional Supplements.* Montvale, NJ: Physicians' Desk Reference, 2001, 575; *Consumer
Lab.* consumerlab.com/answers/is-it-important-to-take-calcium-and-magnesium
-together/calcium_with_magnesium.

185   **Calcium can slightly decrease:** Davidsson L et al., "The effect of individual
dietary components on manganese absorption in humans." *American Journal of Clinical Nutrition* 54, no. 6 (December 1991):1065–70. See also Lutz TA et al., "Effects
of calcium and sugars on intestinal manganese absorption." *Biological Trace Element
Research* 39, no. 2–3 (November–December 1993):221–7.

185   **High intake of sodium:** Pan W et al., "The epithelial sodium/proton exchanger,
NHE3, is necessary for renal and intestinal calcium (re)absorption." *American Journal
of Physiology-Renal Physiology* 302, no. 8 (April 2012):F943–56.

185   **Large doses of calcium can inhibit:** Argiratos V et al., "The effect of calcium
carbonate and calcium citrate on the absorption of zinc in healthy female subjects."

European Journal of Clinical Nutrition 48, no. 3 (March 1994):198–204. See also Jayal-akshmi S et al., "Compromised zinc status of experimental rats as a consequence of prolonged iron and calcium supplementation." *Indian Journal of Medical Research* 143, no. 2 (February 2016):238–44; Spencer H et al., "Effect of zinc supplements on the intestinal absorption of calcium." *Journal of the American College of Nutrition* 6, no. 1 (February 1987): 47–51.

185   **Excessive amounts of the fat-soluble vitamins:** Goncalves A et al., "Fat-soluble vitamin intestinal absorption: absorption sites in the intestine and interactions for absorption." *Food Chemistry* 172 (April 2015):155–60.

185   **Large doses of B9:** Dickinson CJ et al., "Does folic acid harm people with vitamin B12 deficiency?" *QJM: An International Journal of Medicine* 88, no. 5 (May 1995):357–64.

185   **When vitamin C:** Shrimpton DH, "Nutritional implications of micronutrient interactions." *Chemist and Druggist* 15 (2004):38–41. See also Kondo H et al., "Presence and formation of cobalamin analogues in multivitamin-mineral pills." *Journal of Clinical Investigation* 70, no. 4 (October 1982):889–98; Gaby A. *Nutritional Medicine.* Concord, NH: Perlberg, 2011.

186   **Cobalt ions:** Ahmad I et al., "Effect of Riboflavin on the Photolysis of Cyanoco-bolamin in Aqueous Solution" *The Open Analytical Chemistry Journal.* 6 (2012):22–7. https://www.ncbi.nlm.nih.gov/pmc/articles/PMC4137421/#R15

186   **Potassium supplements:** Cox L, "Vitamin B12: deficiency and supplements." *LiveScience.* June 21, 2017. livescience.com/47398-vitamin-b12-deficiency-supplements.html.

186   **Iron can bind with vitamin E:** Omara FO et al., "Vitamin E is protective against iron toxicity and iron-induced hepatic vitamin E depletion in mice." *Journal of Nutrition* 123, no. 10 (October 1993):1649–55. See also Gaby A. *Nutritional Medicine.* Concord, NH: Perlberg, 2011.

186   **Calcium can inhibit the absorption:** Whiting SJ, "The inhibitory effect of dietary calcium on iron bioavailability: a cause for concern?" *Nutritional Review* 53, no. 3 (March 1995):77–80. See also Pallarés I et al., "Effects of iron replenishment on iron, calcium, phosphorus and magnesium metabolism in iron-deficient rats." *International Journal for Vitamin and Nutrition Research* 66, no. 2 (1996):158–65.

186   **Chromium may compete:** Quarles CD et al., "Competitive binding of Fe3+, Cr3+ and Ni2+ to transferrin." *Journal of Biological and Inorganic Chemistry* 16, no. 6 (August 2011):913–21.

186   **Iron inhibits the absorption:** Arredondo M et al., "Inhibition of iron and copper uptake by iron, copper and zinc." *Biological Research* 39, no. 1 (2006):95–102. See also Storey ML et al., "Iron, zinc and copper interactions: Chronic versus acute response of rats." *Journal of Nutrition* 117, no. 8 (August 1987):1434–42.

186   **High levels of iron or manganese:** Rossander-Hulten L et al., "Competitive inhibition of iron absorption by manganese and zinc in humans." *American Journal of Clinical Nutrition* 54, no. 1 (July 1991):152–6.

186   **Iron and molybdenum compete:** Seelig MS, "Proposed role of copper–molybdenum interaction in iron-deficiency and iron-storage diseases." *American Journal of Clinical Nutrition* 26, no. 6 (June 1973):657–72.

186   **Iron and phosphorus compete:** Pallarés I et al., "Effects of iron replenishment on iron, calcium, phosphorus and magnesium metabolism in iron-deficient rats." *International Journal for Vitamin and Nutrition Research* 66, no. 2 (1996):158–65.

186 **Iron adversely affects:** Chareonpong-Kawamoto N et al., "Selenium deficiency as a cause of overload of iron and unbalanced distribution of other minerals." *Bioscience, Biotechnology, and Biochemistry* 59, no. 2 (February 1995):302–6.

186 **Iron and zinc both decrease:** Gaby A. *Nutritional Medicine.* Concord, NH: Perlberg, 2011. See also Solomons NW et al., "Studies on the bioavailability of zinc in humans: effects of heme and nonheme iron on the absorption of zinc." *American Journal of Clinical Nutrition* 34, no. 4 (April 1981):475–82.

186 **Calcium and magnesium compete for absorption:** Hendrix ZJ et al., "Competition between calcium, strontium, and magnesium for absorption in the isolated rat intestine." *Clinical Chemistry* 12 (December 1963):734–44. See also Alcock N et al., "Inter-relation of calcium and magnesium absorption." *Clinical Science* 22 (April 1962):185–93; De Swart PM et al., "The interrelationship of calcium and magnesium absorption in idiopathic hypercalciuria and renal calcium stone disease." *Journal of Urology* 159, no. 56 (May 1998):1650; Giles MM et al., "Magnesium metabolism in preterm infants: effects of calcium, magnesium, and phosphorus, and of postnatal and gestational age." *Journal of Pediatrics* 117, no. 1, part 1 (July 1990):147–54; Gaby A. *Nutritional Medicine.* Concord, NH: Perlberg, 2011; *PDR for Nutritional Supplements.* Montvale, NJ: Physicians' Desk Reference, 2001, 575.

186 **Magnesium intake inhibits:** Cook JD et al., "The effect of red and white wines on nonheme-iron absorption in humans." *American Journal of Clinical Nutrition* 61, no. 4 (1995): 800–4.

186 **Magnesium may decrease:** Greger JL et al., "Effect of dietary protein and phosphorus levels on the utilization of zinc, copper, and manganese by adult males." *Journal of Nutrition* 110(1980):2243–53. See also Gropper SAS, ed. *Advanced Nutrition and Human Metabolism.* Boston: Cengage Learning, 2005, 473–74; Klimis-Tavantzis DJ, ed. *Manganese in Health and Disease.* Boca Raton, FL: CRC Press, 1994), 47–48.

186 **High intake of phosphorus competes:** Brink EJ et al., "Interaction of calcium and phosphate decreases ileal magnesium solubility and apparent magnesium absorption in rats." *Journal of Nutrition* 122, no. 3 (March 1992):580–6.

186 **High zinc intake may decrease:** Spencer H et al., "Inhibitory effects of zinc on magnesium balance and magnesium absorption in man." *Journal of the American College of Nutrition* 13, no. 5 (October 1994):479–84.

187 **Many years ago:** "Multiple vitamin-mineral supplements." *Publix.* http://publix .aisle7.net/publix/assets/generic/multiple-vitamin-mineral-supplements/~default.

188 **The first was published back in 1998:** van den Berg H et al., "Effect of simultaneous, single oral doses of beta-carotene with lutein or lycopene on the beta-carotene and retinyl ester responses in the triacylglycerol-rich lipoprotein fraction of men." *American Journal of Clinical Nutrition* 68, no. 1 (July 1998):82–9.

188 **The study's developer, Edward Paul, OD, PhD:** Warnock S, "Researchers continue to find nutrition's value in preventing—even treating—AMD." *Primary Care Optometry News.* August 2001. healio.com/optometry/retina-vitreous/news /print/primary-care-optometry-news/%7Ba535ed9c-8d7f-4664-b4b4 -765b5a161742%7D/researchers-continue-to-find-nutritions-value-in-preventing —even-treating—amd.

191 **Calcium is required for the proper absorption:** Linus Pauling Institute. lpi.oregonstate.edu/mic/vitamins/vitamin-B12.

191 **Vitamin D increases:** Khazai N et al., "Calcium and vitamin D: skeletal and extraskeletal health." *Current Rheumatology Reports* 10, no. 2 (April 2008):110–7.

See also Heaney RP, "Vitamin D and calcium interactions: functional outcome." *American Journal of Clinical Nutrition* 88, no. 2S (2008):541S–4S.

192 **Vitamin K and calcium:** van Ballegooijen AJ et al., "The synergistic interplay between vitamins D and K for bone and cardiovascular health: a narrative review." *International Journal of Endocrinology* 2017 (September 2017):1–12.

192 **Boron converts vitamin D:** *Vitamin D Council.* vitamindcouncil.org/about -vitamin-d/vitamin-d-and-other-vitamins-and-minerals/#.W_XQbi3MxE4.

192 **Magnesium helps retain:** Lubi M et al., "Magnesium supplementation does not affect blood calcium level in treated hypoparathyroid patients." *Journal of Clinical Endocrinology and Metabolism* 97, no. 11 (November 2012):E2090–2.

192 **Omega-3 increases:** Orchard TS et al., "A systematic review of omega-3 fatty acids and osteoporosis." *British Journal of Nutrition* 107, no. 2 suppl. (2012):S253–60.

192 **High consumption of potassium:** Gaby A. *Nutritional Medicine.* Concord, NH: Perlberg, 2011. See also Turner KM et al., "Sodium and potassium excretion are related to bone mineral density in women with coeliac disease." *Clinical Nutrition* 34, no. 2 (April 2015):265–8.

192 **Dietary silicon helps:** Price CT et al., "Silicon: a review of its potential role in the prevention and treatment of postmenopausal osteoporosis." *International Journal of Endocrinology* 2013 (April 2013):1–6.

192 **Vitamin E helps:** *MedlinePlus.* medlineplus.gov/ency/article/002406.htm.

192 **Calcium and vitamin K:** "Proper calcium use: Vitamin K2 as a promoter of bone and cardiovascular health." *Integrative Medicine (Encinitas)* 14, no. 1 (2015):34–9.

192 **Manganese functions with vitamin K:** Watts DL, "The nutritional relation-ships of manganese." *Journal of Orthomolecular Medicine* 5, no. 4 (1990):219–22.

192 **Vitamin B6 works synergistically:** *Harvard School of Public Health.* www.hsph .harvard.edu/nutritionsource/what-should-you-eat/vitamins/vitamin-b.

192 **Vitamin B9 works synergistically:** *Harvard School of Public Health.* www.hsph .harvard.edu/nutritionsource/what-should-you-eat/vitamins/vitamin-b/.

193 **Vitamin C works with B12:** *MedlinePlus.* medlineplus.gov/ency/article/002408 .htm.

193 **Vitamin E is required:** Pappu AS et al., "Possible interrelationship between vi-tamins E and B12 in the disturbance in methylmalonate metabolism in vitamin E deficiency." *Biochemical Journal* 172, no. 1 (1978):115–21.

193 **Calcium is required:** Bland JS, ed. *Clinical Nutrition: A Functional Approach.* Fed-eral Way, WA: Institute For Functional Medicine, 2004, 120.

193 **Vitamins B9 and B12 and iron:** Mahmood L, "The metabolic processes of folic acid and vitamin B12 deficiency." *Journal of Health Research and Reviews* 1(2014):5–9.

193 **Vitamin A increases:** García-Casal MN et al., "Vitamin A and beta-carotene can improve nonheme iron absorption from rice, wheat and corn by humans." *Journal of Nutrition* 128, no. 3 (March 1998):646–50.

193 **Riboflavin is necessary:** *Linus Pauling Institute.* lpi.oregonstate.edu/mic/vitamins /riboflavin.

193 **Vitamins B9 and B12 and iron:** Mahmood L, "The metabolic processes of folic acid and vitamin B12 deficiency." *Journal of Health Research and Reviews* 1(2014):5–9.

193 **Elevated vitamin C levels:** Cook JD et al., "Effect of ascorbic acid intake on nonheme-iron absorption from a complete diet." *American Journal of Clinical Nutrition* 73, no. 1 (January 2001):93–8.

193 **Copper shares a physiological synergy:** Higdon J, ed. *An Evidence-Based Approach to Vitamins and Minerals: Health Benefits and Intake Recommendations.* New York: Thieme, 2003, 207.

193 **The effects of a deficiency of iodine:** Hess SY, "The impact of common micronutrient deficiencies on iodine and thyroid metabolism: the evidence from human studies." *Best Practice and Research Clinical Endocrinology and Metabolism* 24, no. 1 (February 2010):117–32. See also Higdon J, ed. *An Evidence-Based Approach to Vitamins and Minerals: Health Benefits and Intake Recommendations.* New York: Thieme, 2003, 132.

194 **High amounts of vitamin B6:** Fathizadeh N et al., "Evaluation the effect of magnesium and magnesium plus vitamin B6 supplement on the severity of premenstrual syndrome." *Iranian Journal of Nursing and Midwifery Research* 15, no. 1 suppl. (December 2010):401–5.

194 **Vitamin D slightly increases:** Uwitonze AM et al., "Role of magnesium in vitamin D activation and function." *Journal of the American Osteopathic Association* 118, no. 3 (March 2018):181–9. See also *Linus Pauling Institute.* lpi.oregonstate.edu/mic /minerals/magnesium.

194 **Boron plays an important role:** Naghii MR et al., "The role of boron in nutrition and metabolism." *Progress in Food and Nutrition Science* 17, no. 4 (October–December 1993):331–49.

194 **Magnesium helps retain serum blood calcium:** Higdon J, ed. *An Evidence-Based Approach to Vitamins and Minerals: Health Benefits and Intake Recommendations.* New York: Thieme, 2003, 149.

194 **Potassium and magnesium share a physiological synergy:** Bara M et al., "Regulation of sodium and potassium pathways by magnesium in cell membranes." *Magnesium Research* 6, no. 2 (June 1993):167–77.

194 **Magnesium is required:** *ScienceDirect.* sciencedirect.com/topics/biochemistry -genetics-and-molecular-biology/gamma-linolenic-acid.

194 **According to the late Derek H. Shrimpton, PhD:** Shrimpton DH, "Nutritional implications of micronutrient interactions." *Chemist and Druggist* 15 (2004):38–41.

Chapter 7: Supplementation and Testing Methods Beyond the ABCs

201 research indicates that larger quantities: Cockayne S et al., "Vitamin K and the prevention of fractures: systematic review and meta-analysis of randomized controlled trials." *Archives of Internal Medicine* 166, no. 12 (2006):1256–61.

203 **Studies show that supplementing with GLA:** Kruger MC et al., "Calcium, gamma-linolenic acid and eicosapentaenoic acid supplementation in senile osteoporosis." *Aging* 10, no. 5 (October 1998):385–94.

204 **Remember, free radicals:** Darden AG et al., "Osteoclastic superoxide production and bone resorption: stimulation and inhibition by modulators of NADPH oxidase." *Journal of Bone and Mineral Research* 11, no. 5 (May 1996):671–5. See also Fraser JH et al., "Hydrogen peroxide, but not superoxide, stimulates bone resorption in mouse calvariae." *Bone* 19, no. 3 (September 1996):223–6; Yang S et al., "Nicotinamide adenine dinucleotide phosphate oxidase in the formation of superoxide in

osteoclasts." *Calcified Tissue International* 63, no. 4 (October 1998):346–50; Yang S et al., "A new superoxide-generating oxidase in murine osteoclasts." *Journal of Biological Chemistry* 276, no. 8 (February 2001):5452–8.

204 **Those with the lowest levels:** Nuttall S et al., "Glutathione: in sickness and in health." *Lancet* 351, no. 9103 (1998):645–6.

204 **Build strong bones:** Lean JM et al., "A crucial role for thiol antioxidants in estrogen-deficiency bone loss." *Journal of Clinical Investigation* 112, no. 6 (2003):915–23. See also Rendina E et al., "Dried plum's unique capacity to reverse bone loss and alter bone metabolism in postmenopausal osteoporosis model." *PLoS One* 8, no. 3(2013):e60569.

204 **Build a strong immune system:** Dröge W et al., "Glutathione and immune function." *Proceedings of the Nutrition Society* 59, no. 4 (November 2000):595–600.

204 **Reduce inflammation:** Chatterton DE et al., "Anti-inflammatory mechanisms of bioactive milk proteins in the intestine of newborns." *International Journal of Biochemistry and Cell Biology* 45, no. 8 (August 2013):1730–47. See also Rahman I et al., "Oxidative stress and regulation of glutathione in lung inflammation," *European Clinical Respiratory Journal* 16, no. 3 (September 2000):534–54.

204 **Optimize your central nervous system:** Viña J et al., "Molecular bases of the treatment of Alzheimer's disease with antioxidants: prevention of oxidative stress." *Molecular Aspects of Medicine* 25, no. 1–2 (February–April 2004):117–23.

204 **Fight infections:** Ghezzi P et al. "Role of glutathione in immunity and inflammation in the lung." *International Journal of General Medicine* 4(2011):105–13.

204 **Prevent cancer:** Parodi PW et al. "A role for milk proteins and their peptides in cancer prevention." *Current Pharmaceutical Design* 13, no. 8 (2007):813–28.

204 **Help in the treatment of AIDS:** De Rosa SC et al., "N-acetylcysteine replenishes glutathione in HIV infection." *European Journal of Clinical Investigation* 30, no. 10 (October 2000):915–29.

204 **Detoxify your body:** Farombi EO et al., "The effect of modulation of glutathione levels on markers for aflatoxin B1-induced cell damage." *African Journal of Medicine and Medical Sciences* 34, no. 1 (March 2005):37–43.

205 **Protect your body from alcohol damage:** Matsumoto H et al., "New biological function of bovine alpha-lactalbumin: protective effect against ethanol- and stress-induced gastric mucosal injury in rats." *Bioscience, Biotechnology, and Biochemistry* 65, no. 5 (May 2001):1104–11.

205 **Promote heart health:** Gerdes SK et al., "Bioactive components of whey and cardiovascular health." Applications monograph. *U.S. Dairy Export Council.* 2001; See also Zhang X et al., "Lowering effect of dietary milk-whey protein v. casein on plasma and liver cholesterol concentrations in rats." *British Journal of Nutrition*, 70, no. 1 (July 1993):139–46.

205 **Increase strength and endurance:** Willoughby DS et al., "Effects of resistance training and protein plus amino acid supplementation on muscle anabolism, mass, and strength." *Amino Acids* 32, no. 4 (2007):467–77.

205 **Shift metabolism:** Hyman M, "Essential glutathione: the mother of all antioxidants." drhyman.com/blog/2010/05/19/glutathione-the-mother-of-all-antioxidants /#close.

205 **Flush out heavy metals:** Patrick L, "Mercury toxicity and antioxidants: part 1: role of glutathione and alpha-lipoic acid in the treatment of mercury toxicity." *Alternative Medicine Review* 7, no. 6 (December 2002):456–71. See also Kromidas L et al., "The protective effects of glutathione against methylmercury cytotoxicity." *Toxicology Letters* 51, no. 1 (March 1990):67–80.

205 **Promote longevity:** Lang CA et al., "High blood glutathione levels accompany excellent physical and mental health in women ages 60 to 103 years." *Journal of Clinical and Laboratory Medicine* 140, no. 6 (December 2002):413–7.

206 **high estrogen levels have been associated:** Cassidy A et al., "Biological effects of a diet of soy protein rich in isoflavones on the menstrual cycle of premenopausal women." *American Journal of Clinical Nutrition* 60, no. 3 (September 1994):333–40.

206 **This can result in lower metabolism:** Nienhiser JC, "Studies showing adverse effects of isoflavones, 1950–2013." *Weston A. Price Foundation*. westonaprice.org/health-topics/soy-alert/studies-showing-adverse-effects-of-isoflavones-1950-2010.

208 **The metabolism of an ethyl ester:** Lawson LD et al., "Human absorption of fish oil fatty acids as triacylglycerols, free acids, or ethyl esters." *Biochemical and Biophysical Research Communications* 152, no. 1 (1988):328–35. See also el Boustani, S et al., "Enteral absorption in man of eicosapentaenoic acid in different chemical forms." *Lipids* 22, no. 10 (1987): 711–4; Ikeda I. et al., "Digestion and lymphatic transport of eicosapentaenoic and docosahexaenoic acids given in the form of triacylglycerol, free acid and ethyl ester in rats." *Biochimica et Biophysica Acta* 1259, no. 3(1995):297–304; Krokan HE et al., "The enteral bioavailability of eicosapentaenoic acid and docosahexaenoic acid is as good from ethyl esters as from glyceryl esters in spite of lower hydrolytic rates by pancreatic lipase in vitro." *Biochimica et Biophysica Acta* 1168, no. 1 (1993):59–67; Yang LY et al., "Lipolysis of menhaden oil triacylglycerols and the corresponding fatty acid alkyl esters by pancreatic lipase in vitro: a reexamination." *Journal of Lipid Research* 31, no. 1 (1990):137–47.

208 **The triglyceride form of omega-3 is at least 70 percent better:** Dyerberg J et al., "Bioavailability of marine n-3 fatty acid formulations." *Prostaglandins, Leukotrienes and Essential Fatty Acids* 83, no. 3 (September 2010):137–41.

208 **One study showed the EPA and DHA:** Lawson LD et al., "Human absorption of fish oil fatty acids as triacylglycerols, free acids, or ethyl esters." *Biochemical and Biophysical Research Communications* 152, no. 1 (1988):328–35.

208 **The triglyceride form of omega-3 is far more stable:** Lee H et al., "Analysis of headspace volatile and oxidized volatile compounds in DHA-enriched fish oil on accelerated oxidative storage." *Journal of Food Science* 68, no. 7 (2003):2169–77.

209 **The problem with plant-based omega-3 supplements:** *Linus Pauling Institute*. lpi.oregonstate.edu/mic/other-nutrients/essential-fatty-acids#metabolism-bioavailability.

210 **Scientists agree that separating EPA and DHA:** Peet M. et al., United States Patent #8188146. May 29, 2012. See also Kelly OJ et al., "Long-chain polyunsaturated fatty acids may mutually benefit both obesity and osteoporosis." *Nutrition Research* 33, no. 7 (July 2013):521–33.

210 **When fish oil is oxidized:** García-Hernández VM et al., "Effect of omega-3 dietary supplements with different oxidation levels in the lipidic profile of women:

a randomized controlled trial." *International Journal of Food Sciences and Nutrition* 64, no. 8 (December 2013):993–1000.

210   **New Zealand researchers:** Albert BB et al., "Fish oil supplements in New Zealand are highly oxidised and do not meet label content of n-3 PUFA." *Scientific Reports* 5 (January 2015):7928.

210   **A similar study from South Africa:** Opperman M et al., "Analysis of the omega-3 fatty acid content of South African fish oil supplements: a follow-up study." *Cardiovascular Journal of Africa* 24, no. 8 (September 2013):297–302.

210   **A 2012 study:** Laupsa-Borge J. "Velg ferske og naturlige omega-3 produkter." *Helsemagasinet Vitenskap & Fornuft*, December 9, 2012.<is this available in English? I can't figure out what this is, but the date doesn't match>

210   **a recent Canadian study:** Jackowski SA et al., "Oxidation levels of North American over-the-Counter n-3 (omega-3) supplements and the influence of supplement formulation and delivery form on evaluating oxidative safety." *Journal of Nutritional Science* 4, no. 4 (November 2015):e30.

211   **we recommend taking flaxseed oil:** de Carvalho WF, "The role of mixotrophy in the ecology of marine phytoplankton." Dissertation, University of Kalmar, Faculty of Natural Science, 2007, 1650–2779.

211   **Additionally, research shows:** *Linus Pauling Institute*. lpi.oregonstate.edu/mic/other-nutrients/essential-fatty-acids#metabolism-bioavailability.

212   **You've probably already heard:** Kaunitz H et al., "Coconut oil consumption and coronary heart disease." *Philippine Journal of Internal Medicine* 30 (1992):165–71. See also Baba N, "Enhanced thermogenesis and diminished deposition of fat in response to overfeeding with diet containing medium-chain triglycerides." *American Journal of Clinical Nutrition* 35, no. 4 (April 1982):678–82; Melissa Clark, "Once a villain, coconut oil charms the health food world." *New York Times*, March 1, 2011; Enig MG, "Coconut: In support of good health in the 21st century." Paper presented at the 36th meeting of the Asian Pacific Coconut Community. January 1999; *Thyroid-Info.* thyroid-info.com/articles/ray-peat.htm; Kabara JJ et al., "Fatty acids and derivatives as antimicrobial agents." *Antimicrobial Agents and Chemotherapy* 2, no. 1 (July 1972):23–8; Ogbolu DO et al., "In vitro antimicrobial properties of coconut oil on Candida species in Ibadan, Nigeria." *Journal of Medicinal Food* 10, no. 2 (June 2007):384–7; Ruzin A et al., "Equivalence of Lauric acid and glycerol monolaurate as inhibitors of signal transduction in *Staphylococcus aureus*." *Journal of Bacteriology* 182, no. 9 (May 2000):2668–71.

212   **but peer-reviewed published research:** Dean W et al., "Beneficial Effects on Energy, Atherosclerosis and Aging." *Nutrition Review*, April 22, 2013. See also St-Onge MP, "Weight-loss diet that includes consumption of medium-chain triacylglycerol oil leads to a greater rate of weight and fat mass loss than does olive oil." *American Journal of Clinical Nutrition* 87, no. 3 (March 2008):621–6; Stubbs RJ, "Covert manipulation of the ratio of medium- to long-chain triglycerides in isoenergetically dense diets: effect on food intake in ad libitum feeding men." *International Journal of Obesity and Related Metabolic Disorders* 20, no. 5 (May 1996):435–44.

213   **Recent studies have demonstrated:** Xu X et al., "Intestinal microbiota: a potential target for the treatment of postmenopausal osteoporosis." *Bone Research* 4, no. 5 (October 2017):17046.

213 **One recent study determined:** Nilsson AG et al., "*Lactobacillus reuteri* reduces bone loss in older women with low bone mineral density: a randomized, placebo-controlled, double-blind, clinical trial." *Journal of Internal Medicine* 284, no. 3 (June 2018):307–17.

214 **lactic acid reduces the pH in your gut:** Markowiak P et al., "Effects of Probiotics, Prebiotics, and Synbiotics on Human Health." *Nutrients* 9 no. 9: (September 2017): 1021. https://www.mdpi.com/2072-6643/9/9/1021/htm

214 **Produce short-chain fatty acids:** Serpa J et al., "Butyrate-rich colonic micro-environment is a relevant selection factor for metabolically adapted tumor cells." *Journal of Biological Chemistry* 285, no. 50 (December 2010):39211–23.

214 **Empower your gut cells:** Rao RK et al., "Protection and restitution of gut barrier by probiotics: nutritional and clinical implications." *Current Nutrition and Food Science* 9, no. 2 (2013):99–107.

214 **Reduce the impact of dietary phytates:** Gaón D et al., "[Lactose digestion by milk fermented with Lactobacillus acidophilus and Lactobacillus casei of human origin]." *Medicina (B Aires)* 55, no. 3 (1995):237–42. [Article in Spanish.]; See also LeBlanc JG et al. "Beneficial effects on host energy metabolism of short-chain fatty acids and vitamins produced by commensal and probiotic bacteria." *Microbial Cell Factories* 16, no. 1 (2017):79.

214 **Produce important vitamins:** Ríos-Covián D et al., "Intestinal short chain fatty acids and their link with diet and human health." *Frontiers in Microbiology* 7 (2016):185. See also Rao RK et al., "Protection and restitution of gut barrier by probiotics: nutritional and clinical implications." *Current Nutrition and Food Science* 9, no. 2 (2013):99–107; Markowiak P et al., "Effects of Probiotics, Prebiotics, and Synbiotics on Human Health." *Nutrients* 9, no. 9 (2017).

214 **Reduce stress levels:** Messaoudi M et al., "Beneficial psychological effects of a probiotic formulation (*Lactobacillus helveticus* R0052 and *Bifidobacterium longum* R0175) in healthy human volunteers." *Gut Microbes* 2, no. 4 (July–August 2011):256–61. See also *Nutraceutical Business Review*. nutraceuticalbusinessreview.com/news/article_page/Addressing_stress_and_anxiety_with_probiotics/103853.

216 **One important clinical trial:** Amstrup AK et al., "Melatonin improves bone mineral density at the femoral neck in postmenopausal women with osteopenia: a randomized controlled trial." *Journal of Pineal Research* 59, no. 2 (September 2015):221–9.

216 **Melatonin promotes osteoblast differentiation:** Roth JA et al., "Melatonin promotes osteoblast differentiation and bone formation." *Journal of Biological Chemistry* 274, no. 31 (July 1999):22041–7.

216 **Melatonin has been shown:** Kotlarczyk MP et al., "Melatonin osteoporosis prevention study (MOPS): a randomized, double-blind, placebo-controlled study examining the effects of melatonin on bone health and quality of life in perimenopausal women." *Journal of Pineal Research* 52(2012):414–26. See also Amstrup AK et al., "Melatonin improves bone mineral density at the femoral neck in postmenopausal women with osteopenia: a randomized controlled trial." *Journal of Pineal Research* 59, no. 2 (September 2015):221–9.

216 **One study found that taking a DHEA supplement:** Weiss EP et al., "Dehydroepiandrosterone replacement therapy in older adults: 1- and 2-y effects on bone." *American Journal of Clinical Nutrition* 89, no. 5 (May 2009):1459–67.

216   **Another study found that both men and women:** Villareal DT et al., "Effects of DHEA replacement on bone mineral density and body composition in elderly women and men." *Clinical Endocrinology* 53, no. 5 (November 2000):561–8.

217   **strontium is heavier than calcium:** Mirza FS et al., "Change in bone mineral density with strontium citrate: an illusion or reality." *Journal of Nutritional Health and Food Science* 4, no. 3 (2016):1–3. See also Blaschko SD et al., "Strontium substitution for calcium in lithogenesis." *Journal of Urology* 189, no. 2 (2012):735–9.

218   **Studies have proven that:** Turner MR et al., "Functional vitamin B12 deficiency." *Practical Neurology* 9, no. 1 (February 2009):37–41.

218   **Scientists have determined that:** Duncan A et al., "Quantitative Data on the magnitude of the systemic inflammatory response and its effect on micronutrient status based on plasma measurements." *American Journal of Clinical Nutrition* 95, no. 1 (January 2012):64–71.

Acknowledgments

We would like to thank the brave women and men who have shared their stories of osteoporosis with us, and urged us to write this book. Their pain and frustration concerning the lack of information currently available on scientifically proven, natural methods to prevent and reverse osteoporosis gave us the drive and determination to gather this research and lay it out in an easy-to-follow plan. We would also like to thank all of the medical and health professionals who have been using our micronutrient therapy protocol and our forty healing habits to treat their patients and clients without prescription medications. We are always inspired by your amazing results and greatly respect how you are proactively discussing bone health with younger women, men, and even children as a preventive measure.

Thanks to Celeste and her team of literary agents. You saw our vision and the lack of books addressing this far-reaching, yet preventable health condition, and you allowed us to get the truth out about osteoporosis, a disease so personal to us. To our amazing readers, Jeanne, Jennifer, Denise, and Kevin, all we can say is thank you. . . .

Finally, to all of you who have read this book, and taken the time to share this information with loved ones and friends to help them prevent or reverse osteoporosis, we want you to know that we appreciate you. Your efforts to help us educate others about micronutrient therapy as a safe and effective alternative to drug therapy is key to ultimately beating osteoporosis once and for all. Education and empowerment is a team effort and we are proud to have you on our team.

Index

beverages, 60
buy local and organic, 58
definition of, 57
diet plan, 46–47
Fab 14 and Terrible 20 list, 58
flour alternatives, 59
free-range/pasture-raised poultry and
    eggs, 59
meal plan/meal planning, 229
meats, 59
milk alternatives, 58–59
oils, 59
osteoporosis grocery guide, 229
raw, unpasteurized dairy products, 58
salad dressings and condiments, 59
shopping for, 58–60, 229
stevia, 60
wild fish, 59
xylitol, 60
R-proteins, 77

saccharin, 66
sarcopenia, 107, 217
sauces, 59, 271–277
scurvy, 9
secondary hyperparathyroidism, 19
secondary osteoporosis. See osteoporosis
secondhand smoke, 134
seeds. See nuts and seeds
selective serotonin reuptake inhibitors
    (SSRIs), 143
selenium, 45, 180, 186
serum blood testing, 218–219
shampoos, as toxins, 124
Shrimpton, Derek H., 194
side dishes and wraps, 268–270
silica, as accessory supplement, 202
silicon, 45, 180, 192
Sinister S's. See lifestyle habits
SKINNYFat, 59, 213, 228, 252–255
sleep deprivation, 132–133
smartphones, 137–138
smog, 134–135
smoking, 133–134, 235–236
sodium, 61, 92, 185
sodium lauryl sulfate, 124, 125
soy, 96, 205–206
SpectraCell hormone, thyroid, and adrenal
    test, 221, 226–227

spongy bone. See trabecular bone
statins, 201
stevia, 60
stomach acid, 20, 41
stress
    bone fractures and, 127–128, 129
    bone loss and, 128
    chronic stress, 41
    cortisol and, 129–130
    micronutrient deficiencies and, 18
    omega-3 supplementation, 130
    reduction of, 131–132, 236
    stress eating, 130–131
    vitamins and, 128
stress eating, 130–131
strontium, 217–218
sucralose, 66
sugar, 60–66
sugar substitutes, 64–66
sun exposure, 18
sunscreen, 18, 135–137
supplementation, 130, 169–172,
        180–182, 207–211, 227–228. See
        also micronutrient competitions;
        multivitamin supplements
sustained micronutrient sufficiency, 12
Swanson, Christine, 133
sweat, 138–139
Switzerland, 13

Tagamet, 144
tannins, 81–82
Teflon nonstick coating, 126–127
teriparatide, 31–34
testosterone, 70, 120, 217, 221
thiamine, 9, 41, 128, 173, 185–186
three-step plan, 46–48
thyroid, 221
toothpaste, as toxins, 125
toxic load. See also lifestyle habits
    description of, 118–119
    heavy metals, 121–122
    in household items, 123–127
    industrialization and, 119
    plastics and, 119–120
TOZAL study, 188–189
trabecular bone, 14
transcobalamin-2, 218
triclosan, 126

About the Authors

JAYSON CALTON, PhD, and MIRA CALTON, CN, are among the world's leading experts in micronutrients and dietary supplement science. Fellows of the American Association of Integrative Medicine, board certified in Integrative Health, and on the American Board of Integrated Health, the Caltons operate Calton Nutrition and The Calton Institute of Lifestyle Medicine in Florida, offering training to health professionals through their Certified Micronutrient Specialist program. They are the authors of *The Micronutrient Miracle, Naked Calories,* and *Rich Food Poor Food.* They have been featured in the *Wall Street Journal, First for Women,* and *Prevention,* and on Fox, CNN, and PBS.